CBS—Quick Medical Examination Review Series

PEDIATRICS

FIFTEENTH EDITION

Edited by :
DR. M.S. BHATIA (MD, Dip. WPA, MNAMS)
Professor & Head, Department of Psychiatry
University College of Medical Sciences
&
Guru Teg Bahadur Hospital,
Dilshad Garden, Delhi-110095.

Previously at :
Maulana Azad Medical College and Associated Hospitals, New Delhi.
&
Lady Hardinge Medical College and Associated Hospitals, New Delhi

Contributing Editor :
DR. NIRMALJIT KAUR (MD)
Senior Specialist, Department of Microbiology
Dr. R.M.L. Hospital
New Delhi - 110001

Previously at :
LHMC & Smt. S.K. Hospital, New Delhi

CBS

CBS PUBLISHERS & DISTRIBUTORS PVT. LTD.
NEW DELHI • BANGALORE • PUNE • COCHIN • CHENNAI (INDIA)

ISBN : 978-81-239-1832-7

First Edition : 1992
Second Edition : 1993
Third Edition : 1994
Fourth Edition : 1995
Fifth Edition : 1996
Sixth Edition : 1997
Seventh Edition : 1998
Eighth Edition : 1999
Ninth Edition : 2000
Tenth Edition : 2001
Eleventh Edition : 2002
Twelveth Edition : 2003
Thirteenth Edition : 2004
Fourteenth Edition : 2005
Fifteenth Edition : 2010

Published by Satish Kumar Jain and produced by V.K. Jain for
CBS Publishers & Distributors Pvt. Ltd.,
CBS Plaza, 4819/XI Prahlad Street, 24 Ansari Road, Daryaganj,
New Delhi - 110002, India.
e-mail: cbspubs@vsnl.com, cbspubs@airtelmail.in, delhi@cbspd.com
Website: www.cbspd.com

Branches:

- ***Bangalore:*** Seema House, 2975, 17th Cross, K.R. Road,
  Bansankari 2nd Stage, Bangalore - 560070
  Fax: 080-26771680 • e-mail: bangalore@cbspd.com
- ***Pune:*** Shaan Brahmha Complex, 631/632, Basement, Appa Balwant Chowk,
  Budhwar Peth, Next to Ratan Talkies, Pune - 411002
  Fax: 020-24464059 • e-mail: pune@cbspd.com
- ***Cochin:*** 36/14, Kalluvilakam, Lissie Hospital Road,
  Cochin - 682018, Kerala • e-mail: cochin@cbspd.com
- ***Chennai:*** 20, West Park Road, Shenoy Nagar,
  Chennai - 600030 • e-mail: chennai@cbspd.com

Printed at : Somya Printers, Delhi

DEDICATED TO

READERS WHO READ, UNDERSTAND

&

RECIPROCATE

PREFACE

Life is a continuous learning process. Human beings are born to learn and gain knowledge. Education is a means to acquire knowledge and skills that an individual desires to practise. Examinations are the means to evaluate the knowledge. Though no method of evaluation is without flaw, the process of standardization has resulted in a multiple choice system of examination. This system satisfies the basic qualities of a measuring instrument viz., validity, reliability and objectivity.

Recently, a number of books have been published about these examinations but the **best book still remains that which covers the maximum number of questions, which had been asked in that particular examination,** because the chance of repetition of these questions from so-called **"Question Bank"** remains very high. Recently, it has been observed that many **"Question Banks"** have overlapped. So, it is best to do a book which is complete and covers the **"Question Banks"** of maximum number of examinations. This book is being forwarded in this direction.

This book is designed as a supplement to the standard textbooks. It includes the **Referenced - MCQ's** (of previous years papers) of various PG Medical Entrance and Services Examinations **speciality-wise and Chapter-wise** arranged. The students while preparing the text or just before the examination can quickly go through this book. This will help in detecting the areas of weakness in understanding the text and thus, will improve the skills with multiple choice system of examination. It is a favourite book for **"Paper-setters".**

The importance of doing MCQ's alongwith text has increased tremendously because, recently, it has become a tendency to frame MCQ's usually not covered by the standard textbooks followed at undergraduate level. **"Quick Medical Text Review Series"** can be a useful adjuant to this book.

Beware of the **Fraudulent Books** available in the market, which covers a part of copied '**Question Bank**' from this book, and also, based on '**Constructed**' rather than '**Original**' Question Book. It is suggested not to waste time on these books. Every MCQ matters a lot in a highly competitive exams.

I request the readers not to forget to send their opinions, as also suggestions and contributions if any, about all aspects of this book. It will be of invaluable help in enhancing the utility of the book in future.

All suggestions are welcome and will be duly acknowledged in future editions.

— Editors

A book of the Readers, for the
Readers, by the Readers

NOTE

The MCQ's of multiple response type (i.e. with **more than one correct answer** have been omitted in this Edition. Kindly refer to separate books **(PGI MD Entrance Exam & DNB Entrance Exam.** Part-I) by the same author and Publishers.

ADVICE

Read carefully the suggestions in the beginning of this book.

Prepare text from books suggested in the beginning of each chapter and go through **Referenced MCQ's** of this book. Don't waste time in inexperienced, **incomplete and Fraudulent courses conducted for PG Entrance Medical Examinations.**

ABOUT THE BOOK

This book has been compiled with the main aim to help the students to **quickly revise the Chapter-wise up-to-date referenced questions** asked in various entrance examinations (Years indicated in the brackets).

Quick Medical Examinations Review Series contain Speciality-wise 45,000 MCQ's based on up-to-date papers from 1978 onwards.

The important examinations covered in this book (with code word in the bracket) are :

	Examinations	*Code used*
(A)	***All India level***	
1.	All India Postgraduate Entrance Examination	(AI)
2.	AIIMS MD Entrance Examination	(AIIMS)
3.	PGI MD Entrance Examination	(PGI)
4.	Combined Medical Services Examination by UPSC	(UPSC)
5.	Civil Services Entrance Examination, Part-I (Medicine)	(CS)
6.	Army Medical Corps Entrance Examination	(AMC)
7.	Diplomate of National Board Entrance Examination	(DNB)
8.	NIMHANS PG Entrance Examination	(NIMHANS)
9.	Sanjay Gandhi PG Institute Entrance Examination	(SGPGI)
10.	CIP Ranchi PG Entrance Examination	(CIP)
11.	Manipal Academy of Higher Education PG Entrance	(Manipal/MAHE)
12.	Sree Chitra Tirunal Institute for Medical Science & Technology	(SCTIMST)
13.	Command Hospital, Bangalore	(CH)
14.	Bhabha Atomic Research Centre	(BARC)
15.	Institute of Aerospace Medicine	(IAM)
(B)	***State level***	
16.	Delhi MD Entrance Examination	(Delhi)
17.	Bihar MD Entrance Examination	(Bihar)
18.	JIPMER PG Entrance Examination	(JIPMER)
19.	CMC PG Entrance Examination	(CMC)
20.	Rohtak PG Entrance Examination	(Rohtak)
21.	MP State PG Entrance Examination	(MP)
22.	AP State MD Entrance Examination	(AP)
23.	TN State MD Entrance Examination	(TN)
24.	Karnataka Postgraduate Medical Examination	(Karnataka)
25.	Maharashtra PG Entrance Examination	(Maharashtra)
26.	Kerala State MD Entrance Examination	(Kerala)
27.	Rajasthan Postgraduate Entrance Examination	(Rajasthan)
28.	PG Entrance Examination, Varanasi	(BHU)
29.	Burdwan University	(BU)
30.	Combined Entrance Examination for PG Courses, U.P.	(UP)
31.	Punjab State PG Entrance Examination	(Punjab)
32.	Aligarh Muslim University PG Entrance Examination	(AMU)
33.	Nizam's Institute Entrance Examination, Hyderabad	(Nizam's)
34.	Postgraduate Admission Test, Orissa	(Orissa)
35.	Calcutta University Public Service Commission	(CUPSC)
36.	TN Public Service Commission	(TNPSC)
37.	Calcutta PG Entrance Examination	(Calcutta)
(C)	***Foreign Examinations***	
	PLAB, FCGP, GMC, FLEX, USMLE, MRCP, FRCS, MRCOG, etc.	

Sources of Error (Pediatrics)

Example 1 : **Pellagra is associated with the following except :**

A. Diarrhoea B. Dermatitis
C. Dementia D. Delirium

Answer : All the four choices are correct. (Davidson's as well as Harrison's)

Example 2 : **Which of the following is not seen in Fallot's tetralogy :**

A. ASD B. VSD
C. Pulmonary D. Left ventricular hypertrophy

Answer : Both a and d are correct choices (Tetralogy consists of VSD, PS, RVH and overriding of aorta) (Ghai)

Example 3 : **Commonest valvular lesion in Rheumatic heart disease is :** **UPSC 1985, 87**

A. MS B. MR
C. TS D. TR

Answer : 'b'. (Ghai as well as Harrison) but other books mention —'a' (API)

Example 4 : **Commonest brain tumor in children is :** **AIIMS 1983, 87**

A. Astrocytoma B. Meningioma
C. Medulloblastoma D. Craniopharyngioma

Answer : 'c' (Ghai) but in some books answer is 'a' as even in cerebellum, tumor is usually astrocytoma

Example 5 : **Which of the following cardiac lesion is common in Turner's syndrome :** **AIIMS 1984, Rohtak 1985**

A. Coarctation of aorta B. Pulmonary stenosis
C. ASD D. VSD

Answer : Both a and b (Ghai)

ADVICE

Questions with inaccurate language or wrong choices should better be left unattempted.

IMPORTANT TIPS OF PEDIATRICS

Read

* Read Table of some Pediatric problems and their management from Bhatia's **Quick Medical Text Review Series, Pediatrics.**
* About hypervitaminosis A and D from O.P. Ghai's **Essential Pediatrics.**
* About Apgar scoring from Table in Bhatia's **Quick Medical Text Review Series, Pediatrics.**
* About Milestones of development from Tables in Bhatia's **Quick Medical Text Review Series, Pediatrics.**
* About Reye's syndrome from **Current Pediatric Diagnosis and Treatment** (CPDT).
* About Dentition in Children from Table in Bhatia's **Quick Medical Text Review Series, Pediatrics.**
* About Rheumatic fever from Ghai's **Essential Pediatrics.**
* About Turner's, Down's and Klinefelter's syndrome from Ghai's **Essential Pediatrics.**
* Named Syndromes from Bhatia's **Quick Medical Text Review Series, Pediatrics.**
* About differential diagnosis of short stature from Table in Bhatia's **Quick Medical Text Review Series, Pediatrics.**
* About various reflexes from Table in Bhatia's **Quick Medical Text Review Series, Pediatrics.**
* About CHF and congenital heart disease from Ghai's **Essential Pediatrics.**
* About Rickets from Ghai's **Essential Pediatrics.**
* About hypoxic ischemic encephalopathy from **Current Pediatric Diagnosis & Treatment.**
* About Breastmilk (secretion, composition & storage) from Nelson's **Textbook of Pediatrics.**
* About Grades of Malnutrition from Bhatia's **Quick Medical Text Review Series, Pediatrics.**
* About Respiratory Physiology in neonates from Ghai's **Essential Pediatrics.**
* One must know important points from Bhatia's **Quick Medical Text Review Series, Pediatrics** and Pediatric surgery (especially of GIT) from **Current Pediatric Diagnosis and Treatment.**

IMPORTANT PEDIATRICS TEXT FOR MCQ's

Growth & Development	Assessment of growth (parameters at birth, weight, height, skull circumference change), Important Milestones, Sexual maturation, Behavioural problems (Enuresis, Breath holding spells, Stammering etc.), Development Delay, Short Stature.
Nutrition	Vitamins (sources, amount required, deficiency, Excess of A&D), Energy & Nutrient requirements (with age), Kwashiorkor, Marasmus, Breast feeding, Dehydration.
Newborn	Assessment of maturity (signs, reflexes), Prematurity, IUGR, APGAR score, Hyperbilirubinemia, Resp. distress syndrome, Congenital infections & hypoglycemia, Hypocalcemia malformations
Haematology	Anaemias (Iron deficiency, Megaloblastic, Aplastic, hemolytic), Sickle cell anemia, Thalassemia, Purpura, Hemophilia, DIC, Leukemias, Lymphomas
Immunity & Infections	Immune-deficiency, Immunization, Common infections (TB, Malaria, Leprosy, Diphtheria, Polio, Hepatitis, Typhoid, Dengue), Fluid & Blood requirement
GIT	Congenital lesions (Pyloric stenosis, hiatus hernia, anal atresia, Hirschsprung's disease), Cystic fibrosis, Indian Childhood Cirrhosis, Hepatosplenomegaly.
CVS	Congenital lesions (Cyanotic & acyanotic), CHF, Rheumatic fever, Hypertension, Pericarditis, Normal changes with age
Respiratory Tract	Wheezing, Stridor, Dyspnoea, Asthma, Bronchiolitis, Bronchiectasis, Common Pneumonias, Respiratory Distress Syndrome, Lung Function Test
Urinary Tract	Renal Physiology (function Tests), GN, PN, Nephrotic syndrome, Hemolytic uremic syndrome, ARF, CRF, Hematuria
CNS	Meningitis, Reye's syndrome, SOL (Tumors, Tuberculomas), Neurocysticercosis), Epilepsies, Cerebral Palsy, Mental retardation, Myopathies, Juvenile Rheumatoid arthritis
Endocrine	Cretinism, Hypothyroidism, Diabetes mellitus, Hypoglycemia, Short stature, Congenital adrenal hyperplasia, Precocious & Delayed puberty
Miscellaneous	Syndromes (Down's, Klinefelter, Turner's), Neuroblastoma, Phenylketonuria, Maple Syrup Disease. Homocystinuria, Common Poisonings, Drugs (uses, side effects, teratogenicity)

CONTENTS

1

IMPORTANT TEXT OF GROWTH & DEVELOPMENT

MNEMONICS

Age (months)	0	1	2	3	4	5	6	7	8	9	10	11	12	24	36	48	84	120
Weight (Kg.)	3					x2							x3	x4	x5		x7	x10
Height (cm.)	50												75		90	100		
Head circumference (cm).	35			40									45	48			50	
Chest circumference (cm.)	32													45				

MILESTONES OF DEVELOPMENT

The 'milestones' given here are approximations and to assess any individual child, all types of growth development and behaviour must be taken into account

	Motor development	*Language development*	*Adaptive development*	*Socio-personal development*
6—8 weeks				Looks at mother and smiles
3 months	holds head erect			
4—5 months		listening	begins to reach out for objects	recognises mother
6—8 months	sits without support	experimenting with noises	transfers objects from hand-to-hand	enjoy hide and seek
9—10 months	crawling	increasing range of sounds	releases objects	suspicious of strangers
10—11 months	stands with support	first words		
12—14 months	walks wide base	Two words with meaning	Plays a simple ball	
18—21 months	walks narrow base beginning to run	10 words with meaning		
24 months	runs, walks upstairs	short sentences		
36 months	—	telling a story	—	Knowing gender

APGAR SCORE SYSTEM

Score	*0*	*1*	*2*
1. Respiratory effort	None	Slow, irregular	Good, crying
2. Heart ratio/min	Absent	< 100	> 100
3. Color of the body	Blue or pale	Body pink, extremities blue	Pink
4. Muscle tone	Flaccid	Some flexion	Actively moving the extremities
5. Reflex stimulation (catheter in the nose)	No response	Grimace	Cries, cough

MCQ's OF GROWTH & DEVELOPMENT

What is important in Growth & Development

Assessment of growth (parameters at birth, weight, height, skull circumference change), Important Milestones, Sexual maturation, Behavioural problems (Enuresis, Stammering etc)

1. A 6 years old child with 50% IQ is able to : AI 2007

A. Ride bicycle
B. Draw triangle
C. Read simple sentence
D. Identify colour

2. Which of the following appears 1st in child : AI 2007

A. Creeping
B. Crawling
C. Mirror play
D. Pincer grasp

3. A child has started mouthing objects, shows likes and dislikes and not yet developed stranger anxiety. The age of child is : AI 2007

A. 3 months
B. 5 months
C. 7 months
D. 9 months

4. A female child has recently learned to eat with spoon without spilling; to dress and undress herself with supervision, and to understand that she is a girl. These skills are FIRST mastered between the ages of : AIIMS 2005

A. 2 and 3 years
B. 3 and 4 years
C. 4 and 5 years
D. 5 and 6 years

5. Consider the following milestones: Ability to : UPSC 2000

1. Crawl
2. Indicate desire by pointing
3. Make a tower of four cubes
4. Draw a line with a crayon

Which of the above are the milestones one would expect of a 15-months old baby:

A. 1 and 3
B. 2 and 4
C. 1, 2 and 4
D. 1, 2, 3 and 4

6. A child tells his name & sex accurately. His age is: JIPMER 2000

A. 30 months
B. 36 months
C. 40 months
D. 24 months

7. To assess motor function of a 4 years old child is : UP 1999

A. Hoppes for 15 feets in succession
B. Stands on single leg for 15 seconds
C. Ascends with alternate step from staircase with holding the railing
D. Skips smoothly

8. Developmental examination should be withheld in a child of 12 weeks, if he : AIIMS 2000

A. Does not hold head at 90°
B. Does not vacalise
C. Does not babble
D. Does not change bright red ring from one hand to other even if given in hand

9. The percentage rise in length of infant in first year of life is : DNB 2001, 2004

A. 20%
B. 30%
C. 40%
D. 50%

10. 15 months old child do all except : DNB 2001, 2006

A. Feeds self with spoon
B. Says three words
C. Builds tower of 2 blocks
D. Creeps upstairs

11. At what age does a child sees the toy hidden and then again hides it and gives to mother if she asks for : DNB 2001

A. 6 months
B. 8 months
C. 10 months
D. 12 months

12. Sexual maturity rating in girls includes all except : JIPMER 2002

A. Development of breast
B. Onset of menstruation
C. Pubic hair development
D. Height, weight velocity

13. The following milestones are seen in 16 weeks child, except: JIPMER 2002

A. Kicks the ground on placing it on feet
B. Polysyllobic vowel sounds
C. Brings objects to mouth
D. Laughs loudly

Ans. 1. D 2. C 3. B 4. A 5. D 6. C 7. C 8. A 9. D 10. C 11. D 12. D 13. B

14. A 12 weeks old child should be further evaluated for developmental delay if found to have which of the following defects : AI 2002

A. Failure to raise head to 90 degrees
B. Fails to vocalize
C. Unable to make babbling noises
D. Does not transfer a red ring even when given in hand

15. A girl can walk upstairs, alternating feet, and make a tower of 8 cubes. She refers to herself by the pronount 'I' knows her name, but not her age and gender. The most likely chronological age is : UPSC 2002

A. 24 months B. 30 months
C. 36 months D. 42 months

16. A six weeks infant cannot : UPSC 1985, AIIMS 1992

A. Lift and hold head
B. Turn head towards sound
C. Fix gaze
D. Grasp dangling objects

17. Which is true regarding normal growth curve? AIIMS 1992

A. Growth rate-5 cm/year
B. Spurt in pre-pubertal period
C. Decreased exogenous obesity
D. Entirely influenced by growth Hormone

18. A five years old child can remember numbers upto how many digits? PGI 1993

A. 4 B. 5
C. 6 D. 7

19. Increase of length in the first year of life is : AIIMS 1996

A. 12 cms B. 15 cms
C. 25 cms D. 35 cms

20. Most characteristic behavioural change in pubescent is : PGI 1983; AIIMS 1997

A. Defensive B. Aggressive
C. Antagonistic attitude D. Uncooperative

21. The behaviour of an adolescent is probably best described as being : AIIMS 1993

A. Domineering B. Beligerant
C. Aggressive D. Paradoxical

22. Most significant health problem of adolescent is : PGI 1996

A. Sexual perversions
B. Malnutrition
C. Frequency of serious accidents
D. Myopia

23. Anovulatory menstruation may precede ovulatory menstruation by as much as : AIIMS 1992

A. 2 years B. One month
C. 8 months D. 6 months

24. School phobia is characterized by all, except : AIIMS 1994

A. Dependent child
B. Passive child
C. Usually an overprotective mother
D. Usually a punitive and domineering father

25. A school age child is most apt to have fears about : DNB 1998

A. Snakes B. High places
C. Loud noises D. Death or injury

26. What is catch-up delay : UPSC 1990

A. Normal growth velocity but growth prolonged beyond the usual time.
B. Supranormal growth velocity but growth decelerated beyond the usual time.
C. Normal growth velocity but growth accelerated beyond time.
D. None of the above.

27. By age, definition of delayed eruption of first decidious teeth means : AIIMS 1993

A. 8 months B. 10 months
C. 12 months D. 20 months

28. Waking up at night, screaming with fear, at 2.5 years age, is generally a manifestation of : PGI 1990

A. Organic illness
B. Normal development pattern
C. Castration anxiety
D. Separation anxiety

29. During first year of life, most of increase in body length is due to growth of : AMU 1992

A. Legs B. Trunk
C. Neck D. Head

30. The first decidious teeth usually appear : UPSC 1994

A. On stop age of nipple feedings
B. At 9-12 months
C. At 5-9 months
D. Before 5 months

31. Child changes Rattle from one hand to another at the age of : AIIMS 1992

A. 3 months B. 6 months
C. One year D. Two years

32. To avoid displacement of permanent teeth, finger sucking should be terminated by : AIIMS 1990

A. 8 years B. 5 years
C. 4 years D. 2 years

33. Which of the following is of little value in curing a crossed eye : AIIMS 1995

A. Corrective lenses
B. Orthoptics
C. Surgery on eye muscles
D. Patching of turning eye

Ans.									
14. A	15. B	16. D	17. B	18. B	19. C	20. C	21. D	22. C	23. A
24. D	25. D	26. B	27. C	28. D	29. B	30. C	31. B	32. B	33. B

34. Macular vision is completed by the age of : AMU 1999

A. 1 year B. 3 years
C. 5 years D. 9 years

35. Single most common cause of visual loss in children is : AMU 1999

A. Venous thrombosis B. Nystagmus
C. Amblyopia D. Cataracts

36. Visual acuity reaches adult acuity by the age : DNB 1999

A. 7 years B. 9 years
C. 5 years D. 3 years

37. Probable cause for delayed puberty of a 14 yr old child : Kerala 1998

A. Starvation B. Hypothyroidism
C. Cushing's D. Familial

38. A child is able to ride a tricycle, build tower of 9 cubes, gives his sex and name and copy a circle by the age of : UPSC 1995

A. 1 year B. 2 years
C. 3 years D. 4 years

39. "Hutchinson's teeth" usually involves : DNB 1990

A. Permanent upper molars
B. Permanent upper incisors
C. Permanent lower incisors
D. Temporary upper molars only

40. What are sex dimorphic features of children : DNB 1990

A. Length of bones and thickness of cortex
B. Female with wider Hips
C. Males with shoulder breadth
D. All the above

41. Child smiles at familiar persons at the age of : UPSC 1999

A. 1 month B. 2 months
C. 4 months D. 6 months

42. A 8 months old child will be able to do which of the following : PGI 1990

A. Pincer grasp
B. Sitting stably
C. Stand without support
D. Say mama-baba
E. Tells when he is wet

43. Disease common in first male child is : AIIMS 1996

A. Congenital hydronephrosis
B. Congenital hypertrophic pyloric stenosis
C. Volvulus of ileum
D. Duodenal atresia

44. Normal stage of hyperactivity is seen in age group (years) : DNB 1990

A. 1-2 B. 2-3
C. 3-5 D. 9-12

45. Precocious puberty is only diagnosed if age is below: AIIMS 1996

A. 8 years B. 10 years
C. 11 years D. 12 years

46. In a 2 years old child, head circumference (cm) is about : DNB 1991

A. 40 B. 45
C. 48 D. 52

47. The mean stem stature index at 3 years of age is : AIIMS 1997

A. 66% B. 58%
C. 61% D. 52%

48. The number of permanent teeth in a 12 years old child is : UPSC 1985; AMC 1995

A. 20 B. 24
C. 28 D. 30

49. A child hold spoon without spilling at the age of : UPSC 1993

A. 12 months B. 15 months
C. 18 months D. 24 months

50. The age group commonly affected by breath holding spells are : AIIMS 1994

A. 6 months to 5 years B. 2 to 8 years
C. 4 to 9 years D. 8 to 12 years

51. Growth in children occurs in : UPSC 1983; AMC 1986, 97

A. Linear fashion B. Inverse linear fashion
C. Spurts D. Any of the above

52. Which of the following is wrong about 7 months old child : UPSC 1983; Delhi 1983, 87

A. Weight 7 Kg
B. Head circumference - 41 cm
C. Crawling
D. Sitting

53. A child can sit with good coordination, says, 'peak-a-boo'. His age is : AIIMS 1983, 87; UPSC 1984, 85, 88; Delhi 1984; ESI 1999

A. 28 weeks B. 32 weeks
C. 36 weeks D. 40 weeks

54. A child learns to walk on tip toes at the age of —— years : DNB 1994

A. 1.5 B. 2.0
C. 2.5 D. 3.5

55. Weight of 1 year old child is : Delhi 1995

A. 100 gm/week gain
B. 10 kg
C. Gained after one month
D. Fall till one month

Ans.										
	34. C	35. C	36. A	37. D	38. C	39. B	40. D	41. B	42. B	43. B
	44. C	45. A	46. C	47. B	48. C	49. B	50. A	51. C	52. C	53. C
	54. C	55. B								

56. In anthropometry of 1 year old child, head circumference is : Delhi 1998
A. More than that of chest
B. Equal to chest
C. Less than that of chest
D. May be more or less

57. Most unreliable milestone is : Delhi 1990
A. Teething B. Social smile
C. Neck holding D. Pincer reflex

58. A child aged one year weights 5 Kg. He suffers from: UPSC 1995
A. Marasmus B. Marasmic kwashiorkor
C. Kwashiorkor D. Underfeeding

59. A child climbs up the stairs in a coordinated manner at —— years of age : AIIMS 1999
A. 1.5 B. 2
C. 2.5 D. 3

60. A child should be able to pull up to a standing position by age : UPSC 1993
A. 16 weeks B. 28 weeks
C. 40 weeks D. 52 weeks

61. A full-term infant will generally double its birth weight by : UPSC 1984, 96
A. 1 month B. 3 months
C. 5 months D. 7 months

62. A child can run well by : UPSC 1994
A. 7-9 months of age B. 9-12 months of age
C. 12-15 months of age D. 18-24 months of age

63. An infant can transfer objects from one hand to the other by age : UPSC 1982; AIIMS 1996
A. 2 months B. 4 months
C. 6 months D. 8 months

64. The commonest cause of delayed speech is : UPSC 1993
A. Mental retardation B. Congenital deafness
C. Chronic otitis media D. Tongue tie
E. Cleft palate

65. A newborn weight 3 kg and is 50 cms in length. Her head circumference will be : AIIMS 1982, 95
A. 33-35 cms B. 36-48 cms
C. 40-42 cms D. 50-52 cms

66. At one year of age, an infant weights 9.75 kgs and has a head circumference of 46 cms. The child has : UPSC 1994
A. Hydrcephalus B. A normal sized head
C. Microcephaly D. Down's syndrome
E. Maternal rubella syndrome

67. 4 months infant : Rajasthan 1998
A. Differentiates humans and animals
B. Differentiates male & female
C. Tries to grasp a rattle dangling
D. Enjoys watching his own image

68. Control of bladder in the day time : WB 1994
A. 1.5 years B. 2.5 years
C. 3.5 years D. 6 years

69. Late onset of puberty in male is defined after : AIIMS 1994
A. 16 years B. 17 years
C. 18 years D. 21 years

70. Precuseus puberty is commonly caused by : Delhi 1994
A. Idiopathic causes
B. Neurogenic causes
C. Hypothyroidism
D. McCune Albright syndrome

71. Number of teeth in a 15 months old child is : Delhi 1995
A. 8 B. 10
C. 12 D. 16

72. Short stature is —— percentile of height : Delhi 1996
A. Ist B. 2nd
C. 3rd D. 98th

73. Head control by a child is at —— weeks of age : Delhi 1996
A. 2-4 B. 4-6
C. 6-8 D. 12-14

74. Two carpal bones are radiologically seen in the wrist X-ray of most of the children by the end of : UPSC 1996
A. 1 year B. 2 years
C. 3 years D. 4 years

75. In a term neonate, sitting height is : UPSC 1996
A. 55% of the total length
B. 60% of the total length
C. 65% of the total length
D. 70% of the total length

76. Delayed eruption of teeth occurs in all of the following conditions except : UPSC 1996
A. Malnutrition
B. Achondroplasia
C. Hypothyroidism
D. Rickets

77. Infants can enjoy mirror at the age of : PGI 1995
A. 4 months B. 6 months
C. 9 months D. 10 months

78. A child triples weight at the age of —— months : AIIMS 1996
A. 9 B. 12
C. 15 D. 18

79. In boys, order of development of secondary sexual characteristics : PGI 1996
A. ↑ Testes, ↑ Penis, Pubic hair appear
B. Pubic hair appear, ↑ Penis, ↑ Testes
C. Pubic hair dark, ↑ Testis, ↑ Penis
D. ↑ Penis, ↑ Testes, Pubic hair appear

Ans.									
56. B	57. B	58. D	59. D	60. C	61. C	62. D	63. C	64. A	65. A
66. B	67. C	68. B	69. B	70. A	71. A	72. C	73. D	74. B	75. C
76. D	77. B	78. B	79. A						

80. During first 3 months of life head circumference grows about : Rajasthan 1994

A. 2 cms B. 4 cms
C. 5 cms D. 6 cms

81. The use of one hand (Handedness) is first evident by : Kerala 1997

A. 6 months B. 1 yr
C. 2 yrs D. 3 yrs.

82. Which of the following is not a development milestone: Delhi 1997

A. Social smile
B. Motor manipulative abilities
C. Language and behaviour development
D. Head circumference

83. A child holds a inkpot without touching the medial side of the palm at ——— months : JIPMER 1997

A. 4 B. 6
C. 9 D. 12

84. A child is able to reach for objects, sit with minimal support, roll over from supine to prone position but has no pincer grasp. His age is —— months : Manipal 1998

A. 4 B. 6
C. 9 D. 12

85. The prime principles of growth and development include all of the following except : Karnataka 1998

A. Growth is a continous process from conception to adolescence.
B. It follows the same pattern in all human beings.
C. Growth and development go hand-in-hand.
D. Development occurs in Caudo-cephaloid fashion.

86. The upper segment : lower segment ratio at 2 years of age in a normal child is : Karnataka 1996

A. 1.8:1 B. 1.5:1
C. 1.25:1 D. 1.12:1

87. Mental retardation is present in all except : AIIMS 1993

A. Protein energy malnutrition
B. Cretinism
C. Cerebral palsy
D. Mongolism

88. Earliest indication of sexual maturation in a girl is: AIIMS 1985, 86, 89, 92

A. Manarche B. Pubarche
C. Thelarche D. Maturation of breasts

89. The first permanent teeth to erupt are usually the : AIIMS 1981

A. Lateral incisors B. Central incisors
C. Second molars D. First molars

90. A child can copy a circle first at the age of : UPSC 1996

A. 2 years B. One and half year
C. 4 years D. 3 years

91. Vocabulary of a child at 18 months of age is : UPSC 1997

A. 3 words B. 5 words
C. 10 words D. 100 words

92. Sitting height of a newborn is roughly equal to the : AIIMS 1993

A. Upper segment B. Lower segment
C. Chest circumference D. Head circumference

93. Delayed speech in a 5 years old child with normal motor and adaptive development is most likely due to : AIIMS 1996

A. Mental retardation B. Cerebral palsy
C. Kernicterus D. Deafness

94. A 5 year old child is assessed to have developmental age of one year. His developmental quotient would be : AIIMS 1984, 97

A. 100 B. 80
C. 60 D. 20

95. Which of the following acts can a one year old child perform ? UPSC 1985, AIIMS 1983, 95

A. Sits down from standing position
B. Drinks from cup
C. Speaks one or two words with meaning
D. Rings bell purposefully

96. Head control is possible in an infant by ——— months : JIPMER 1997

A. 1 B. 2
C. 3 D. 6

97. A child starts crawling at : JIPMER 1987; DNB 1993

A. 5 months B. 7 months
C. 8 months D. 9 months

98. Which of the following would be considered normal in a 4 years child ? AIIMS 1991

A. Articulatory deficiencies
B. Stammering
C. Lisping
D. All of the above

Ans.									
80. C	**81. A**	**82. D**	**83. C**	**84. B**	**85. D**	**86. D**	**87. A**	**88. C**	**89. D**
90. D	**91. C**	**92. D**	**93. D**	**94. D**	**95. C**	**96. C**	**97. C**	**98. D**	

99. An infant sits with support at the age of——— months: **Delhi 1992**

A. 1-3 B. 3-5
C. 6-8 D. 10-12

100. Which causes concern : **AI 1993**

A. Delayed development of teeth upto 9 months
B. Slurred speech at 3 yrs
C. Social smile absent at 10 weeks
D. No walking till 1 yr.

101. A two-month old child is able to : **AI 2004**

A. Show a positive parachute protective reflex.
B. Hold head steady in a seated position.
C. Lift head and chest off a flat surface.
D. Sustain head level with the body when placed in ventral suspension.

102. Consider the following statements : **UPSC 2004**

On an average, healthy babies gain weight as follows :
1. Double their birth weight by 5 to 6 months
2. Triple their birth weight by two years
3. Quadruple their birth weight by two years
4. Triple their birth weight by one year

Which of the statements given above is/are corret:

A. 1, 2 and 3 B. 1, 3 and 4
C. 1 and 2 D. 2 only

103. Consider the following statements : **UPSC 2004**

A. 16-weeks old child
1. Makes polysyllabic vowel sounds
2. Gets excited at sight of food
3. Enjoys mirror
4. Laughs out loud

Which of the statements given above is/are correct ?

A. 1 only
B. 1 and 2
C. 2 and 4
D. 1, 2, 3 and 4

104. Majority of the adolescent girls attain menarche when the sexual maturity rating (SMR) is : **Karnataka 1998**

A. SMR-I B. SMR-II
C. SMR-III D. SMR-IV

105. 15th percentile of head circumference (HC) means : **AIIMS 1999**

A. 15% of children have HC more than that
B. 15% will have HC less than that
C. 15% will have same HC
D. None of the above

106. Infant with no social smile and no eyebrow : **TN 1999**

A. Cretinism
B. Down's
C. Mucopolysaccharidosis
D. Rickets

107. A normal infant sits briefly leaning forward on her hands, reaches for and grasp a cube and transfers it from hand-to-hand. She babbles but cannot wave bye-bye nor can she grasp objects with the finger and thumb. Her age is: **UPSC 2000**

A. 4 months B. 7 months
C. 10 months D. 14 months

108. Which of the following tanner SMR stage correspond to maximum or highest increase in height in a boy? **Maharashtra-2006**

A. G4PH3 B. PH2, B2
C. G3PH1 D. G1PH2

109. Integrated management of childhood illness includes except : **AI 2009**

A. ARI B. Malaria
C. Diarrhea D. TB

Ans. 99. C 100. C 101. D 102. B 103. C 104. D 105. B 106. A 107. B 108. A 109. D

EXPLANATIONS OF GROWTH & DEVELOPMENT

1. Ans.— D. Identify colour
2. Ans.— C. Mirror play
3. Ans.— B. 5 months

   Ghai - "Child shows stranger anxiety at the age of 7-8 months".

   Nelson- "Child starts getting everything in mouth at the age of 6 months".

   As the child has not yet developed stranger anxiety, the age should be less than 7 months, ideally 6 months.

   Age of 6 months is not provided in the option. So, go confidently with option (B) i.e. 5 months.
4. Ans.— A 2 and 3 years

   * A child learn to feed himself with spoon without spilling its content—> By 15 months.
   * A child knows his gender —> At the age of 3 years.
   * A child can dress or undress himself completely —At the age of 3 years.
5. Ans.— D. 1, 2, 3 and 4
6. Ans.— C. 40 months
7. Ans.— C. Ascends with alternate step from staircase with holding the railing
8. Ans.— A. Does not hold head at 90°
9. Ans.— D. 50%
10. Ans.— C. Builds tower of 2 blocks
11. Ans.— D. 12 months
12. Ans.— D. Height, weight velocity
13. Ans.— B. Polysyllobic vowel sounds
14. Ans.— A. Failure to raise head to 90 degrees

    It indicates developmental delay.
15. Ans.— B. 30 months
16. Ans.— D. Grasp dangling objects
17. Ans.— B. Spurt in pre-pubertal period
18. Ans.— B. 5
19. Ans.— C. 25 cms

    Baby measures 50 cm at birth, 60 cm at 3 months, 70 cm at 9 months, 73 to 75 cm at 1 year of age. Average height of a 2 years old child is 90 cm.
20. Ans.— C. Antagonistic attitude
21. Ans.— D. Paradoxical
22. Ans.— C. Frequency of serious accidents
23. Ans.— A. 2 years
24. Ans.— D. Usually a punitive and domineering father
25. Ans.— D. Death or injury
26. Ans.— B. Supranormal growth velocity but growth decelerated beyond the usual time.
27. Ans.— C. 12 months
28. Ans.— D. Separation anxiety
29. Ans.— B. Trunk
30. Ans.— C. At 5-9 months

    Among temporary teeth the lower central incisors appear first between the ages of 5 and 8 months. The upper central incisors appear 3 months later. Among permanent teeth, 1st molar at 6 years, central and lateral incisors 6 to 8 years, canines and premolars 9 to 12 years, second molars 12 years and third molars 18 years or later.
31. Ans.— B. 6 months
32. Ans.— B. 5 years
33. Ans.— B. Orthoptics
34. Ans.— C. 5 years
35. Ans.— C. Amblyopia
36. Ans.— A. 7 years

    And macular vision is completed by 5 years of age.
37. Ans.— D. Familial
38. Ans.— C. 3 years

39. Ans.— B. Permanent upper incisors

40. Ans.— D. All the above

41. Ans.— B. 2 months

42. Ans.— B. Sitting stably

43. Ans.— B. Congenital hypertrophic pyloric stenosis

44. Ans.— C. 3-5 years

45. Ans.— A. 8 years

46. Ans.— C. 48

47. Ans.— B. 58%

48. Ans.— C. 28

49. Ans.— B. 15 months

50. Ans.— A. 6 months to 5 years

51. Ans.— C. Spurts

52. Ans.— C. Crawling

Crawling is seen around the age of 8 months.

53. Ans.— C. 36 weeks

54. Ans.— C. 2.5

55. Ans.— B. 10 kg

56. Ans.— B. Equal to chest

57. Ans.— B. Social smile

58. Ans.— D. Underfeeding

59. Ans.— D. 3

60. Ans.— C. 40 weeks

61. Ans.— C. 5 months

If weight at birth is 3 kg, it doubles at 5 months of age, triples at 12 months, quadruples at one year, 5 times at 36 months and 6 times at 60 months.

62. Ans.— D. 18-24 months of age

63. Ans.— C. 6 months

64. Ans.— A. Mental retardation

65. Ans.— A. 33-35 cms

66. Ans.— B. A normal sized head

67. Ans.— C. Tries to grasp a rattle dangling

68. Ans.— B. 2.5 years

In mentally retarded, age is relaxed by about 2 years.

69. Ans.— B. 17 years

70. Ans.— A. Idiopathic causes

71. Ans.— A. 8

72. Ans.— C. 3rd

73. Ans.— D. 12-14

74. Ans.— B. 2 years

75. Ans.— C. 65% of the total length

76. Ans.— D. Rickets

77. Ans.— B. 6 months

78. Ans.— B. 12

79. Ans.— A. ↑ Testes, ↑ Penis, Pubic hair appear

80. Ans.— C. 5 cms.

Head circumference at birth is 35 cms, 40 cm by 3 months, 45 cm at 1 year, 48 cm at 2 years, 50 cms at 84 months, 52 cms at 120 months.

81. Ans.— A. 6 months

82. Ans.— D. Head circumference

83. Ans.— C. 9

84. Ans.— B. 6

85. Ans.— D. Development occurs in Caudo-cephaloid fashion.

86. Ans.— D. 1.12:1

87. Ans.— A. Protein energy malnutrition

88. Ans.— C. Thelarche

Sexual development in girls occur in the following order —breast development (thelarche), development of pubic hair, peak growth velocity, further development of breast and pubic hair, menarche usually starts two years after the pubic hair start appearing and further development of breast and pubic hair.

89. Ans.— D. First molars

90. Ans.— D. 3 years

91. Ans.— C. 10 words

92. Ans.— D. Head circumference

93. Ans.— D. Deafness

94. Ans.— D. 20

95. Ans.— C. Speaks one or two words with meaning

96. Ans.— C. 3

97. Ans.— C. 8 months

98. Ans.— D. All of the above

99. Ans.— C. 6-8

By age of 8 months, he can maintain steady sitting position with straight back. By the age of 10 months, he can pull himself up from supine to sitting position.

100. Ans.— C. Social smile absent at 10 weeks

It is also associated with epiphyseal dysgenesis, mental retardation, hypotony, shade like hands, thick lips, constipation and delayed milestones (= cretinism).

101 Ans.— D. Sustain head level with the body when placed in ventral suspension.

- **From the age of 4 weeks to 12 weeks, the infant learns to lift and control his head in the horizontal plane and then above the horizontal plane on ventral suspension.**
- **The infant gradually gains control of his head between the age of 12 and 20 weeks on supine position.**
- **By 6 months, child can lift his head and greater part of his chest while supporting weight on extended arms.**

102. Ans.— B. 1, 3 and 4

103. Ans.— C. 2 and 4

104. Ans.— D. SMR-IV

Menarche usually starts two years after the pubic hair start appearing (mean 12.5 years).

105. Ans.— B. 15% will have HC less than that

106. Ans.— A. Cretinism

By age of 8 to 10 weeks, a cretin has coarse facial features of hyperthyroidism such as pully face, swollen eyelids, widely separated eyes, narrow palpebral pressure, broad nose and depressed bridge.

107. Ans.— B. 7 months

108. Ans.— A. G4PH3

109. Ans.— D. TB

IMNCI is Indian adaptation of Global Programme of WHO and UNICEF to reduce childhood morbidity and mortality.

Given the fact that majority of the infant deaths occur in the first week of birth, the "integrated Management of Childhood Illnesses (IMCI)" was adapted to include the care of children from 0-7 days renaming it as IMNCI where "N" is for newborn care.

The Government of India recognizes that IMNCI is a superior approach to newborn and child survival and health.

Specific Elements of IMNCI Clinical Protocols (Indian Pediatrics, 2007: 44:169-171)

For newborns and young Infants (under 2 montsh)	*For infants and young children (2 months to 5 years)*
* Early initiation of breast- and counselling exclusive breastfeeding	* Identification and classification of common illnesses. Diarrhea, acute respiratory infections (pneumonia), malaria, measles, ear infection, and malnutrition for home treatment and/or referral
* Cord, skin and eye care	* Prevention and management of iron and vitamin A deficiency
* Counselling to keep the child warm	* Counselling on feeding for all children below 2 years (exclusive breastfeeding and complementary feeding)
* Idenitification and classification of newborn illness for home treatment and/or referral	* Immunization
* Immunization	

2

IMPORTANT TEXT OF NUTRITION

SOME COMMON INDICES USED IN CLINICAL PRACTICE

	Normal	*Severely malnourished*
$\frac{\text{Weight Kg}}{(\text{Height cm})^{1.6}} \times 100$	0.88-0.97	0.79
$\frac{\text{Weight in Kg}}{(\text{Height cm})^{2}} \times 100$	0.15-0.16	0.14
$\frac{\text{Midarm circumference cm}}{\text{Head circumference in cm}}$ or sneezes	0.32-0.33	0.25

MCQ's OF NUTRITION

What is important in Nutrition

Vitamins (sources, amount required, deficiency), Energy and Nutrient requirements (with age), Kwashiorkor, Marasmus

1. **Administration of glucose solution is prescribed for all of the following situations except :** **AIIMS 2006**
   A. Neonates
   B. Child of a diabetic mother
   C. History of unconsciousness
   D. History of hypoglycemia

2. **A child presents with diarrhea and peripheral circulatory failure. The arterial pH is 7.0, PCO_2 15 mmHg, and PO_2 76 mm Hg. What will be the most appropriate therapy :** **AIIMS 2005, 2007**
   A. Sodium bicarbonate infusion
   B. Bolus of Ringers lactate
   C. Bolus of hydroxyethyl starch
   D. 5% Dextrose infusion

3. **Kwashiorkor versus marasmus :** **Delhi 1995, 99**
   A. ↓ Serum Essential amino acids
   B. ↓ Serum Fatty acids x cholesterol
   C. ↓ GH
   D. ↓ Insulin

4. **A 10-months old baby is brought to the hospital with signs of dehydration. Pulse volume and blood pressure are maintained without the loss of skin turgor. The most likely cause is :** **UPSC 1996**
   A. Hyponatremic dehydration
   B. Hypernatremic dehydration
   C. Isonatremic dehydration
   D. Shock and dehydration

5. **Shakir's tape is used to monitor :** **Delhi 1996**
   A. Nutritional status B. Growth of skull
   C. Height D. Ascites

6. **Vitamin-D resistant Rickets is not seen in :** **Kerala 1997**
   A. Fanconi's syndrome
   B. De Toni-Fanconi Debree's syndrome
   C. Renal tubular acidosis
   D. Malabsorption

7. **Convulsions in a child with dehydration and vomiting may be due to :** **Kerala 1997**
   A. ↑ Na B. ↓ Na
   C. ↑ K+ D. ↓ Mg
   E. ↓ K+

8. **Hypernatremic dehydration in a child is suggested by :** **JIPMER 1998**
   A. Irritability B. Lethargy
   C. Anuria D. Convulsions

9. **Commonest vitamin deficiency seen in immuno-compromised children is :** **Delhi 1997**
   A. Thiamine B. Biotin
   C. Vitamin-E D. Vitamin-C

10. **Poor prognostic factors in a child with Kwashiorkor include all of the following except :** **Karnataka 1996**
    A. Hypothermia B. Hepatomegaly
    C. Purpura D. Dermatosis

11. **Breast feeding is contraindicated in all except :** **Kerala 1999**
    A. HIV B. CMV
    C. Active TB D. Active herpes genitalis

12. **Supine feeding at the age of 4 months predisposes to following except :** **Kerala 1999**
    A. Bilateral bronchitis B. Sleep apnoea
    C. Bottle caries D. Middle ear infection

13. **A common finding in osteomalacia is :** **PGI 1999**
    A. Low serum phosphate
    B. Normal level of 1,25 di-hydroxy Vit. D3
    C. Low serum calcium
    D. Increased hydroxy proline in urine

14. **Grade-III malnutrition according to IAP is :** **PGI 1999**
    A. 50% B. 51-60%
    C. 61-80% D. 81-100%

Ans. 1. C 2. B 3. C 4. C 5. A 6. D 7. B 8. A 9. B 10. B 11. D 12. C 13. A 14. A

15. **Indicator of moderate to severe malnutrition is : PGI 1999**
A. ↓ Serum transferrin 160 B. ↓ Body mass index 19
C. ↓ Albumin 2.1 mg/dL D. ↓ Transthyretin

16. **Which of the following is caused in an infant feeding on cows milk : JIPMER 2000**
A. Diarrhoea
B. Pulmonary haemosiderosis
C. Microcytic hypochromic anaemia
D. Jaundice

17. **When infant is given with cow milk, he presents with following except : JIPMER 2000**
A. Mucous and bloody diarrhoea
B. Pulmonary haemosiderosis
C. Hypergomma globulinemia
D. None of the above

18. **Which one of the following is the best source for essential fatty acids for infants? Kerala 2000**
A. Ghee B. Coconut oil
C. Ground Nut oil D. Breast Milk
E. Sunflower oil

19. **A baby presents with tetany, first thing to be given is : AIIMS 2000**
A. Diazepam B. Calcitonin
C. Calcium gluconate D. Vitamin-D

20. **In ORT all can be used except : Rohtak 2001**
A. Rice with salt B. Sugar & salt
C. ORS D. Glucose without salt

21. **In a newborn being exclusively fed with goats milk will develop which of the following as compared to being fed with breast milk : SGPGI 2002**
A. Scurvy
B. Rickets
C. Microcytic anemia
D. Megaloblastic anemia

22. **A neonate on breast feeding presents with golden yellow stools on the 10th day. Treatment is : AIIMS 2002**
A. Stop breast feeding for 3 days
B. Reassurance to the mother
C. Investigate the child
D. Substitute breast milk with cow's milk

23. **Kwashiorkor is characterized by all except : BHU 2002**
A. Flag sign B. Liver changes
C. Weight loss D. Apathy

24. **The most important fac'or to overcome PEM in children of 3 years is : TN 1993; AIIMS 1983, 94**
A. Supply of subsidized food
B. Early solid food supplementation
C. Immunization of child
D. Treatment of anemia and pneumonia

25. **Signs and symptoms of thiamine deficiency include all, except : UPSC 1994**
A. Oedema
B. Anaemia
C. Sensory and motor neuritis
D. Heart enlargement

26. **Calcium requirement of a growing school age child is about : UPSC 1996**
A. 10 Gm/day B. 0.1 Gm/day
C. 1.0 Gm/day D. 2.0 Gm/day

27. **Percentage of protein present as phenylalanine is : PGI 1993**
A. Greater in human milk
B. Greater in Cow's milk
C. Similar in both milks
D. So variable as to defy comparison

28. **A 17 months child, whose diet is almost exclusively milk, is very likely to have : AMU 1994**
A. Iron deficiency anaemia
B. Decreased serum proteins
C. Systemic hypertension
D. Elevated blood urea nitrogen

29. **In Hypervitaminosis D, following may be used : AIIMS 1997**
A. BAL B. EDTA
C. Sodium versenate D. Sodium thiosulphate

30. **The earliest indicator of PEM is : PGI 1984, 97**
A. Hair changes B. Edema
C. Underweight for age D. Restlessness

31. **Which of the following trace element is found in abundance in human body and is next to iron : Bihar 1990**
A. Ca++ B. Cu++
C. Mb D. Zn

32. **Children with long straight black hair may show a pale band across the hair ('flag sign'), corresponding to an earlier episode of : UPSC 1985; JIPMER 1987; DNB 1999**
A. Marasmus B. Kwashiorkor
C. Pellagra D. Obesity

33. **What is the normal average stool sodium content in a new born who is fed on breast milk alone : PGI 1997**
A. 19 mEq/L B. 26 mEq/L
C. 22 mEq/L D. 27 mEq/L

34. **Late CNS changes of Niacin deficiency include following except : AMU 1999**
A. Demyelinisation of Ant. columns of spinal cord.
B. Degeneration of the ganglion cells of the spinal cord.
C. Patchy areas of Demyelinisation of cerebral cortex.
D. Demyelinisation of post and lateral columns of spinal cord.

Ans.									
15. C	16. C	17. A	18. D	19. C	20. D	21. D	22. B	23. C	24. C
25. B	26. C	27. C	28. A	29. C	30. C	31. B	32. B	33. A	34. A

35. Vitamin B_6 corrects the following derangements except: **Kerala 1999**
A. Xanthurinic Aciduria B. Cystathioninuria
C. Homocystinuria D. Porphyria

36. Which of the following is not a sign of scurvy : **AIIMS 1984, 87; PGI 1983, 87, 2000**
A. Irritability B. Pseudoparalysis
C. Red rosary D. Craniotabes

37. Kwashiorkor is characterized by all of the following except : **AIIMS 1984; Delhi 1993**
A. Apathy
B. Liver changes
C. Decreased body weight
D. Flag sign

38. Daily protein requirement in a 6-9 months old child is: **AIIMS 1996**
A. 3.2 gms B. 2.4 gms
C. 1.2 gms D. 0.8 gms

39. Phrynoderma is seen in : **AIIMS 1999**
A. Niacin deficiency
B. Vitamin-A deficiency
C. Hypervitaminosis-D
D. Vitamin-D resistant rickets

40. Prevalence of undernutrition in Preschool children is : **AIIMS 1986, 97**
A. 0.1% B. 1.8%
C. 5% D. 15%

41. Pseudoparalysis in an infant is suggestive of : **AIIMS 1996**
A. Acute Rheumatic fever B. Vitamin-D deficiency
C. Vitamin-E deficiency D. Vitamin-C deficiency

42. All of the following clinical features are found in a child with severe dehydration except : **Karnataka 1998**
A. Fluid loss is more than 100 ml/kg.
B. Pulses are thready.
C. Capillary refill time is more than 5 sec.
D. Patient can be treated with oral rehydration therapy. 100 ml/kg. in 6-8 hours.

43. All of the following of Kwashiorkor may be seen in marasmus except : **AIIMS 1997**
A. Growth retardation B. Low weight
C. Anasarca D Hepatomegaly

44. Hypervitaminosis-A is characterised by all except : **AIIMS 1997**
A. Alopecia B. Bone swelling
C. Anorexia D. Peripheral neuritis

45. Grade of malnutrition in 2 years old child wt. 6.4 kg with Vitamin-A deficiency is : **AIIMS 1987; UPSC 1993**
A. I B. II
C. III D. IV

46. ICMR recommendation for protein intake per kg in 1-3 years is : **AIIMS 1997**
A. 1.8 gms B. 1.3 gms
C. 2.3 gms D. 3.0 gms

47. All of the following endocrinal changes are seen in protein energy malnutrition except : **PGI 1986, 97**
A. Cortisol B. ↑GH
C. ↑ Insulin D. ↓ Somatomedin

48. Oral rehydration therapy will prevent : **TN 1998**
A. Vomiting B. Diarrhoea
C. Dehydration D. Acute renal failure

49. "Casal's Necklace" and "Crazy pavement" is seen in : **AIIMS 1991**
A. Beri-Beri B. Scabies
C. Pityriasis rosea D. Pellagra

50. Scrotal dermatitis is caused by : **UPSC 1996**
A. Scurvy
B. Essential fatty acids deficiency
C. Riboflavin deficiency
D. Vitamin-A deficiency

51. Vitamin-C is least in : **Delhi 1997**
A. Milk B. Amla
C. Citrus fruits D. Guava

52. Rickets is differentiated from Achondroplasia by : **Delhi 1983, 96**
A. Increase in epiphyseal space and fraying of distal ends
B. ↑ Bone length
C. ↑ Bone thickening
D. ↑ Alkaline phosphatase

53. A baby who is given nothing but boiled cow's milk is likely to develop : **Delhi 1998**
A. Rickets B. Scurvy
C. Vitamin-A deficiency D. Angular stomatitis
E. Beri-Beri

54. An infant aged one year who has a widely open fontanelle, widened epiphysis and beading of the ribs has : **AMC 1995**
A. Vitamin A deficiency B. Pellagra
C. Scurvy D. Rickets
E. Congenital syphilis

55. Deficient mineralisation in epiphyseal growth cartilage is seen in : **AI 1999**
A. Rickets B. Osteomalacia
C. Scurvy D. Hyperparathyroidism

56. Excess of vitamin-K in a newborn causes : **AIIMS 1999**
A. Bleeding tendencies B. Hyper-bilirubinemia
C. Vomiting D. Hemolysis

57. Keshan disease is due to deficiency of : **DNB 1994**
A. Cu B. Mn
C. Se D. Ni

Ans.									
35. D	36. D	37. C	38. C	39. B	40. B	41. D	42. D	43. C	44. D
45. C	46. B	47. C	48. C	49. D	50. C	51. A	52. A	53. B	54. D
55. A	56. B	57. C							

58. **Following are seen in Kwashiorkor except : AI 1999**
A. Depigmented areas
B. Oedema
C. Fatty infiltration of liver
D. Fatty infiltration of pancreas

59. **Which is not an early sign of copper deficiency : AIIMS 1990**
A. Neutropenia
B. Flaring of long bone metaphysis
C. Hypochromic anemia
D. Osteoporosis

60. **Energy requirement of an infant is : UPSC 1991**
A. 70-90 Kcal/Kg. B. 50-60 Kcal/Kg.
C. 60-70 Kcal/kg. D. 110-120 Kcal/kg.

61. **One year old baby exclusively breast fed has 1 cm hepatomegaly, severe pallor and no spleen. The most importan investigation is : AIIMS 1986, 99**
A. B_{12} estimation
B. Serum iron estimation
C. Folic acid estimation
D. Fetal hemoglobin estimation

62. **Perioral rash, pigmentation of skin increases and neuritis is seen in deficiency of : AIIMS 1982, 99**
A. Zinc B. Copper
C. Magnesium D. Biotin

63. **Pyridoxine deficiency in infants will be associated with the following except : Karnataka 1999**
A. Generalised seizures.
B. Gastrointestinal distress and an aggravated startle response.
C. Peripheral neuropathy during INH therapy.
D. Macrocytic anemia.

64. **Hartnup disease is a vitamin dependent state of : Karnataka 1994**
A. Vitamin-A B. Pyridoxine
C. Vitamin-E D. Niacin

65. **The daily requirement of zinc for a one-year old child is : Karnataka 1994**
A. 1 mg/day B. 5 mg/day
C. 10 mg/day D. 20 mg/day

66. **In PEM, all of the following are altered except : Delhi 1994**
A. Phagocytosis B. Chemotaxis
C. Immunoglobulins D. Cellular immunity

67. **Recommended daily dietary allowance of Vitamin-A for an infant is : UPSC 1994**
A. 1000 IU B. 500 IU
C. 200 IU D. 1500 IU

68. **B_6 deficiency will result in : AMU 1997**
A. Normocytic anaemia B. Megaloblastic anaemia
C. Dimorphic anaemia D. Microcytic anaemia

69. **Drug therapy with the following anticonvulsant drugs can lead to rickets except : TN 1991**
A. Phenobarbitone B. Phenytoin
C. Ethosuximide D. Sodium valproate

70. **Young infants can not digest : AIIMS 1994**
A. Starches B. Dextrin
C. Disaccharides D. Monosaccharides

71. **A blood gas estimation in a child revealed, pH = 7.21. PaO2 = 68, PaCO2 = 36 and HCO3 = 20 with a base deficit of 18. The most likely diagnosis is : UPSC 1997**
A. Metabolic acidosis B. Respiratory alkalosis
C. Metabolic alkalosis D. Respiratory acidosis

72. **Infantile marasmus is characterized by all except : BHU 1996**
A. Decreased physical activity
B. Malabsorption and hunger stools
C. High mortality when untreated
D. Raised serum potassium levels

The following given item (Ques. 73) consists of two statements, one labelled the 'Assertion A' and the other labelled the 'Reason R'. You are to examine these two statements carefully and decide if the Assertion A and the Reason R are individually true and if so, whether the Reason is a correct explanation of the Assertion. Select your answer to these items using the codes given below and mark your answer sheet accordingly : UPSC 1998

Codes :
A. Both A and R are true and R is the correct explanation of A.
B. Both A and R are true but R is not a correct explanation of A.
C. A is true but R is false.
D. A is false but R is true.

73. **Assertion (A) : About 30% of newborn babies born in India are low birth weight babies.**
Reason (R) : The majority of the low birth weight babies are preterm babies.

74. **Fluid requirement in a 4 months old 5 kg baby with severe dehydration in 1st 30 minutes : WB 1998**
A. 75 ml B. 100 ml
C. 125 ml D. 150 ml

75. **In rickets due to kidney disease, vitamin-D is given in the form of : DNB 1998**
A. Cholecalciferol
B. 25-hydroxycholecalciferol
C. 1, 25 dihydroxycholecalciferol
D. Any of the above

Ans.									
58. D	59. B	60. D	61. B	62. A	63. D	64. D	65. C	66. A	67. D
68. D	69. D	70. A	71. D	72. D	73. D	74. A	75. C		

76. Consider the following statements about kwashiorkor: **CSE 1997**
1. It often occurs in the second year of life
2. It is caused by a diet low in proteins and calories
3. Liver enlargement is characteristic

Of these statements
A. 1, 2 and 3 are correct B. 1 and 3 are correct
C. 2 and 3 are correct D. 1 and 2 correct

77. From which of the following, the highest percentage of iron is absorbed : **UPSC 1985, AIIMS 1983, 95**
A. Spinach B. Soyabean
C. Mutton D. Egg

78. Vitamin-D-deficiency rickets is confirmed by demonstration of all except : **PGI 1986, AIIMS 1983, 97**
A. Epiphyseal changes in X-ray.
B. Hypocalcemia and hypophosphatemia.
C. Raised serum alkaline phosphatase.
D. Healing with physiologic doses of Vitamin-D.

79. The most important anthropometric characteristic of nutritional dwarfism is : **AIIMS 1983, 92**
A. Normal weight for chronological age
B. Normal birth weight and subsequent retardation of growth
C. Normal weight for height
D. Normal weight for chronological age

80. In Fanconi syndrome, following are not reabsorbed from renal tubules except : **DNB 1995**
A. Sodium B. Glucose
C. Amino acids D. Phosphates

81. Costochondral junction swelling are seen in : **JIPMER 1998**
A. Scurvy B. Rickets
C. Chondrodystrophy D. All of the above

82. Fraying at the ends of long bones is seen in : **Delhi 1987, 93**
A. Rickets
B. Scurvy
C. Osteogenesis imperfecta
D. Congenital syphilis

83. The fatty acids required during 0-6 months of age is: **JIPMER 1992**
A. Linolic acid B. Linolenic acid
C. Palmitic acid D. Arachidonic acid

84. All the following vitamins are required for epiphyseal growth except : **AIIMS 1986, JIPMER 1992**
A. A B. B
C. C D. K

85. Which vitamin deficiency is not seen in newborn : **AIIMS 1992**
A. E B. C
C. D D. K

86. Which is not true of Vitamin-D resistant rickets: **AIIMS 1992**
A. Normal parathromone levels
B. Craniotabes
C. Hypotonia
D. Renal tubular defects

87. The normal calorie requirement for a 5 years old child is : **PGI 1993**
A. 1000 Cal B. 1500 Cal
C. 5000 Cal D. 2500 Cal

88. Harlequin Skin Change in the newborn is seen in : **JIPMER 1993**
A. Icthyosis B. Polycythemia
C. Septicemia D. Autonomic dysfunction

89. Vitamin-K deficiency occurs in following except : **JIPMER 1993**
A. Malabsorption states B. Biliary obstruction
C. Oral antibiotic therapy D. Artificial milk feeds

90. Which one of the following is not associated with childhood obesity : **UPSC 2004**
A. Wilson-Mikity syndrome
B. Cushing's syndrome
C. Frohlich's syndrome
D. Laurence-Moon Bardet-Biedl syndrome

91. Oral rehydration mixture contains glucose and sodium because both of them : **AIIMS 2004**
A. Are needed to maintain the plasma osmolality.
B. Are prominent energy sources for the body.
C. Facilitate the transport of each other from the intestinal mucosa to the blood.
D. Are required for the activation of sodium potassium ATPase.

92. Mental changes, skin changes and diarhoea are the manifestations of : **UPSC 1994**
A. Vit. A deficiency
B. Riboflavin deficiency
C. Niacin deficiency
D. Cyanocobalamin deficiency

93. In severe kidney disease, synthesis of which vitamin is decreased : **PGI 1994**
A. Vit-A B. Vit-D
C. Vit-B D. Vit-E

94. In Kwashiorkor, the letter 'K' is postfixed to indicate: **Maharashtra 2006**
A. Edema B. Skin changes
C. Weight for height D. Muscle wasting

95. Nutrition in community is assessed by all/except : **AI 2009**
A. Hb < 11.5 gm% in 3rd trimester pregnancy
B. Increased 1-4 years mortality rate
C. Height and weight of children
D. BW < 2500 gm

Ans.										
	76. A	77. C	78. D	79. B	80. A	81. D	82. A	83. B	84. D	85. A
	86. A	87. B	88. A	89. D	90. A	91. C	92. C	93. B	94. A	95. A

EXPLANATIONS OF NUTRITION

1. Ans.— C History of Unconsciousness

Neonates are susceptible for developing hypoglycemia during the first 2-4 years of life.

If the breast-feeding is not started within 1/2 an hour of birth about 10% of normal neonates are likely to develop hypoglycemia.

This hypoglycemia is corrected either by starting breast-feeding or by administration of glucose.

In certain conditions neonates are at more risk for developing hypoglycemia than others, these conditions are :

* Hyperinsulinism e.g. infant of diabetic mother.
* Increased utilization or decreased production of glucose e.g.

- Prematurity	- Exchange transfusion
- IUGR	- Polycythemia
- Delayed feeding	- Various inborn errors of metabolism
- Perinatal stress	- Maternal beta-blockers therapy

2. Ans.— B Bolus of Ringers lactate

It is a case of metabolic acidosis (lactic acidosis) due to peripheral circulatory failure (It is a common knowledge that in cases of peripheral circulatory failure metabolic acidosis occurs due to production of lactic acid). In moderate or mild cases of metabolic acidosis i.e., when the pH is > 7.2 metabolic acidosis needs no specific t/t. T/T of the underlying cause is sufficient. (it will correct the acidosis).

Once the underlying cause (here tissue perfusion) is corrected the pH will return to normal.

But when the pH is < 7.2 specific bicarbonate therapy is warranted because this degree of acidosis may depress cardiac contractility.

According to Harrison :

"In general severe acidosis (pH < 7.20) warrant the intravenous administration of 50-100 meq of NaHCO3 over 30-45 minutes during the initial, 1 to 2 hours of therapy".

3. Ans.— C. ↓ GH
4. Ans.— C. Isonatremic dehydration
5. Ans.— A. Nutritional status
6. Ans.— D. Malabsorption
7. Ans.— B. ↓ Na
8. Ans.— A. Irritability
9. Ans.— B. Biotin
10. Ans.— B. Hepatomegaly

    Hepatomegaly is not the very poor prognostic feature.
11. Ans.— D. Active herpes genitalis
12. Ans.— C. Bottle caries

    Bottle caries is not linked to supine position.
13. Ans. A. Low serum phosphate

    Alkaline phosphate is high and serum phosphatase is low.
14. Ans.— A. 50%
15. Ans.— C. ↓ Albumin 2. 1mg/dL
16. Ans.— C. Microcytic hypochromic anaemia
17. Ans.— A. Mucous and bloody diarrhoea
18. Ans.— D. Breast Milk
19. Ans.— C. Calcium gluconate
20. Ans.— D. Glucose without salt
21. Ans.— D. Megaloblastic anemia
22. Ans.— B. Reassurance to the mother
23. Ans.— C. Weight loss
24. Ans.— C. Immunization of child
25. Ans.— B. Anaemia

    Anaemia is due to iron, polato and cyanocobalamin deficiency.

26. Ans.— C. 1.0 Gm/day

27. Ans.— C. Similar in both milks

28. Ans.— A. Iron deficiency anaemia

29. Ans.— C. Sodium versenate

30. Ans.— C. Underweight for age

Weight for age is one of the best indicator.

31. Ans.— B. Cu++

32. Ans.— B. Kwashiorkor

33. Ans.— A. 19 mEq/L

34. Ans.— A. Demyelinisation of Ant. columns of spinal cord.

35. Ans.— D. Porphyria

36. Ans.— D. Craniotabes

Craniotabes is seen in rickets. Delayed wound healing, petechiae and epiphyseal windowing are also seen.

37. Ans.— C. Decreased body weight

38. Ans.— C. 1.2 gms

39. Ans.— B. Vitamin-A deficiency

40. Ans.— B. 1.8%

41. Ans.— D. Vitamin-C deficiency

42. Ans.— D. Patient can be treated with oral rehydration therapy. 100 ml/kg. in 6-8 hours.

43. Ans.— C. Anasarca

Edema is not seen in Kwashiorkor.

44. Ans.— D. Peripheral neuritis

45. Ans.— C. III

46. Ans.— B. 1.3 gms

47. Ans.— C. ↑ Insulin

48. Ans.— C. Dehydration

49. Ans.— D. Pellagra

50. Ans.— C. Riboflavin deficiency

51. Ans.— A. Milk

52. Ans.— A. Increase in epiphyseal space and fraying of distal ends.

53. Ans.— B. Scurvy

Vitamin-C content is very low.

54. Ans.— D. Rickets

55. Ans.— A. Rickets

On X-ray, there is an irregular mosaic formation of 'haversian system and trabecular halos' of low density bone

56. Ans.— B. Hyper-bilirubinemia

57. Ans.— C. Se

58. Ans.— D. Fatty infiltration of pancreas

Skin may show hyperpigmentation and hyperperatosis, raw areas and infection and Casal's pigmentation dermatosis

59. Ans.— B. Flaring of long bone metaphysis

It is called Wilson's disease

60. Ans.— D. 110-120 Kcal/kg.

61. Ans.— B. Serum iron estimation

62. Ans.— A. Zinc

63. Ans.— D. Macrocytic anemia

64. Ans.— D. Niacin

65. Ans.— C. 10 mg/day

66. Ans.— A. Phagocytosis

67. Ans.— D. 1500 IU

68. Ans.— D. Microcytic anaemia

Vitamin B_6 deficiency causes dermatitis, diarrhoea and dementia.

69. Ans.— D. Sodium valproate

70. Ans.— A. Starches

71. Ans.— D. Respiratory acidosis

72. Ans.— D. Raised serum potassium levels

73. Ans.— D. A is false but R is true

74. Ans.— A. 75 ml

75. Ans.— C. 1, 25 dihydroxycholecalciferol

76. Ans.— A. 1, 2 and 3 are correct

77. Ans.— C. Mutton

In spinach it is bound whereas in soyabean and eggs not much iron.

78. Ans.— D. Healing with physiologic doses of Vitamin-D

79. Ans.— B. Normal birth weight and subsequent retardation of growth.

80. Ans.— A. Sodium

81. Ans.— D. All of the above

82. Ans.— A. Rickets

83. Ans.— B. Linolenic acid

84. Ans.— D. K

85. Ans.— A. E

86. Ans.— A. Normal parathromone levels

In Vitamin-D resistant rickets, there is severe muscular weakness, RTA, recurrent nausea vomiting diarrhoea, lethargy, MR, buphthalmos etc.

87. Ans.— B. 1500 Cal

88. Ans.— A. Icthyosis

89. Ans.— D. Artificial milk feeds

90. Ans.— A. Wilson-Mikity syndrome

91. Ans.— C. Facilitate the transport of each other from the intestinal mucosa to the blood.

The transport of most hexoses is uniquely affected by the amount of Na+ in the intestinal lumen; a high concentration of Na+ on the mucosal surface of the cells facilitates and a low concentration inhibits sugar influx into the epithelial cells. This is because glucose and Na+ share the same cotransporter, or symport, the sodium-dependent glucose transporter (SGLT, Na+ glucose cotransporter).

92. Ans.— C. Niacin deficiency

Delirium or dementia may be seen.

93. Ans.— B. Vit-D

94. Ans.— A. Edema

95. Ans.— A. Hb < 11.5 gm% in 3rd trimester pregnancy

Malnutrition in community is measured by :

1. Anthropometric Parameters like
   * Weight for age
   * Height for age
     - Weight for height
     - AC or AC/CC
2. Morbidity and mortality parameters like :
   * Av birth weight in the community
   * Infant mortality rate
   * Under 5 mortality rate
   * Prevalence of anemia in community

In pregnancy anemia is defined as Hb < 10 g in all trimesters of pregnancy, not < 11.5 g% thus this is thew most appropriate choice.

3

IMPORTANT TEXT OF NEWBORN

BREATH HOLDING SPELLS (BHS) VERSUS GRAND MAL EPILEPSY (GME)

		BHS	*GME*
1.	Age of onset	Often infancy	Rarely
2.	Family history	+	Often ±
3.	Precipitating factor	Usually+	±
4.	Occurrence during sleep	—	+
5.	Sequence	Long cry or single cry - cyanosis or pallor - Unconsciousness —Opisthotones- Clonic Jerks rarely	Singly cry usually absent - Tonic clonic phase - cyanosis may occur later in attack
6.	Perspiration	Cold sweat	Warm sweat
7.	Heart rate	Markedly increased, asystole	Increased
8.	Average duration	<1 minute	>1 minute
9.	Incontinence and tongue biting	Uncommon	Common
10.	Postictal phase	Rare	Drowsiness common
11.	Ictal EEG pattern	Isoelectric preceded and followed by diffuse high voltage delta waves	Generalized high voltage polyspike discharge gradually subsiding into slow waves and depression for several minutes
12.	Interictal EEG	Normal	Bilateral discharges
13.	Oculocardiac activation	About 50% develop asystole > 2 sec.	No response. In 7% asystole of <4 sec.

CAUSE OF GIT OBSTRUCTION PRESENTING IN THE NEONATAL PERIOD

Anatomical	*Functional*
Oesophageal atresia	Pyloric stenosis
Duodenal atresia	Hirschsprung's disease
Jejunal atresia	Meconium plug syndrome
Volvulus due to malrotation	Meconium ileus
Colon atresia	
Stricture secondary to necrotizing enterocolitis	

CAUSES OF STRIDOR

Congenital	*Acquired*
Laryngomalacia	Acute laryngotracheobronchitis
Laryngeal web	Acute epiglottis
Laryngeal cleft	Subglotitic stenosis
Haemangioma	Allergic laryngeal oedema
Bilateral vocal cord palsy	Diphtheria
	Foreign body
Subglottic stenosis	Laryngeal papilloma

MCQ's OF NEWBORN

What is important in Newborn

Assessment of Maturity (signs, reflexes), Prematurity, IUGR, APGAR score, Hyperbilirubinemia, Resp. Distress Syndrome, Congenital Malformations

1. A newborn baby presented with prouse bleeding from umbilical stump after birth. Probably diagnosis is : AIIMS 2007

A. Factor-XIII deficiency
B. Glanzmann thrombothenia
C. vWF Deficiency
D. Bernord Soulier syndrome

2. Bart's hydrops fetalis is lethal because : AIIMS 2007

A. Hb Bart's cannot bind oxygen.
B. The excess α-globin form insoluble precipitates.
C. Hb Bart's cannot release oxygen to fetal tissues.
D. Microcytic red cells become trapped in the placenta.

3. The protective effects of breast mild are known to be associated with : AI 2005

A. IgM antibodies B. Lysozyme
C. Mast cells D. IgA antibodies

4. For fetal paternity, most reliable test is : Rohtak 2001

A. DNA finger printing B. Major blood group
C. Minor blood group D. All of the above

5. The most important cause of under 5 mortality is : DNB 2001

A. Diarrhoea B. Malnutrition
C. Respiratory Infections D. Trauma

6. All of the following are used to assess IUGR except : DNB 2001

A. Fetal movements B. Head size
C. Fundus height D. Liquor volume

7. Congenital toxoplasmosis is diagnosed by demonstration of : AIIMS 2002

A. IgM in mother B. IgM in baby
C. IgG in mother D. IgG in fetus

8. Cyanosis in newborn is due to : Delhi 2002

A. Hypocalcemia
B. Sepsis
C. Ventricular septal defect
D. Polycythemia

9. A large for date newborn presents with hypoglycemia which of the following is most likely cause : Delhi 2002

A. TGA B. Hypothyroidism
C. Beckwith syndrome D. Hypocalcemia

10. Average weight of newborn in India is (in kg) : Maharashtra 2000

A. 2.5 B. 2.8
C. 3 D. 3.5

11. Average length of newborn in India is (in cm) : Maharashtra 2000

A. 35 B. 50
C. 55 D. 70

12. New born gains normal weight after what days of delivery : CMC 2001

A. 2 B. 5
C. 10 D. 15
E. 30

13. All features help to decide about maturity of newborn except : CMC 2001

A. Breast nodule B. Anterior fontanelle
C. Planter creases D. Scrotal rugae

14. Pincer grasp without ulnar deviation indicate age of how many months ? CMC 2001

A. 6 B. 8
C. 12 D. 15

15. True about neonatal resuscitation is : BHU 2002

A. Wrapping in a wet towel
B. Place the baby on the back
C. Suction of the nose is done first then the mouth
D. All of the above

16. All of the following groups of newborns are at an increased risk of hypoglycemia except : AIIMS 2002

A. Birth asphyxia
B. Respiratory distress syndrome
C. Maternal diabetes
D. Post-term infant

Ans.

1. C	2. C	3. A	4. A	5. C	6. A	7. B	8. D	9. C	10. B
11. B	12. C	13. B	14. C	15. D	16. D				

17. **Infant born to a diabetic mother is at risk for all of the following except : UPSC 2002**
A. Neonatal hepatitis
B. Polycythemia
C. Hypoglycemia
D. Congenital malformations

18. **A newborn baby had normal APGAR score at birth and developed excessive frothing and choking on attempted feeds. The investigation of choice is: AIIMS 2003**
A. Esophagoscopy
B. Bronchoscopy
C. MRI chest
D. X-ray chest and abdomen with the red rubber catheter passed per or

19. **A new born baby has been referred to the casualty as a case of congenital diaphragmatic hernia. The first clinical intervention is to: AIIMS 2003**
A. Insert a central venous pressure line
B. Bag and mask ventilation
C. Insert a nasogastric tube
D. Ventilate with high frequency ventilator

20. **Not true about sudden infant death syndrome : Kerala 1997**
A. Common in male child
B. Allergy to animal milk
C. Seen in premature babies
D. Cause is prolonged breast feeding

21. **99% of the Neonates void within : AMU 1998**
A. 24 hrs B. 38 hrs
C. 8 hrs D. 12 hrs

22. **At birth the normal heart rate is : Bihar 1991**
A. 60-80 B. 80-110
C. 70-120 D. 110-150

23. **Which of the following statements about human colostrum is not true : AMU 1994**
A. Contains antibodies
B. Is almost sodium free
C. Contains more protein than natural milk
D. Is secretion of breast during first day of lactation

24. **Which of the following chronic diseases is transmitted transplacentally : AMU 1997**
A. Syphilis
B. Malaria
C. Listeria monocytogenes
D. All the above

25. **Infants weighing less than 2.5 kgs at birth are best labelled as : UPSC 1996**
A. Low birth weight B. Pre-term
C. Under grown D. Premature

26. **The gestational age of the preterm baby is : UPSC 1996**
A. Less than 28 weeks B. Less than 30 weeks
C. Less than 37 weeks D. Less than 35 weeks

27. **All the following statements regarding neonatal mortality are true except : AP 1991**
A. Acrocyanosis
B. Birth asphyxia
C. Birth injuries
D. Congenital malformation

28. **Immediately after birth, the baby is given stomach wash with normal saline routinely in the following situations except : Rohtak 1995**
A. Heart rate is more than 100
B. Babies born by cesarean section
C. Severely asphyxiated baby
D. Meconium stained liquor

29. **The following babies should be given special care except : Rohtak 1995**
A. Birth weight of less than 2000 mgs
B. Birth asphyxia
C. Respiratory distress in the baby
D. Baby with cephalhaematoma

30. **Within a few hours after birth, the skin is : Orissa 1991**
A. Quite pale B. Quite red
C. Oedematous D. Scaly and dry

31. **Which of the following organ in a fetus is not affected by intrauterine malnutrition : AIIMS 1995**
A. Liver B. Spleen
C. Brain D. Adrenals

32. **Which of the following drug will increase lactation if given to a nursing mother : AMU 1996**
A. Metaclopropamide B. Hydrocortisone
C. Iron preparations D. Propranolol

33. **At what point of infancy, intracellular and extracellular fluid volumes are equal : AIIMS 1990**
A. One month B. Three months
C. Five months D. Nine months

34. **The most common organism causing neonatal septicemia in most of the neonatal unit is : AIIMS 1991**
A. Staph aureus B. Staph albus
C. Klebsiella D. E. coli

35. **The bacteriologically confirmed causes of neonatal septicemia should receive antibiotic therapy for : AIIMS 1990**
A. 7 days B. 10 days
C. 20 days D. 28 days

36. **Osteomyelitis in a neonate should be treated for at least : AIIMS 1996**
A. 10 days B. 21 days
C. 14 days D. 28 days

Ans.										
	17. A	18. A	19. C	20. B	21. D	22. D	23. B	24. D	25. A	26. C
	27. A	28. A	29. D	30. B	31. C	32. A	33. B	34. C	35. B	36. B

37. **Which of the following situation in tetanus neonatorum carries a bad prognosis:** **Rohtak 1995**
A. High grade fever.
B. Onset of symptoms within first week of life.
C. Interval between lockjaw and onset of spasms of less than 48 hours.
D. All the above these.

38. **Chloramphenicol is particularly hazardous in premature infant because of the risk of :** **UPSC 1993**
A. Jaundice
B. Cardiovascular collapse
C. Thrombocytopenia
D. Pancytopenia

39. **In a newborn, enzymes system shows deficiencies of :** **AIIMS 1993**
A. Carbonic anhydrase
B. Glucuronyl transferase
C. Triphosphopyridine nucleotide
D. All of the above

40. **A hymenal tag in a newborn is best treated by :** **PGI 1991**
A. Steroids B. Surgery
C. Leaving it alone D. None of the above

41. **The number of fontanelles presents in new born child is :** **AMC 1997**
A. 1 B. 2
C. 4 D. 6

42. **The composition of breast milk, per 100 ml :** **UPSC 1994**
A. 67 calories, 3.5 g protein, 3.5 g fat and 4.5 g carbohydrate.
B. 67 calories, 1.2 g protein, 4 g fat and 4.5 g carbohydrate.
C. 67 calories, 3.5 g protein, 4 g fat and 7 g carbohydrate.
D. 100 calories, 3.5 g protein, 4 g fat and 7 g carbohydrate.

43. **Breast fed babies as compared to artificially fed babies have all the following benefits except :** **PGI 1992**
A. Lower incidence of diarrhoea episodes
B. Lower incidence of respiratory infection
C. Lower incidence of late onset tetany
D. Lower incidence of future obesity

44. **A mother is preparing to breast feed her infant, it would be of value to her, if she were acquainted with:** **PGI 1981; AIIMS 1993**
A. Moro's reflex B. Rooting reflex
C. Grasp reflex D. Cough reflex

45. **All are commonly observed in postmature infant, except :** **AIIMS 1993**
A. Long nails
B. Increased alertness
C. Abundance of lanugo
D. Abundance of scalp hair

46. **All are characteristics of premature infants, except :** **PGI 1990**
A. Hypotonic muscles
B. Thin extremities
C. Minimal subcutaneous fat
D. Breast engorgement

47. **Breast feeding should begin —— hours after delivery:** **AIIMS 1994**
A. 2 B. 4
C. 8 D. 24

48. **Breast milk jaundice is due to :** **UPSC 1993**
A. Pregnandiole B. Vitamin-K excess
C. Excessive calcium D. Cause not known

49. **In an infant with galactosemia —— should be avoided:** **PGI 1991**
A. Gluten B. Egg
C. Milk D. Rice

50. **90% of the milk is obtained by the breast feeding infant in :** **PGI 1997**
A. 20 minutes B. 10 minutes
C. 7 minutes D. 4 minutes

51. **Defect most commonly occurring in congenital rubella is :** **AIIMS 1991**
A. Cataract B. Deafness
C. Microcephaly D. Blindness

52. **Vocabulary of 1.5 year old child is :** **AMU 1996**
A. 1-10 words B. 10-20 words
C. 20-30 words D. 30-40 words

53. **Infant with extrahepatic biliary atresia, jaundice usually develops at about :** **AIIMS 1996**
A. 1-2 days of age B. 3-6 days of age
C. 3-6 weeks of age D. 6-12 weeks of age

54. **In amniotic fluid, the finding of the following helps to determine fetal maturation :** **UPSC 1991**
A. Creatinine/Lecithin ratio
B. Bilirubin
C. Urea
D. DNA and amino acids

55. **Epstein's pearls on the hard palate should be treated with the following except :** **AIIMS 1990**
A. Topical antibiotics B. Topical steroids
C. No therapy needed D. Systemic steroids

56. **The diapers of newborns may be normally stained faintly red by the decomposition of :** **AIIMS 1990**
A. Ammonia B. Bilirubin
C. Urates D. Oxalates

57. **In an infant exclusively fed on breast milk has pallor, hepatomegaly but no splenomegaly, investigation of choice is :** **AIIMS 1997**
A. Serum iron levels B. HbF levels
C. Serum B_{12} levels D. Serum folic acid levels

Ans.	37. D	38. B	39. D	40. C	41. D	42. C	43. D	44. B	45. C	46. D
	47. A	48. A	49. C	50. D	51. B	52. A	53. B	54. A	55. C	56. C
	57. A									

58. **In cold injury to preterm infant, following are seen except : AIIMS 1997**
A. Shivering B. Scleroma
C. Bradycardia D. Metabolic acidosis

59. **Normal reflex patterns at birth may include : AMC 1992**
A. Grasp reflex
B. Moro reflex
C. Seeking or rooting reflex
D. All of the above

60. **If a normally developing infant just acquires a pincer grasp, which of the following would be his recently acquired gross motor milestones: UPSC 1997**
1. Ability to sit without support
2. Ability to pull to stand
3. Ability to crawl on the floor

Select the correct answer using the codes given below:
Codes :
A. 2 and 3 B. 1 and 2
C. 1 and 3 D. 1, 2, and 3

61. **What will be the Apgar score of new born infant who is pink in colour, with regular respiration, pulse rate above 100/minute, good muscle tone and the infant responding well to external stimuli: UPSC 1997**
A. 5 B. 6
C. 7 D. 8
E. Exactly 10

62. **New borns may be particularly susceptible to gram-negative infections because they have : AMU 1990**
A. Low levels of IgM B. High levels of IgE
C. Optimum level of IgM D. All of the above

63. **True undescended testicle should be brought surgically into scrotum : Delhi 1998**
A. Just after puberty B. Just before puberty
C. At 4-6 years of life D. During first year of life

64. **Long term complication of infant born to IDDM mother is : AI 1995**
A. DM B. Ketotic hypoglycemia
C. Obesity D. Hyperthyroidism

65. **Which of the following reflex is absent at birth : DNB 1990**
A. Laughing B. Moro
C. Startle D. Sucking

66. **Umbilical cord usually falls after : DNB 1991**
A. 5-10 days B. 15-20 days
C. 1-5 days D. None of the above

67. **Children above 6 years of age usually get acute otitis media due to : AIIMS 1996**
A. Haemophilus influenzae type
B. Staphylococcus aureus
C. Streptococcus pneumoniae
D. Klebsiella sp.

68. **With the first breath of a newborn what is true : UPSC 1998**
A. Pulmonary resistant falls to one tenth of its value.
B. Aspiration of amniotic fluid occurs.
C. Intra-pleural pressure reaches 60 cms of water.
D. Ductus arteriosus closes.

69. **Continuous pharyngeal suction in an asphyxiated infant is not recommended because it may lead to : Delhi 1998**
A. Vomiting B. Seizures
C. Bradycardia D. All of the above

70. **A child with blue sclera and multiple fracture has : AIIMS 1982, 94**
A. Rickets
B. Scurvy
C. Osteogenesis imperfecta
D. Achondroplasia

71. **Possetting is treated by : AIIMS 1986; Delhi 1996**
A. Putting the child in a prone position
B. Carminative
C. Burping
D. Honey

72. **Neonatal septicemia is most commonly caused by : AIIMS 1986, 98**
A. Streptococcus viridans
B. Streptococcus pyogenes
C. Group-B streptococcus
D. Staphylococcus viridans

73. **The commonest symptoms in the children with spread of infection from CSOM to brain is : UPSC 1986; AIIMS 1996**
A. Vomiting B. Chronic deep headache
C. Vertigo D. Focal paralysis

74. **All of the following are characteristics of cephalo-haematoma except : UPSC 1995**
A. Does not increase in size while crying.
B. The swelling is pulsatile.
C. It is benign, self-limiting and resolves in a few weeks's time.
D. Does not cross suture line.

75. **A child with purpuric rash, irritability, high grade fever is suffering from : UPSC 1995**
A. Pneumococcal pneumonia
B. Addison's disease
C. Mumps
D. Meningococcal meningitis

76. **In a new born, liver is 1 cm enlarged. The child has : AIIMS 1996**
A. Hemolytic disease B. Malaria
C. Nutritional cirrhosis D. Normal

77. **Tongue tie is best corrected at : AIIMS 1997**
A. Birth B. 1-2 years
C. 3-4 years D. Puberty

Ans.									
58. C	59. D	60. D	61. E	62. A	63. C	64. D	65. A	66. A	67. C
68. A	69. C	70. C	71. C	72. D	73. B	74. A	75. D	76. D	77. C

78. Long standing unconjugated jaundice of newborn is caused by all except : AIIMS 1986, 90

A. Criggler Najjar syndrome
B. Breast milk jaundice
C. Cretinism
D. Septicemia

79. Hematoma of the sternomastoid muscle detected in a 16 days old infant requires : UPSC 1996

A. Immediate surgical evacuation
B. Surgical intervention within 2 weeks
C. Prophylactic antibiotic therapy
D. No immediate therapy

80. Infant born to HbS Ag positive mother : AP 1993

A. Should only be observed for any development of hepatitis.
B. Hepatitis vaccine alone is sufficient.
C. Gammaglobulin should be administered.
D. Hepatitis-B immunoglobin and Hepatitis vaccine should be administered immediately.

81. Physiological Icterus usually appears on the —— and regresses by the —— : AIIMS 1981, 83, 96

A. First day and third day
B. Third day and seventh day
C. Third day and ninth day
D. Ninth day and eleventh day

82. Breast milk is adequate in all of the following nutrients for normal infants growth, except : Karnataka 1994

A. Proteins B. Vitamin-A
C. Vitamin-D D. Copper

83. The following finding is of serious pathological significance in infants : PGI 1999

A. Loss of weight
B. Palpable kidney
C. Palpable spleen
D. Deviation of trachea from midline

84. Slate-blue areas over buttocks of newborn indicates : PGI 1999

A. Mongolian spots
B. Acrocyanosis
C. Peripheral cyanosis
D. Harlequein colour change

85. Hair on end appearance of skull is due to : PGI 1990

A. Haemolytic anaemias
B. Sturge-Weber syndrome
C. Multiple myeloma
D. Rickets
E. ↑ I.C.T. (Intracranial tension)

86. At birth, the number of ossification centres are approximately : AIIMS 1992

A. 2-3 B. 3-4
C. 5-6 D. 7-9

87. Resuscitation of baby starts with : WB 1998

A. Nasal & oral suction
B. Cleaning-up of baby
C. Placed in trendelenburg position
D. Radiant heat

88. A one-day-old neonate, who was born by a difficult forceps delivery, is alert and active. However, she does not move her left arm. The left arm lies by her side, internally rotated with the forearm extended and pronated. She does not even move the arm during a Moro reflex. The remainder of her physical examination is unremarkable. Which of the following diagnosis is strongly suggested by the clinical picture : MAHE 1992

A. Fracture of the left clavicle
B. Left-sided Erb-Duchenne paralysis
C. Left-sided Klumpke's paralysis
D. Spinal injury with left hemiparesis

89. Which of the following is not a cause of Jaundice in first week of birth : AIIMS 1982, 86, 87; Delhi 1984, 87, 89; AMC 1987, 99

A. Physiological B. Hemolytic
C. Biliary atresia D. Septicemia

90. Which of the following is not present in full term infant: AIIMS 1983; UPSC 1995

A. Moro's reflex
B. Tonic neck reflex
C. Tonic labyrinthine reflex
D. All of the above

91. Bilateral absence of Moro's reflex is seen in : AIIMS 1983; ESI 1988, 99

A. Clavicle fractures B. Erb's palsy
C. Prematurity D. Cranial trauma

92. Prematurity in a child is diagnosed by all except : Delhi 1999

A. Single-sole crease
B. Descending testis
C. Breast nodule at 32-34 weeks
D. Hair texture

93. Peak level of bilirubin is reached on the -------- day in physiological jaundice : Delhi 1999

A. 1-2 B. 2-3
C. 4-5 D. 6-7

94. Moro's reflex is abnormal after : AIIMS 1983, 84; Delhi 1998

A. 4 weeks B. 10 weeks
C. 12 weeks D. 20 weeks

95. Commonest correctable anomaly in neonates is : Delhi 1997

A. Intestinal obstruction
B. Anal atresia
C. Spina bifida
D. Congenital heart disease

Ans.									
78. D	79. D	80. D	81. B	82. D	83. A	84. A	85. A	86. C	87. C
88. B	89. C	90. C	91. D	92. C	93. C	94. C	95. B		

96. India has to achieve Infant Mortality rate (by 2,000 A.D.) below : AIIMS 1988, 91, 92, 93; UPSC 1989, 92, 93
A. 82 B. 75
C. 60 D. 45

97. In an obese child, true is : Delhi 1985, 90
A. Low muscle mass B. Short stature
C. Increased Bone age D. Delayed Milestones

98. In iodine deficiency, which is not seen : TN 1998
A. Goitre
B. Low IQ
C. Melaena
D. Retarded physical growth

99. In a 4 years old child with ASOM, the infecting organism is likely to be : AI 1999
A. Pneumococcus B. H. influenzae
C. Streptococcus D. Staphylococcus

100. Acute osteomyelitis in infants is best diagnosed by : PGI 1983, 94
A. History and high degree of suspicion
B. X-ray
C. Blood culture
D. Elevated WBC count

101. Syphilis attack the fetus after the —— months of gestation: JIPMER 1987, 99
A. 2nd B. 3rd
C. 4th D. 7th

102. Intrauterine growth retardation can be caused by all except : AIIMS 1984, 97
A. Nicotine B. Alcohol
C. Propranolol D. Phenathiazine

103. A 8 months old child will be able to do which of the following : PGI 1982, 97
A. Pincer grasp B. Sitting stably
C. Stand without support D. Tells when he is wet

104. Physiological Jaundice : AIIMS 1993
A. Lasts longer in the premature.
B. Can cause clay-coloured stools.
C. Result from decreased activity of uridine diphospho glucoronyl.
D. Can cause kernicterus.

105. The steps required to be taken to resuscitate a new-born who does not cry spontaneously are indicated below : CSE 1996
1. Expand the neck of the baby about 30°.
2. Clear mouth and throat with a mucus extractor.
3. Stimulate the baby by flicking the soles withfingers two or three times.
4. Give assisted ventilation.

The correct sequence of these steps is :
A. 1,2,3,4 B. 1,2,4,3
C. 2,1,3,4 D. 2,1,4,3

106. Following are early manifestations of congenital syphilis except : Delhi 1990
A. Hutchinson's teeth B. Interstitial keratitis
C. Nephritis D. Clutton's joints

107. A mother kissing her baby find that baby's skin is slaty, the diagnosis is : Delhi 1985; TN 1990
A. Fanconi's syndrome B. Thalassemia
C. Cystic fibrosis D. Niemann Pick disease

108. All of the following are transmitted from mother to neonate during delivery except : AMU 1986; PGI 1987, 98
A. H. simplex B. Toxoplasmosis
C. Salmonella D. C. trachomatis

109. Breast feeding is contraindicated if the mother is taking : AIIMS 1981; PGI 1985, 99
A. Propranolol
B. Broad spectrum antibiotics
C. Sulfonyl ureas
D. Insulin

110. Commonest cause of pathological hyperbilirubinemia in India is : AMC 1982; PGI 1986, 99
A. ABO incompatibility B. Rh incompatibility
C. Septicemia D. G-6-P-D deficiency

111. Which of the following consist of the correct set of strategies for improved neonatal survival : CSE 1996
1. Early registration and antenatal care of all pregnant women, promoting safe delivery.
2. Maintaining newborn's warmth, giving bottle feeding advice, preventing infections.
3. Promoting early exclusive breast feeding, early detection of high risk newborns and referral promoting birth spacing.
4. Giving lacteal feeds, making mother aware of danger of dehydration, giving vitamin drops to the neonate.

Select the correct answer
A. 2 and 4 B. 1 and 3
C. 1,2 and 3 D. 2,3 and 4

112. Neonatal hypocalcemia to produce seizures is below serum level of ——— mg% : Orissa 1998
A. 7 B. 8
C. 9 D. 10

113. Which is high risk neonate : PGI 1983, 99
A. Less than 1500 gms
B. Previous neonatal death
C. Less than 37 weeks
D. All of the above

114. Lecithin-sphingomyelin ratio of more than atleast indicates full maturation of lungs : AIIMS 1986, 89, 92
A. 1.0 B. 1.5
C. 2.0 D. 3.0

Ans.										
	96. C	97. B	98. E	99. B	100. A	101. C	102. D	103. B	104. A	105. A
	106. C	107. C	108. C	109. C	110. B	111. C	112. B	113. D	114. C	

115. In physiological jaundice in full term infants serum bilirubin does not generally exceed : AIIMS 1983, 97

A. 5 mg% B. 10 mg%
C. 15 mg% D. 20 mg%

116. High Risk Baby is all except : AIIMS 1993

A. Born to a working mother
B. Mother with H/O abortion
C. Death of 2, sibling death within 2 months
D. Low birth wt.

117. True about neonatal sepsis is : AI 1996

A. Infection through umbilical cord
B. Infection by GUT bacteria
C. Infection through respiratory tract
D. Not very common

118. With exclusive breast milk feeding, growth is normal in a full term child, till : Karnataka 1994

A. 2 months B. 4 months
C. 8 months D. 12 months

119. About teething, all are true except : Delhi 1994

A. Upper incisors are first to appear
B. All upper teeth appear earlier
C. All evolve by 24 months
D. Ist molars evolve by 12-14 months

120. The significance of single umbilical artery is that one should : Delhi 1994

A. Look for congenital abnormalities
B. Look for malignancies
C. Look for mental retardation
D. Normal variation

121. An infant dies at the age of six months. At post-mortem examination, extensive granulomatous destruction of the brain is noticed. The lesions showed a protozoan in macrophages. The mother had a mild febrile illness with enlarged palpable cervical lymph nodes three months before the birth of the child. The protozoan involved is most probably : UPSC 1994

A. Entamoeba histolytica
B. Leishmania donovan
C. Plasmodium falciparum
D. Toxoplasma gondii

122. The amino acid in breast milk that is claimed to promote neurological development in infants is : UPSC 1994

A. Valine B. Tyrosine
C. Taurine D. Leucine

123. A 5-months old boy weighing 6 kgs has a cleft lip and cleft palate. What will be the most appropriate advise regarding surgical correction of this congenital deformity : UPSC 1994

A. Surgical correction of the cleft lip and palate immediately.
B. Surgical correction of the cleft lip immediately and palate at the age of 1-1.5 years.
C. Surgical correction of cleft palate immediately and the lip at the age of one year.
D. Surgery after the child has started talking well.

124. A neonate with scaphoid abdomen with respiratory distress has : AI 1994

A. Congenital Pyloric stenosis
B. Diaphragmatic hernia
C. Volvulus
D. Scurvy

125. The use of steroids in a neonate is required in : AI 1994

A. Bronchial aplasia
B. Congenital Polycystic disease
C. Meconium aspiration syndrome
D. Phenylketonuria

126. New born child not passed urine for 36 hours. Investigation of choice is : AIIMS 1995

A. Ultrasound of Kidney & Bladder
B. X-ray pelvis
C. Cystoscopy
D. CT Scan

127. Child (Breast fed) at 30 hours of life develops yellowing of face, palms & sole which is not true : AIIMS 1995

A. Is physiological jaundice
B. Is due to septicemia
C. Breast milk jaundice
D. Congenital obliteration of bile duct

128. Consider the following statements about Sudden Infant Death Syndrome : UPSC 1995

1. It occurs in apparently healthy infants
2. Familial recurrences are known
3. The peak incidence is at five to six months of age
4. Greatest number of deaths occur between midnight and 9 a.m.

Of these statements :

A. 1, 2 and 4 are correct B. 1, 3 and 4 are correct
C. 2, 3 and 4 are correct D. 1, 2 and 3 are correct

129. Bedside investigation in a newborn with septicemia are all except : AI 1996

A. Micro ESR
B. Leucocytosis
C. ↑ CR protein
D. Toxic granulated multilobulated nuclei

130. Growth chart is an epidemiological tool in detection of : Delhi 1996

A. Short stature B. Malnutrition
C. Endocrinal disorders D. Health status of country

Ans.									
115. B	116. A	117. A	118. B	119. A	120. A	121. D	122. C	123. B	124. B
125. A	126. A	127. A	128. C	129. C	130. B				

131. A six-months old infant has crying spells followed by passage of bloody stools. On examination of abdomen, a sausage shaped mass is palpable around the umbilicus. The investigation of choice in this case would be : UPSC 1996

A. Sigmoidoscopy B. Gastroscopy
C. Barium meal D. Barium enema

132. Which one of the following is the cause of neonatal jaundice with cutaneous rashes and intracranial calcification: UPSC 1996

A. Cytomegalic virus B. Congenital syphilia
C. Herpes simplex D. Rubella syndrome

133. The following conditions are associated with prolonged unconjugated hyperbilirubinemia in the newborn, except : UP 1996

A. Breast milk jaundice
B. Hypothyroidism
C. Criggler Najjar syndrome
D. Septicemia

134. Absence of nail in a new born indicates : Kerala 1996

A. Yellow nail syndrome
B. Nail patella syndrome
C. Ecto dermal dysplasia
D. Prematurity

135. A newborn with goitre, following may be the causes except : PGI 1995

A. Mother has hyperthyroidism
B. Mother has hypothyroidism
C. Mother taking antithyroid drugs
D. None of the above

136. A child breast fed, had cataracts hyperbilirubinemia and convulsions, has : AIIMS 1996

A. Breast milk jaundice B. Gala
C. D. Tetany

137. Vomiting in a neonate is due to : AI 1997

A. Oesophageal atresia B. Pyloric stenosis
C. Aerophagy D. Amnion gastritis

138. A baby was intubated thrice for meconium. After full spiration there were no breathing movements. Next management is : AI 1997

A. Tactile stimulation
B. Cardiac compression
C. Intubation + Ventillation mask
D. Ventillator

139. 8 days old neonate with extensor posture : TN 1999

A. Cerebral palsy
B. Hypoxic ischemic encephalopathy
C. Malnutrition
D. Infection

140. Increased release of cortisol in a fetus just before delivery helps in : Kerala 1999

A. Initiating uterine contraction
B. Placental separation
C. Lung maturation
D. Liver maturity

141. MC cause of apnoea in a neonate is : Kerala 1999

A. Prematurity B. Sleep apnoea
C. Pulmonary hypoplasia D. Maternal sedation

142. All are complications of supine self-feeding except : Kerala 1999

A. Chronic bronchitis B. Bottle caries
C. Apnoea D. Otitis media

143. Complication of full term small for gestation age baby is : AI 2000

A. Intraventricular haemorrhage
B. PDA
C. Acidosis
D. Hypoglycemia

144. Apnoeic spells, convulsions, tachycardia, cyanotic episodes, hypothermia, lethargy and limpness in a neonate suggest : UPSC 2000

A. Hypoglycaemia B. Hypocalcaemia
C. Sepsis D. Apnea of prematurity

145. A male baby aged 6/12 is brought with a history of retarded milestones in every aspect of motor activity, physical and mental development with refractory constipation and anaemia. The most likely diagnosis is: UPSC 2000

A. Down's syndrome
B. Congenital hypothyroidism
C. 18-Trisomy
D. 13-Trisomy

146. A newborn, tachypnoea is defined as respiratory rate more than ——per min : Delhi 2000

A. 30 B. 50
C. 60 D. 80

147. What is warm chain ? TNPSC 1998

A. It is important in maintaining vaccines.
B. It is an important Microbiological Culture Technique.
C. It is important for maintenance of Newborn temperature from birth.
D. It is important in ELISA Technique.

148. The following may be physiological in newborn, except : TNPSC 2000

A. May not pass urine in first 24 hours of birth.
B. May not pass motion within 24 hours of birth.
C. Has greyish blue pigmentation of back.
D. Has a small subconjunctival haemorrhage.

Ans. 131. D 132. A 133. D 134. C 135. A 136. B 137. B 138. A 139. B 140. C
141. D 142. A 143. D 144. D 145. B 146. C 147. C 148. A

149. **In neonatal herpes, true is : PGI 2000**
A. Cause by HSV-II
B. Hepatosplenomegaly diagnosis
C. Spontaneous recovery occurs
D. If not treated, disseminates

150. **Cong. rubella manifestations are following except : PGI 2000**
A. Rash appears first on trunk
B. Pre-auricular L. nodes
C. Arthralgia
D. Retinopathy

151. **Which of the following findings in a newborn would indicate that he was mature (40 weeks) : UPSC 1993**
A. Head circumference over 34 cm
B. Sole of foot covered with creases
C. Presence of 2 mm breast nodule
D. Presence of ear cartilage

152. **Maternal characteristics suspected of causing reduction in foetal growth include all of the following, except : UPSC 1990**
A. Living at high altitude
B. Small heart volume
C. Heavy smoking, primiparity
D. Prediabetic state

153. **All are true about neonatal osteomyelitis, except : UPSC 1991**
A. Surgical drainage not always required
B. Rarely spread into the joint space
C. Uncommonly high fever
D. Rarely development of chronic osteomylitis

154. **Oral candidiasis in the newborn generally : PGI 1992**
A. Required systemic therapy with Amphotericin-B.
B. Requires both local (mycostatin) and systemic (amphotericin) therapy
C. Responds well to oral therapy with mycostatin.
D. None of the above.

155. **Posterior fontanelle is closes by : AMC 1985, 96**
A. 4 months B. 6 months
C. 16 months D. 24 months

156. **All of the following are usually associated with infants of diabetic mothers, except : AIIMS 1993**
A. Moon facies B. Respiratory alkalosis
C. Hypoglycaemia D. Clinical signs of tetany

157. **Yellow colour of skin of an infant at birth is probably due to : PGI 1991**
A. Carotenemia B. Meconium staining
C. Infective hepatitis D. Hyperbilirubinemia

158. **Caput succedaneum disappears within : PGI 1983; UPSC 1996**
A. 1-6 months B. 1-2 weeks
C. 3-5 weeks D. 5-7 weeks

159. **Cephalhematoma usually disappears within : UPSC 1992**
A. 3-5 months B. 2-5 weeks
C. 3-5 weeks D. 5-7 weeks

160. **The bone most frequently fractured during delivery is the : PGI 1992**
A. Radius B. Clavicle
C. Humerus D. Ulna

161. **During a cry of baby, mother wakes up in night because: Delhi 1993**
A. She has developed a conditioned reflex.
B. It is a congenital reflex.
C. Mother with a new born is not able to sleep comfortably.
D. Baby's cry in high pitched.

162. **APGAR score of a child born blue with HR 70/mt. floppy with feeble cry with grimacing on nasal suction is : Delhi 1993**
A. 3 B. 2
C. 4 D. 5

163. **Regarding cretinism which of the following is not true: AP 1997**
A. Diminished reflexes B. Difficulties in feeding
C. Baby hyperactive D. Growth retardation

164. **Moro's reflex is abolished by the age of ——— months: Delhi 1992**
A. 3 B. 1
C. 6 D. 0.25

165. **Following are features of Congenital syphilis except : UPSC 1983; JIPMER 1992**
A. Bone within bone appearance
B. Osteochondritis occurs after 6 months
C. Negative serology indicates absence of disease
D. Severe periostitis can occur

166. **Pincer grasp is seen at : AIIMS 1986; PGI 1993**
A. 4 weeks B. 6 weeks
C. 16 weeks D. 36 weeks

167. **Abstract thinking develops at the age of : DNB 1990, JIPMER 1993**
A. 3 years B. 6 years
C. 9 years D. 12 years

168. **Which of the following is not a normal finding in the newborn : UPSC 1986; JIPMER 1993**
A. Peripheral cyanosis B. Central cyanosis
C. Systolic murmur D. Pulse rate 100/min

169. **Increased age of the mother is associated with : JIPMER 1993**
A. Twins B. Down's syndrome
C. Anencephaly D. Gastroschisis

Ans. 149. A 150. A 151. B 152. D 153. B 154. C 155. B 156. B 157. B 158. B
159. D 160. B 161. A 162. A 163. C 164. A 165. C 166. D 167. A 168. B
169. B

170. A five days old, full term male infant was severely cyanotic at birth. Prostaglandin E was administered initially and later balloon atrial septostomy was done which showed improvement in oxygenation. The most likely diagnosis of this infant is: AI 2004
A. Tetralogy of fallot
B. Transposition of great vessels
C. Truncus arteriosus
D. Tricuspid atresia

171. A 10 months old child presents with two weeks' history of fever, vomiting and alteration of sensorium. Cranial CT Scan reveals basal exudates and hydrocephalus. The most likely etiological agent is: AI 2004
A. Mycobacterium tuberculosis
B. Cryptococcus neoformans
C. Listeria monocytogenes
D. Streptococcus pneumoniae

172. Consider the following : UPSC 2004
A. Respiratory distress syndrome
B. Intraventricular haemorrhage
C. Infections
D. Necrotizing enterocolitis

Which of the above is/are the major cause/causes of mortality in pre-term babies:
A. 1 only
B. 2 and 3
C. 1, 2 and 3
D. 1, 2, 3 and 4

173. The appropriate approach to a neonate presenting with vaginal bleeding on day 4 of life is : AI 2005
A. Administration of vitamin-K
B. Investigation for bleeding disorder
C. No specific therapy
D. Administration of 10ml/kg of fresh frozen plasma over 4 hours

174. The protective effects of breast milk are known to be associated with : AI 2005
A. Igm antibodies B. Lysozyme
C. Mast cells D. IgA antibodies

175. Blood specimen for neonatal thyroid screening is obtained on : AI 2005
A. Cord blood B. 24 hours after birth
C. 48 hours after birth D. 72 hours after birth

176. Non-immune hydrops is not a feature of which of the following : AIIMS 2000
A. Chromosomal abnormalities
B. Alpha thalassemia
C. Renal malformation in fetus
D. Fetal cardiac abnormalities

177. Which of the following is true regarding cretinism : AI 2001
A. Short limbs compared to trunk
B. Proportionate shortening
C. Short limb and short stature
D. Short limb long stature

178. Which is not indicated in primary apnea of newborn: Kerala 2001
A. Adrenaline
B. Initial steps
C. Tactile stimulation
D. Bag and mask ventillation

179. Marasmus is characterized by all except : UPPGME-2006
A. Growth retardation B. Distended abdomen
C. Fatty liver D. Emaciation

180. Most common inherited childhood tumor is : AIIMS 2008
A. Leukemia B. Neuroblastoma
C. Retinoblastoma D. Wilm's tumor

181. Most common sign of acute hypoxia in neonates : AI 2009
A. Tachycardia
B. Bradycardia
C. Cardiac arrest tachypnea
D. Ventricular arrhythmia

Ans. 170. B 171. A 172. D 173. C 174. D 175. A 176. C 177. C 178. A 179. C 180. C 181. B

EXPLANATIONS OF NEWBORN

1. Ans.— A **Factor XIII syndrome**

   Glanzman's thrombasthenia is an extremely rare disorder of the blood, in which the platelets lack glycoprotein IIb/IIIa. Hence, no fibrinogen bridging can occur, and bleeding time is significantly prolonged. Characteristically, there is increased mucosal bleeding :

   * Epistaxis
   * Menorrhagia
   * Increased bleeding post-operatively.

2. Ans.— C **Hb Bart's cannot release oxygen to fetal tissues**

   "In the foetus excess gammaglobin chains form tetramers (Hb Barts) with such high affinity for oxygen that they deliver almost no oxygen to tissues" - *Robbins*

3. Ans.— D. **IgA antibodies**

   Although, antibodies and Lysozyme, both are important for protective effects of breast milk, antibodies play the major role. Out of IgM and IgA antibodies, breast milk is especially rich in secretory IgA which is the single best answer here.

   Human milk contains bacterial and viral antibodies including high concentration of secretory IgA, that prevents microorganisms from adhering to intestinal mucosa. These secretory antibodies provide local gastrointestinal immunity, against organisms entering the body via this route. They probably account atleast partially for lower incidence of diarrhea as well as otitis media, pneumonia, bacteremia and meningitis during the first year of life — Nelson.

4. Ans.— A. **DNA finger printing**
5. Ans.— C. **Respiratory Infections**
6. Ans.— A. **Fetal movements**
7. Ans.— B. **IgM in baby**
8. Ans.— D. **Polycythemia**
9. Ans.— C. **Beckwith syndrome**
10. Ans.— B. **2.8**
11. Ans.— B. **50**
12. Ans.— C. **10**
13. Ans.— B. **Anterior fontanelle**
14. Ans.— C. **12**
15. Ans.— D. **All of the above**
16. Ans.— D. **Post-term infant**
17. Ans.— A. **Neonatal hepatitis**
18. Ans.— A. **Esophagoscopy**
19. Ans.— C. **Insert a nasogastric tube.**
20. Ans.— B. **Allergy to animal milk**
21. Ans.— D. **12 hrs**
22. Ans.— D. **110-150**
23. Ans.— B. **Is almost sodium free**
24. Ans.— D. **All the above**
25. Ans.— A. **Low birth weight**

    Very low birth weight baby is any neonate weighing 1500 gms or less at birth irrespective of gestational age.

26. Ans.— C. **Less than 37 weeks**

    Stillborn is a dead neonate born at a gestational age of 28 weeks or more or weighing more than 1 kg. Term baby is any neonate born between 37 to 42 weeks of pregnancy irrespective of birth weight. Very premature baby is any neonate born in the late second trimester (20-27 weeks) and weighing at least 500 g at birth.

27. Ans.— A. **Acrocyanosis**
28. Ans.— A. **Heart rate is more than 100**
29. Ans.— D. **Baby with cephalhaematoma**
30. Ans.— B. **Quite red**
31. Ans.— C. **Brain**
32. Ans.— A. **Metaclopropamide**

33. Ans.— B. Three months
34. Ans.— C. Klebsiella
35. Ans.— B. 10 days
36. Ans.— B. 21 days
37. Ans.— D. All the above
38. Ans.— B. Cardiovascular collapse
39. Ans.— D. All of the above
40. Ans.— C. Leaving it alone
41. Ans.— D. 6
42. Ans. — C. 67 calories, 3.5 g protein, 4 g fat and 7 g carbohydrate
43. Ans.— D. Lower incidence of future obesity
44. Ans.— B. Rooting reflex

The full term infant suck vigorously when the breast is brought into contact with infant's cheek he or she seeks the nipple (rooting reflex). The reflex is weak, not synchronized with swallowing at 28 weeks of gestation. It is stronger and well synchronized at 32 weeks.

45. Ans.— C. Abundance of lanugo
46. Ans.— D. Breast engorgement
47. Ans.— A. 2
48. Ans.— A. Pregnandiole
49. Ans.— C. Milk
50. Ans.— D. 4 minutes
51. Ans.— B. Deafness
52. Ans.— A. 1-10 words
53. Ans.— B. 3-6 days of age
54. Ans.— A. Creatinine/Lecithin ratio
55. Ans.— C. No therapy needed

Epstein pearl are — palatal (histopathologically described as epithelial inclusion cysts, these appear as whitish spots on hard palate or on either side of median raphe no treatment is needed) or prepucial (they are infrequent, white in colour, rounded in shape, 1-2 mm on diameter and usually situated on the tip of the prepace at 6' clock position.

56. Ans.— C. Urates
57. Ans.— A. Serum iron levels
58. Ans.— C. Bradycardia
59. Ans.— D. All of the above

Grasp reflex and Moro's reflex usually disappear after the age of 12 weeks.

60. Ans.— D. 1, 2, and 3
61. Ans.— E. Exactly 10
62. Ans.— A. Low levels of IgM
63. Ans.— C. At 4-6 years of life
64. Ans.— D. Hyperthyroidism
65. Ans.— A. Laughing
66. Ans.— A. 5-10 days
67. Ans.— C. Streptococcus pneumoniae
68. Ans.— A. Pulmonary resistant falls to one tenth of its value.
69. Ans.— C. Bradycardia
70. Ans.— C. Osteogenesis imperfecta

In osteogenesis imperfecta, the bones are fragile and easily fractured. Deafness, metabolic disorder of collagen and its derivatives (sclera, bones and ligaments) are affected. It is autosomal dominant with variable expression. Autosomal variety is lethal in neonatal period.

71. Ans.— C. Burping
72. Ans.— D. Staphylococcus viridans
73. Ans.— B. Chronic deep headache
74. Ans.— A. Does not increase in size while crying.
75. Ans.— D. Meningococcal meningitis
76. Ans.— D. Normal
77. Ans.— C. 3-4 years

Otherwise it results in stuttering.

78. Ans.— D. Septicemia
79. Ans.— D. No immediate therapy
80. Ans.— D. Hepatitis-B immunoglobin and Hepatitis vaccine should be administered immediately.
81. Ans.— B. Third day and seventh day
82. Ans.— D. Copper
83. Ans.— A. Loss of weight
84. Ans.— A. Mongolian spots
85. Ans.— A. Haemolytic anaemias

In thalassemia, there is retangular shape of small bones of hands, thinning of cortex, diploic spaces in skull, widened bossing, thickening of frontal bones and pneumatization of sinuses is delayed.

86. Ans.— C. 5-6
87. Ans.— C. Placed in trendelenburg position
88. Ans.— B. Left-sided Erb-Duchenne paralysis

89. Ans.— C. Biliary atresia

90. Ans.— C. Tonic labyrinthine reflex

91. Ans.— D. Cranial trauma

92. Ans.— C. Breast nodule at 32-34 weeks

93. Ans.— C. 4-5

94. Ans.— C. 12 weeks

95. Ans.— B. Anal atresia

96. Ans.— C. 60

97. Ans.— B. Short stature

98. Ans.— D. Retarded physical growth

99. Ans.— B. H. influenzae

100. Ans.— A. History and high degree of suspicion

101. Ans.— C. 4th

102. Ans.— D. Phenathiazine

103. Ans.— B. Sitting stably

104. Ans.— A. Lasts longer in the premature

Physiological jaundice in term newborn appears after 30 hours. Peak level of bilirubin is maximum of 12 mg/dL is reached on 4 to 6 days and icterus disappears by 7-14 days. In premature babies, maximum bilirubin level reaches 15 mg/dL on 5th to 7th day and icterus disappears by 14 days to a month.

105. Ans.— A. 1, 2, 3, 4

106. Ans.— C. Nephritis

107. Ans.— C. Cystic fibrosis

108. Ans.— C. Salmonella

109. Ans.— C. Sulfonyl ureas

110. Ans.— B. Rh incompatibility

111. Ans.— C. 1, 2 and 3

112. Ans.— B. 8

113. Ans.— D. All of the above

114. Ans.— C. 2.0

115. Ans.— B. 10 mg%

116. Ans.— A. Born to a working mother

117. Ans.— A. Infection through umbilical cord

Findings include jaundice, hepatosplenomegaly, fever, temperature lability, apnoeic spells, irritability, failure to suck, meningitis, pneumonia, PN, metabolic acidosis, DIC, shock and death may develop.

118. Ans.— B. 4 months

119. Ans.— A. Upper incisors are first to appear

Lower central incisors are first to appear between 5 to 7 months.

120. Ans.— A. Look for congenital abnormalities

121. Ans.— D. Toxoplasma gondii

122. Ans.— C. Taurine

123. Ans.— B. Surgical correction of the cleft lip immediately and palate at the age of 1-1.5 years.

124. Ans.— B. Diaphragmatic hernia

Chest appears ballooned up, breath sounds are absent, Plain X-ray abdomen is diagnostic Bochdalek type (Posterior defect) is most common (on left side).

125. Ans.— A. Bronchial aplasia

126. Ans.— A. Ultrasound of Kidney & Bladder

127. Ans.— A. Is physiological jaundice

128. Ans.— C. 2, 3 and 4 are correct

SIDS is more common in infants with more than 2 severe apparent life threatening events, prematurity with apnea, family history of more than 2 SIDS and infants with alveolar hypoventilation.

129. Ans.— C. ↑ CR protein

130. Ans.— B. Malnutrition

131. Ans.— D. Barium enema

132. Ans.— A. Cytomegalic virus

133. Ans.— D. Septicemia

134. Ans.— C. Ecto dermal dysplasia

135. Ans.— A. Mother has hyperthyroidism

136. Ans.— B. Gala

In galactosemia there is oil drop cataract.

137. Ans.— B. Pyloric stenosis

Vomiting is usually seen in 2-4 weeks of age and in about 10% at birth.

138. Ans.— A. Tactile stimulation

Intubation and ventilation should be undertaken for signs of respiratory failure.

139. Ans.— B. Hypoxic ischemic encephalopathy

140. Ans.— C. Lung maturation

141. Ans.— D. Maternal sedation

142. Ans.— A. Chronic bronchitis

143. Ans.— D. Hypoglycemia

144. Ans.— D. Apnea of prematurity

145. Ans.— B. Congenital hypothyroidism

146. Ans.— C. 60

147. Ans.— C. It is important for maintenance of Newborn temperature from birth.

148. Ans.— A. May not pass urine in first 24 hours of birth.

149. Ans.— A. Cause by HSV-II

150. Ans.— A. Rash appears first on trunk

151. Ans.— B. Sole of foot covered with creases

152. Ans.— D. Prediabetic state

153. Ans.— B. Rarely spread into the joint space

154. Ans.— C. Responds well to oral therapy with mycostatin.

155. Ans.— B. 6 months

156. Ans.— B. Respiratory alkalosis

157. Ans.— B. Meconium staining

158. Ans.— B. 1-2 weeks

159. Ans.— D. 5-7 weeks

Cephalhematoma occurs in 0.5 to 2.5% of all births. Cephalhematoma is subperiosteal haemorrhage usually involving parietal and temporal lobes. Rim around hemotoma disappears by six months.

160. Ans.— B. Clavicle

161. Ans.— A. She has developed a conditioned reflex

162. Ans.— A. 3

163. Ans.— C. Baby hyperactive

164. Ans.— A. 3

165. Ans.— C. Negative serology indicates absence of disease.

166. Ans.— D. 36 weeks

167. Ans.— A. 3 years

168. Ans.— B. Central cyanosis

Moro's reflex can be elicited in preterm infant after 28 weeks of gestation but abduction component of the reflex is weak. The reflex is complete after 32 weeks of gestation. An asymmetric response is seen in Erb's palsy: spastic hemiplegia and fracture of humerus or clavicle. The reflex disappears by the age of 12 weeks.

169. Ans.— B. Down's syndrome

Down's syndrome is commonest chromosomal disorder occurring with a frequency of 1 : 700 newborns. The risk is 1 : 1550 of maternal age is between 25 and 29 years, 1:800 at 30-34 years, 1:270 at 35 to 39 years, 1: 100 at 40 to 44 years and 1:50 after 45 years.

170. Ans.— B. Transposition of great vessels

Cyanosis may be present from birth in all given diseases but improvement in oxygenation after balloon atrial septostomy is in favour of TGV.

Transposition of great vessels (TGV):

- Patients of complete TGV with intact ventricular septum are cynotic at birth.
- Aorta arising from right ventricle and pulmonary artery from left ventricle.
- Chest X-ray shows cardiomegaly with narrow base and plethoric lung field.
- The cardiac silhouette has "egg on side" appearance.
- Oxygenation can hardly be improved by administering oxygen even using oxygen tent
- Balloon atrial septostomy gives temporary relief by providing better mixing as well as reducing the left atrial pressure.
- Infusion of PGE, should be initiated immediately to maintain the patency of ductus arteriosis and to improve oxygenation.

171. Ans.— A. Mycobacterium tuberculosis

Basal exudates and hydrocephalus on CT scan is catch point for diagnosis of TBM.

CT scan finding of TBM :

- Basal exudates
- Inflammatory granuloma
- Hypodense lesions or infarcts
- Hydrocephalus

Tubercular meningitis may occur at any age, but is most common between 6 and 24 months of age.

172. Ans.— D. 1, 2, 3 and 4

173. Ans.— C. No specific therapy

"Vaginal bleeding - Menstrual-like bleeding may occur from the third to seventh day (here 4th day) of life."

- This is attributed withdrawal of maternal hormones after birth.
- The bleeding would subside after 2-3 days and no therapy is required.

174. Ans.— D. **IgA antibodies**

"Breast milk contains antimicrobial factors such as macrophages lymphocytes, secretory IgA, anti-streptococcal factor, Lysozyme and lactoferring which provide considerable protection not only against diarrhoeal diseases and necrotising enterocolitis, but also against respiratory infections in the first month of life."

* **Lower risk of infection with breast milk :**

- **High concentration of secretory IgA, IgM, Lysozyme, anti-staphylococcal factor and specific inhibitory substance against viral infection.**
- **Lactoferrin (less than 50% saturated with iron) not suitable for bacterial growth.**
- **High level of bifidus factor protects from E. coli.**
- **PABA provides protection against malaria.**
- **Colostrum has living phagocytic macrophage and lymphoid cells.**
- **Breast - fed babies have less diarrhea, fewer RTI and middle ear infection.**

Human milk contains bacterial and viral antibodies, including relatively high concentration of secretory IgA

- **Prevents micro-organism from adhering to the intestinal mucosa.**
- **Provide local gastrointestinal immunity against organisms entering the body via this route.**
- **They probably account, at least partially for the lower incidence of diarrhea as well as otitis media, pneumonia, bacteriemia and meningitis during the first year of life.**

So, the best answer is choice D (i.e. IgA antibodies.)

175. Ans.— A. **Cord blood**

"Availability of highly sensitive radioimmunoassay method for the measurement of blood T4 and TSH launched the newborn thyroid screening programs using cord blood samples obtained on filter paper."

* **"Most of the blood specimen for screening are collected on the first day of life."**

176. Ans.— C. **Renal malformation in fetus**

177. Ans.— C. **Short limb and short stature**

Congenital hypothyroidism results due to (a) aplasia/hypolasia or associated with maldescent of thyroid (b) familial iodine induced goitre secondary to metabolic inborn disorders or (c) Maternal ingestion of medications in pregnancy.

178. Ans.— A. **Adrenaline**

179. Ans.— C. **Fatty liver**

180. Ans.— C. **Retinoblastoma**

Though we could not find any straightforward documented evidence in support for our answer; almost every resident or student we discussed with was of opinion that Retinoblastoma should be the answer.

About 40% cases of retinoblastoma are hereditary.

181. Ans.— B. **Bradycardia**

Among the choices given above the most common sign is Bradycardia

Hypoxia in the newborn period is characterized by :

* **Pallor,**
* **Cyanosis,**
* **Apnea,**
* **A slow heart rate,**
* **Unresponsiveness to stimulation, and**
* **Remain hypotonic or change from hypotonic to hypertonic.**

SHORT TEXTBOOK OF PSYCHIATRY
(Aids to Psychiatry)

About this Book (New Edition)

- This new book is specificially written for easy grasping of Psychiatry in a clearent, pointwise, simple and easy understandable language and is exlusively based on the ***examination oriented*** pattern.
- A list of headings important for ***Undergraduate*** and ***Postgraduate examinations*** are given at the starting
- Various ***Question Papers*** of Psychiatry from previous years of many national undergraduate examinations have been added at the end of book.
- ***Multiple Choice Questions (MCQ's)***, asked on various Undergraduate and Postgraduate Examinations have been added at the end of book
- Each chapter ends with ***important points*** enlisted in abox
- A section on the general principles of Psychiatry with a special emphasis on the Historical aspects (indian/Western), ***Symptomatology*** and Psychiatric Examination has been included.
- An updated section on Psychiatric Treatments including newer advances and list of all ***Psychotropic Drugs*** in alphabetically order (according to trade names) have been added.
- Important detailed chapters on Indian Psychiatry (Contributions of Indian Psychiatrists, Epidemiology of various disorders, National Mental Health Programme of India, Forensic Psychiatry, Indian culture bound syndromes etc).
- An important list of appendices include ***Psychiatric Glossary,*** list of ***Psychological Tests, Psychiatric Side effects of Medical Drugs*** etc.
- Useful book for various Medical Competitive and Undergraduate Examination; Civil Services Examinations
- Edited by : ***Dr. M.S. Bhatia*** (M.D., Dip. W.P.A.) an experienced teacher and examiner, associated with editing of many popular books on undergraduate and Postgraduate Examinations.

CBS Publishers & Distributors Pvt. Ltd.

NEW DELHI • BANGALORE • PUNE • CHENNAI • COCHIN (INDIA)

4

IMPORTANT TEXT OF HAEMATOLOGY

ABNORMAL HUMAN HAEMOGLOBINS

* Sickle cell haemoglobinopathy — 22 6 val
* Haemoglobin C —$\alpha_2\beta_2$ $^{6\ val}$
* Haemoglobin E $\alpha_2\beta_2$ $^{26\ lys}$
* Haemoglobin S β_2 $^{6\ val\text{-}glu}$
* Haemoglobin H—B_4
* Haemoglobin Barts —γ_4

Eponymous Anaemias :

* ***Cooley's anaemia*** — (Thalassemia major) :
— A familial, haemolytic, erythroblastic anaemia which occurs usually in families of Mediterranean stock. Homozygous β-thalassemia usually becomes symptomatic severe, progressive during second 6 months of life and show developmental retardation, splenomegaly, skeletal changes, with a hypochromic microcytic anaemia & mongoloid facies.
* ***Cooley's anaemia trait*** (Thalassemia minor) :
— Heterozygous β-thalassemia is associated with mild anaemia.
* ***Cyerny's anaemia :***
— A deficiency anaemia seen in infants on defective or inadequate diets.
* ***Fanconi's anaemia :***
— Familial, usually fatal, anaemia of the aplastic or hypoplastic type with certain endocrine changes & develops in the first decade of life. And associated with high frequency of spontaneous chromosomes breakages & rearrangement.
* ***Jaksch's anaemia (anaemia pseudoleukaemica infantum) :***
— Seen in children < 3 years, considered 25 as symptoms complex; associated with malnutrition, tuberculosis, GIT disorders & many infections leading to severe anaemia; leukocytosis, relative lymphocytosis, splenomegaly, hepathmegaly & lymphadenopathy (Gaucher's & Niemann-Pick diseases were originally in this group).
* ***Leaderer's anaemia :***
— An acute haemolytic anaemia

MCQ's OF HAEMATOLOGY

What is important in Haematology

Anaemias (Iron deficiency, Megaloblastic, Aplastic, Hemolytic), Sickle Cell Anaemia, Thalassemia, Purpura, Hemophilia

1. **The coagulation profile in a 13-years old girl with Menorrhagia having von Willebrands disease is : AI 2005**
   A. Isolated prolonged PTT with a normal PT
   B. Isolated prolonged PT with a normal PTT
   C. Prolongation of both PT and PTT
   D. Prolongation of thrombin time
2. **The most common leukocytoclastic vasculitis affecting children is : AI 2005, 2007**
   A. Takayasu disease
   B. Mucocutaneous lymph node syndrome (Kawasaki disease)
   C. Henoch Schonelin purpura
   D. Polyarteritis nodosa
3. **Diagnosis of β Thalassemia is established by : AI 2005, 2009**
   A. NESTROFT Test
   B. HbA1 C estimation
   C. Hb electrophoresis
   D. Target cells in peripheral smear.
4. **Best prognosis is seen in which AML : SGPGI 2002, 2003**
   A. M6 B. M1
   C. M7 D. M3
5. **Poor prognostic indicator of ALL is : AIIMS 2002**
   A. Female sex
   B. Age > 1 yr
   C. Leucocyte count < 50,000/mm3
   D. Hypoploidy
6. **A child died soon after birth. On examination there was hepatosplenomegaly. The most probable diagnosis is : AIIMS 2002**
   A. α-thalassemia
   B. Homozygous β-thalassemia
   C. Hereditary spherocytosis
   D. Sickle cell anemia
7. **True statement about acute lymphoblastic leukemia is : Delhi 2002**
   A. Lymphoblasts show azurophilic granules in cytoplasm
   B. Usually are of B cell origin
   C. TDt is present in 5% of ALL
   D. Prognosis is good for surface Ig positive B cell ALL.
8. **In which one of the following conditions Dactylitis can not be seen : UPSC 2002**
   A. Sickle-cell anemia
   B. Beta thalassemia
   C. Congenital syphilis
   D. Tuberculosis
9. **Spleen is palpable in all haemolytic anemias in a child of 8 years of age, except in : UPSC 2002**
   A. Thalassemia
   B. Spherocytosis
   C. Sickle-cell anemia
   D. Haemolysis in malaria
10. **A couple with a family history of beta thalassemia major in a distant relative, has come for counseling. The husband has HbA2 of 4.8% and the wife has HbA2 of 2.3%. The risk of having a child with beta thalassemia major is : AI 2003**
    A. 50% B. 25%
    C. 5% D. 0%
11. **Which of the following drugs will prevent platelet aggregation : AMC 1999**
    A. Paracetamol B. Sulfonamides
    C. I.N.H. D. Aspirin
12. **A positive coomb's test in absence of haemolysis, may be seen with administration of : UPSC 1995**
    A. Cephalothin B. Ampicillin
    C. Nalidixic acid D. Carbenicillin
13. **Major indication for intrauterine transfusion of foetus is : AIIMS 1982, 92**
    A. Bradycardia and foetal distress
    B. Sickle cell anaemia
    C. Erythroblastosis foetalis
    D. None of the above

Ans.	1. A	2. C	3. C	4. D	5. D	6. A	7. B	8. B	9. C	10. D
	11. D	12. A	13. C							

14. **Most common complication of intrauterine transfusion is : PGI 1983, 99**
A. Graft versus host reaction
B. Premature onset of labour
C. Transfusion reaction
D. None of the above

15. **Breakdown of 1 gm of haemoglobin yields about : AIIMS 1986, 90**
A. 20 mg bilirubin B. 35 mg bilirubin
C. 5 mg bilirubin D. 1 mg bilirubin

16. **Ideally, children with thalassemia should be transfused with : UPSC 1983; AIIMS 1993**
A. Packed RBC B. Platelet rich plasma
C. Washed RBC D. Blood of polycythemic

17. **Hazards of exchange transfusion include following, except : AIIMS 1993**
A. Oligaemic shock B. Citrate tetany
C. Cardiac arrest D. Hypokalaemia

18. **Foetal blood in the maternal circulation is detected by : AIIMS 1982, 88, 90; Delhi 1983; ESI 1994**
A. Hemoglobin estimation B. Optic density
C. Spectrophotometer D. Kleihauer test

19. **The least common leukaemia in a child is : UPSC 1983, 88; AIIMS 1999**
A. Acute lymphacytic leukaemia
B. Acute myloblastic leukaemia
C. Acute non-lymphocytic leukaemia
D. Chronic myeloid leukaemia

20. **The word, "thalassemia" literally means : AMC 1994**
A. Fatal illness B. Great curse
C. Great sea D. Punishment

21. **Structural haemoglobinopathy is : Delhi 1996**
A. β-Thalassemia B. α-Thalassemia
C. Hb-H disease D. Sickle cell anemia

22. **Hemophilia is because of deficiency of : Delhi 1996**
A. Factor-VIII B. Factor-IX
C. ↑ Bleeding time D. ↑ Prothrombin time

23. **Hypertransfusion in Thalassemia is given by : Delhi 1990**
A. 6 gm% B. 8 gm%
C. 10 gm% D. 12 gm%

24. **Anaphylactoid purpura : AIIMS 1992**
A. Is the same enity as idiopathic thrombocy-topenic purpura.
B. Is the same entity as Henoch-Schonlein purpura.
C. Is the same entity as black measles.
D. May cause acute chest pain.

25. **Lymphocytosis is seen in except : Rajasthan 1998**
A. TB B. Typhoid
C. Brucellosis D. Infant

26. **Thrombocytopenia is seen in following except : AIIMS 1998**
A. Hemolytic uremic syndrome
B. Immune thrombocytopenia
C. Henoch-Schonlein purpura
D. Thrombocytopenic purpura

27. **A 5 years old child has anaemia of long duration. The investigation to be done is : AIIMS 1987, 98**
A. Estimation of Hb% B. RBC count
C. Peripheral smear D. PVC

28. **A child with congenital haemolytic anaemia will show all these features, except : AIIMS 1992**
A. Hepatosplenomegaly
B. Low haemoglobin
C. Low reticulocyte count
D. Hypercellular bone marrow
E. Normal platelet count

29. **Which of the following is affected in sickle cell anaemia: AI 1994**
A. α chain B. β chain
C. γ chain D. Bart's syndrome

30. **The absolute contraindication of phototherapy is : AIIMS 1985, 96**
A. Hereditary spherocytosis
B. Idiopathic thrombocytopenic purpura
C. Severe Rh incompatibility
D. Severe ABO incompatibility

31. **Aminocaproic acid would be recommended for a hemophiliac child with : AIIMS 1991**
A. Epistaxis B. Haematuria
C. Oral bleeding D. Hamarthrosis

32. **What is the role of corticosteroid in the management of idiopathic thrombocytopenic purpura ? Bihar 1991**
A. Prevent progression to pancytopenia
B. Prevent CNS haemorrhage
C. Prevent fatal exanguination
D. Reduce spleen size

33. **All these features suggest acute non-lymphocytic leukaemia except : AIIMS 1999**
A. Presence of periorbital swelling with proptosis (chloroma).
B. Gingival hyperplasia.
C. Blasts are peroxidase negative.
D. Features of disseminated intravascular coagulation present.

34. **Most frequent cause of neonatal thrombocytopenic purpura is : AIIMS 1993**
A. Infection B. Drug idiosyncrasy
C. Erythroblastosis D. Large haemangiomas

Ans.									
14. C	15. B	16. A	17. D	18. D	19. D	20. C	21. D	22. A	23. C
24. B	25. D	26. C	27. C	28. C	29. B	30. B	31. C	32. B	33. C
34. A									

35. **The following conditions are associated with hypochromic microcytic anaemia except : AMU 1997**
A. Iron deficiency B. B_6 deficiency
C. Vit. C deficiency D. Thalassemia major

36. **The type of blood to use if time does not permit adequate cross-matching in an emergency is : AMU 1995**
A. O, Rh negative B. O, Rh positive
C. B, Rh positive D. A, Rh negative

37. **Physiologic anemia of newborn is most severe at the age : Rohtak 1999**
A. 4 months B. 2 months
C. 4 weeks D. 2 weeks

38. **Paroxysmal haemoglobinuria is associated with : AMC 1991**
A. Syphilis B. Chloromycetin toxicity
C. Mongolism D. Ingestion of lead

39. **Commonest cause of anemia during childhood is : AMC 1991**
A. Vitamin B_{12} deficiency B. Folic acid deficiency
C. Pyridoxine deficiency D. Iron deficiency

40. **Characteristic features of acute lymphoblastic leukaemia include : AIIMS 1996**
A. Tumour cells which react with antisera raised against B-lymphocytes.
B. Better prognosis when the white cell count at presentation is very high.
C. Massive splenomegaly.
D. Spread to the meninges unless prophylactic treatment to the central nervous system is given.

41. **Prednisone is the treatment of choice in a haemophilic with : AMU 1998**
A. Spontaneous haematuria
B. Gingival bleeding
C. Traumatic hemarthrosis
D. None of the above

42. **In hemophilia, which of the following is abnormal : DNB 1993**
A. BT B. PT
C. PTT D. None of the above

43. **Poor prognosis in acute lymphatic leukaemia is indicated by all, except : UPSC 1999**
A. Intrathoracic mass
B. Children between 2 & 10 years
C. Cranial secondaries
D. WBC around 10000/mm

44. **Haemorrhagic disease of the newborn most commonly appears in : AP 1999**
A. Haemophilic diseased infants
B. Thrombocytopenic infants
C. Breast-fed infants
D. Early artificial milk-fed infants

45. **Hereditary spherocytosis is : AIIMS 1983, 94**
A. Autosomal dominant B. Autosomal recessive
C. Sex-linked recessive D. Sex-linked dominant

46. **Bronze baby syndrome is a complication of : AIIMS 1984, 96**
A. ABO incompatibility B. Rh incompatibility
C. Chloromycetin toxicity D. Phototherapy

47. **True about spherocytosis is all of the following except: AIIMS 1984, 96**
A. Gall stones
B. Positive Coomb's test suggests immuno-hemolytic anaemia
C. Splenomegaly
D. ↑ MCH and MCHC

48. **Serum iron is raised in : AIIMS 1995**
A. Chronic renal failure B. Thalassemia
C. Iron deficiency anaemia D. Viral hepatitis

49. **A 6-years-old child with petechiae, most commonly has: AIIMS 1983; UPSC 1994**
A. Leukaemia
B. Scurvy
C. Idiopathic thrombocytic purpura
D. Aplastic anaemia

50. **The best investigation to establish diagnosis of thalassemia is : AIIMS 1985, 97**
A. Osmotic fragility B. Coomb's test
C. Hb A2 estimation D. Hb F estimation

51. **Which of the following is not seen in aplastic anaemia: AIIMS 1985; PGI 1995**
A. Anaemia B. Purpura
C. Haemorrhage D. Splenomegaly

52. **In-G-6-P-D deficiency, RBC's hemolysis is induced by: AIIMS 1986, 88; PGI 1990**
A. Erythromycin B Dapsone
C. Chloromycetin D. Levamisol

53. **True about idiopathic thrombocytopenic purpura is : AIIMS 1986; UPSC 1996**
A. It is diagnosed by poor clot retraction
B. Splenomegaly is present in a majority
C. Remits of its own without any treatment in all
D. Decrease in number of megakaryocytes in bone marrow

54. **Sideroblastic anaemia may be caused by all of the following except : AIIMS 1996**
A. Lead poisoning
B. Collagen-vascular disease
C. Cutaneous porphyria
D. Iron deficiency

55. **Which of the following drug may be useful in agranulocytosis : DNB 1992**
A. Cyclosporine B. Azathioprine
C. Lithium D. ACTH

Ans. 35. C 36. A 37. B 38. D 39. D 40. D 41. A 42. C 43. D 44. C
45. A 46. D 47. D 48. B 49. C 50. C 51. D 52. B 53. C 54. C
55. C

56. Pancytopenia is associated with : AIIMS 1987, 90

A. PNH (Paroxysmal Nocturnal hemoglybinuria)
B. Paroxysmal cold hemoglobinuria
C. Thalassemia
D. Hereditary spherocytosis

57. Haemolytic uremic syndrome in children is not associated with : UPSC 1996

A. Changes in the shape of the R.B.C. (Burr cells).
B. Thrombocytopenia.
C. Essential changes involving venous inflammation and subsequent thrombosis.
D. Severe haemolytic anaemia.

58. Treatment of acute lymphoblastic leukaemia in child with CNS manifestations is : AIIMS 1988; UPSC 1991

A. Intrathecal methotrexate
B. Vincristine and prednisolone
C. Intrathecal vincristine
D. Intrathecal steroids and vincristine

59. Regarding hereditary spherocytosis, true is : AIIMS 1990

A. ↓ Osmotic fragility
B. Enzyme deficiency present
C. Choice of Treatment-Splenectomy
D. Moderate splenomegaly found

60. Palpable purpura is seen in all except : AIIMS 1990

A. ITP
B. Drug induced
C. Mixed essential cyroglobulinemia
D. Vasculitis

61. Majority of chronic lymphocytic leukemia is of ——— type : PGI 1986; AIIMS 1996

A. T-cell B. B-cell
C. Null cell D. Mixed B-cell and T-cell

62. Haemoglobin F is : PGI 1998

A. $\alpha_2\beta_2$ B. $\alpha_2\gamma_2$
C. $\alpha_2\delta_2$ D. $\alpha_1\beta_1$

63. 'Warm' type of hermolytic anaemia is caused by all except : PGI 1994

A. Mycoplasma
B. Methyldopa
C. Leukemia (chronic lymphatics)
D. Hodgkin's lymphoma
E. SLE

64. Iron deficiency anaemia in children is characterised by all of the following except : UPSC 1996

A. Microcytic hypochromic red cell morphology
B. Decreased serum ferritin
C. Decreased iron binding capacity
D. Decreased serum iron levels

65. Disseminated intravascular coagulation is common in: PGI 1998

A. Acute lymphocytic leukaemia
B. Acute myelocytic leukaemia
C. CML (chronic myeloid leukaemia)
D. CLL (chronic lymphocytic leukaemia)
E. None of the above

66. Increased fetal Hb is seen in : AIIMS 1997

A. Juvenile CML
B. Pure red cell aplasia
C. Hereditary Spherocytosis
D. Polycythemia vera

67. In Erthroblastosis fetalis not involved is : AIIMS 1997

A. Anti C B. D
C. E D. Anti Lewis

68. Microcytic Hypochromic blood picture is not seen in : AIIMS 1997

A. Thalassemia Major B. Thalassemia Minor
C. Iron deficiency anemia D. Fanconi's anemia

69. A 2-years old healthy child is brought with history of accidental ingestion of some tablets. He is cyanosed but without any respiratory distress. The most likely diagnosis is : UPSC 1997

A. Polycythemia
B. Methemoglobinemia
C. Haemoglobinemia
D. Congenital cyanotic heart disease

70. True about Henoch Schonlein purpura is all except : PGI 1984, 85, 90

A. Purpura on lower limb B. Arthritis
C. Thyromboembolism D. Hematuria
E. Anemia

71. Dactylitis is seen in : UPSC 1997

A. ITP B. Sickle cell anemia
C. HbD disease D. Alpha thalassemia
E. Aplastic anemia

72. Consider the following statements : CSE 1997
Tolerance of infants to blood loss is poor because :

1. A small amount of lost blood represents a sizeable fraction of cardiac output.
2. Of poor defence mechanism to blood loss as the peripheral circulatory resistance is high.
3. Of ineffective vasoconstriction of peripheral vessels.

Of these statements

A. 1,2 and 3 are correct B. 1 and 2 are correct
C. 2 and 3 are correct D. 1 and 3 are correct

73. Foetal acidosis is pH less than : Rajasthan 1998

A. 7.0 B. 7.2
C. 7.3 D. 7.4

Ans.										
	56. A	57. C	58. A	59. C	60. A	61. B	62. B	63. A	64. C	65. B
	66. A	67. D	68. D	69. B	70. C	71. B	72. A	73. B		

74. **A 9-years old child has pallor, fever, pain all over the body. CNS examination and hemogram are normal. GPE shows proptosis. Diagnosis is : AIIMS 1983, 85; UPSC 1986; ESI 1999**
A. Purpura
B. Leukaemia
C. Neuroblastoma
D. Cavernous sinus thrombosis

75. **Treatment of choice in child with Hb-5 gm%, anisocytosis, poikilocytosis and hypochromic microcytic picture is : Delhi 1993**
A. Iron dextran B. Blood transfusion
C. Packed cells D. Oral iron therapy

76. **Punctate basophilia with anaemia is seen in : UPSC 1987; JIPMER 1992**
A. PEM B. Lead poisoning
C. Measles D. Aspirin poisoning

77. **In Hemochromatosis, iron accumulates maximally in : AIIMS 1986; JIPMER 1992**
A. Bone B. Kidneys
C. Liver D. Spleen

78. **Following are true of childhood ITP except : UPSC 1987; AIIMS 1992**
A. Prolonged clotting time
B. Preceding viral infection
C. Decreased bone marrow megakaryocytes
D. Splenectomy for chronic cases

79. **If a one year old on breast milk, develops severe pallor with hepatomegaly but no splenomegaly. The investigation of choice would be : AIIMS 1992**
A. Serum iron estimation B. Fetal Hb estimation
C. Serum Vit-B_{12} level D. Serum folic acid level

80. **The opportunistic infection most commonly seen in children with neutropenia is : JIPMER 1993**
A. Staphylococcal B. Pneumococcal
C. Streptococcal D. Gram negative rods

81. **The Hb to appear first in the fetus is : TN 1993**
A. HbA B. HbA2
C. HbF D. Hb Gower

82. **The major site of active haemopoesis in a foetus of 5 months is : TN 1993**
A. Spleen B. Liver
C. Lymph nodes D. Bone marrow

83. **The percentage of foetal haemoglobin at birth is : Bihar 1999**
A. 90% B. 20%
C. 70% D. 100%

84. **Megaloblastic anaemia is most likely to occur in infant being fed : PGI 1986**
A. Goat's milk B. Soya formulae
C. Human milk D. Cereals before 6 months

85. **Large doses of Vitamin-K administered to a new-born may result in : AIIMS 1992**
A. Hypothyroidism B. RBC destruction
C. Bulging of fontanelles D. Prolonged bilirubinemia

86. **Bone marrow transplantation is not indicated in : AP 1993**
A. Sickle cell anaemia B. Multiple myeloma
C. Leukaemia D. Metastasis

87. **Philadelphia chromosome is : AP 1993**
A. t (8; 22) B. t (8; 21)
C. t (15; 17) D. t (8; 14)

88. **Sickling of red blood cells occurs in : PGI 1993**
A. Eight per cent of whites
B. Megaloblastic anemia
C. Only in sickle cell anemia, not sickle cell trait
D. Thalassemia and sickle cell trait occurring together

89. **Absolute lymphocytosis occurs in all except : AIIMS 1984, 95**
A. Mumps
B. Whooping cough
C. Enteric fever
D. Infectious mononucleosis

90. **In alpha-thalassemia, HbH is formed by chains of ——: DNB 1990**
A. α_3, β_1 B. α_4
C. α_1, β_3 D. β_4

91. **The commonest cause of aplastic anaemia is : AIIMS 1979, 93**
A. Idiopathic B. Chloramphenicol
C. Phenylbutazone D. Petroleum products

92. **Normal infant has ——— mg of iron at the time of birth: DNB 1991**
A. 100—200 B. 250—300
C. 500—600 D. 900—1000

93. **The following are the correct facts in relation to haemorrhage disease of new born except : Karnataka 1999**
A. Self limited bleeding disorder.
B. Results from deficiency of coagulation factors dependent on Vitamin-K.
C. More common in formula fed infants.
D. In most cases, haemorrhagic manifestations become evident for the 2nd and 3rd day of life.

94. **Autoimmune hemolytic anaemia is seen in : AIIMS 1994**
A. AML B. CLL
C. Multiple myeloma D. Sickle anaemia

Ans.										
	74. C	75. C	76. B	77. C	78. C	79. A	80. A	81. C	82. B	83. C
	84. A	85. D	86. A	87. A	88. D	89. C	90. D	91. A	92. B	93. C
	94. B									

95. All of the following are true for sickle cell anaemia except : AIIMS 1994
A. Leukopenia
B. Enlarged heart
C. Fish vertebra
D. Pulmonary arterial hypertension

96. In children, disseminated intravascular coagulation is associated with : UPSC 1994
A. Thrombocytopaenia
B. Normal thrombin time
C. Polycythemia
D. Generalised or fulminant gram negative septicaemia

97. All of the following are known complications of neonatal polycythaemia except : UPSC 1994
A. Renal vein thrombosis
B. Hyperbilirubinaemia
C. Necrotising enterocolitis
D. Hyaline membrane disease

98. Which of the following are poor prognostic factors in acute lymphoblastic leukemia in children : UPSC 1994
A. Total below 2 years
B. Total leucocyte count above 25,000/cu mm
C. Central nervous system involvement
D. Null cell type leukaemia

99. Juvenile myeloid leukemia is associated with all except : AI 1994
A. Philadelphia chromosome
B. Significant lymphadenopathy
C. Marked pallor
D. Raised fetal hemoglobin

100. Polycythemia in infants will cause the following except: AI 1994
A. Increased physiological jaundice
B. Cerebral ischemia
C. CHF
D. Vitamin-E related anemia

101. Henoch Schonlein Purpura is characterized by all except : AI 1994
A. Thrombocytopenia B. Arthralgia
C. Glomerulonephritis D. Abdominal pain

102. The beta thalassemia (Homozygotic), is characterized by all except : AIIMS 1986, 87; AI 1994
A. Increased HbA2 B. Increased HbF
C. ↑ Adult Hb D. Reduced haematocrit

103. Commonest haematological malignancy in children is: Kerala 1994
A. CLL B. CML
C. AML D. ALL

104. Indication for exchange transfusion at birth is : Delhi 1995
A. Cord Hb < 16 gm%
B. Cord bilirubin —3 mg%
C. Cord bilirubin —5 mg%
D. Mother antibody titre > 1 : 64

105. A five-years old child is brought with fever and pallor. On examination he is found to have anaemia, petechial haemorrhages, lymphadenopathy, tenderness of the bones and hepatosplenomegaly. The most likely diagnosis is : UPSC 1995
A. Acute rheumatic fever
B. Infectious mononucleosis
C. Idiopathic thrombocytopenic purpura
D. Acute leukaemia

106. In new born baby, thrombocytopenia is caused by : AIIMS 1999
A. ABO incompatibility
B. Isoimmune thrombocytopenia
C. Auto-immune thrombocytopenia purpura
D. SLE

107. An infant with history of diarrhoea 5 days back has urea 200 mg% and creatinine 5 mg%. The platelet count is 90000. Fragmented RBC's are found in the peripheral smear. The most possible diagnosis is : AIIMS 1999
A. HUS
B. DIS
C. Microangiopathic hemolytic anemia
D. Porphyria

108. A 4 years old child presented with anemia and splenomegaly. Blood smear showed target cells. There is similar history in the family. The best investigation is: AIIMS 1999, 2001; AI 2001
A. Hemoglobin electrophoresis
B. Osmotic fragility
C. Corrected reticulocyte count > 25%
D. Osmotic fragility of RBC's

109. Coomb's positive hemolytic anemia occurs in : PGI 1999
A. SLE B. ITP
C. CML D. Rifampicin intake

110. 6 months old baby with severe pallor and hepatosplenomegaly. Similar history with the sibling. Investigation of choice is : TN 1999
A. Bone marrow biopsy B. Hb. electrophoresis
C. Hb. estimation D. Platelet count

111. Fetal Hb equals adult Hb at : TN 1999
A. Birth B. 2 months
C. 4 months D. 6 months

Ans.										
	95. A	96. D	97. C	98. C	99. A	100. D	101. A	102. C	103. D	104. C
	105. D	106. B	107. A	108. A	109. A	110. A	111. B			

112. Serum Iron level in child -------- mgm: **TN 1999**

A. 20-50 B. 100-200
C. 50-100 D. 200 - 350

113. The following laboratory parameter does not carry a bad prognosis in acute lymphocytic leukaemia : **AIIMS 1990**

A. Presence of anaemia
B. Low initial platelet count
C. Initial WBC count more than 1 lakh/cubic mm
D. L2 cell morphology

114. All are seen in juvenile CML except : **Kerala 1999**

A. Thrombocytopenia B. Monocytosis
C. ↑ fetal Hb D. pH chromosome

115. Drug of choice in the treatment of idiopathic thrombocytopenic purpura is : **Rohtak 1997**

A. Oestrogen B. Nitrogen mustard
C. Amethopterin D. Corticosteroids

116. Acute idiopathic thrombocytopenic purpura can follow: **AIIMS 1991**

A. Mumps B. Rubella
C. Chickenpox D. All of the above

117. During the process of coagulation, the platelets release—which promotes vasoconstriction : **AIIMS 1991**

A. Serotonin B. Fibrinogen
C. Thromboplastin D. Hyaluronidase

118. The bone marrow in idiopathic thrombocytopenic purpura on examination, exhibits : **AIIMS 1993**

A. Foam cells
B. Aplasia of all elements
C. Absence of megakaryocytes
D. Normal or increased number of megakaryocytes

119. A leukaemoid reaction with a predominance of lymphocytes occurs in : **AMU 1997**

A. Chicken pox B. Leukaemia
C. Ulcerative colitis D. Acute tuberculosis

120. Peak age of idiopathic thrombocytopenic purpura is ——— years : **DNB 1990**

A. 1—3 B. 2—8
C. 8—12 D. 12—16

121. In ABO hemolytic disease of the newborn direct Coomb's test is : **UPSC 1984, 87**

A. Usually negative
B. Usually mild positive
C. Usually strongly positive
D. Positive in cases where peripheral smear shows microspherocytosis

122. O +ve mother delivers A-ve baby. Which of the following blood will be ideal if the baby needs exchange blood transfusion : **Rohtak 1984, 97**

A. O -ve
B. A +ve
C. A -ve
D. O -ve cells suspended in AB plasma

123. A 5 years old girl came with history of progressively increasing pallor since birth and hepatosplenomegaly. Which of the following is the most relevant test for achieving diagnosis: **AI 2004**

A. Hb electrophoresis
B. Peripheral smear examination
C. Osmotic fragility test
D. Bone marrow examination

124. A 5 years old child presents with history of fever off and on for past 2 weeks and petechial spots all over the body and increasing pallor for past 1 month. Examination reveals splenomegaly of 2 cms below costal margin. The most likely diagnosis is: **AI 2004**

A. Acute leukemia
B. Idiopathic thrombocytopenic purpura
C. Hypersplenism
D. Aplastic anaemia

125. A nine months old boy of Sindhi parents presented to you with complaints of progressive lethargy, irritability and pallor since 6 months of age. Examination revealed sever Pallor. Investigations showed Hb- 3.8 gm%, MCV - 58 fl, MCH - 19.4 pg/cell. Blood film shows osmotic fragility is normal (target cells and normoblasts). X-ray skull shows expansion of erythroid marrow. Which of the following is the most likely diagnosis: **AI 2004**

A. Iron deficiency anaemia
B. Acute lymphoblastic anaemia
C. Hemoglobin-D disease
D. Hereditary spherocytosis

126. Treatment of choice for Thalassemia Major is : **UPSC 2004**

A. Blood transfusion and iron therapy
B. Folic acid and desferrioxamine
C. Blood transfusion and desferrioxamine
D. Iron, blood transfusion and desferrioxamine

127. When does switch over from fetal to adult hemoglobin synthesis begin : **AI 2005**

A. 14 weeks gestation B. 30 weeks gestation
C. 36 weeks gestation D. 7-10 days postnatal

Ans.									
112. D	113. A	114. D	115. D	116. D	117. A	118. D	119. A	120. B	121. A
122. D	123. D	124. A	125. C	126. C	127. A				

128. The most common leukocytoclastic vasculitis affecting children is : **AI 2005**

A. Takayasu disease.

B. Mucocutaneous lymph node syndrome (Kawasaki disease).

C. Henoch Schonlein purpura.

D. Polyartheritis nodosa.

129. Following are seen in G-6-P-D deficiency except : **Delhi 2000**

A. Hemolysis B. Jaundice

C. Anuria D. Seizures

130. Adult hemoglobin at birth is ——— % : **Delhi 2000**

A. 10 B. 20

C. 30 D. 80

131. The following are features of D+HVS (Diarrhea & Hemolytic uremic syndrome) except : **JIPMER 2002, 2005**

A. Negative coomb's test B. Low platelet

C. Low complement level D. Fall in hematocrit

132. Hallmarks of the hemophillia is : **UPPGME 2006**

A. Epistaxis B. Hemarthrosis

C. Abdominal pain D. Anaemia

133. Absent thumb, radial deviation of wrist, bowing of forearm with thrombocytopenia which investigation need not to be done ? **AIIMS 2008**

A. Echocardiography

B. Boen marrow examination

C. Platelet count

D. Karyotyping

Ans. **128. C** **129. D** **130. B** **131. C** **132. B** **133. A**

EXPLANATIONS OF HAEMATOLOGY

1. Ans.— A Isolated prolonged PTT with a normal PT

Von Willebrand's factor acts as a plasma carrier of factor-VIII and circulates in the blood as factor-VIII-VWF complex. Its deficiency therefore impairs the intrinsic pathway of coagulation and prolongs the GPTT as the intrinsic pathway of coagulation remains unimpaired, PT is not altered.

2. Ans.— C Henoch Schonlein purpura

"Henoch Schonlein purpura' is the most common of childhood vasculitides with an estimated incidence of 13.5 : 100,000. Pathologically HSP causes a leukocytoclastic vasculitis — Forfur & Arncil's

3. Ans.— C Hb electrophoresis

'The diagnosis of thalassemia syndromes is best established by Hb electrophoresis.'

Thalassemia is a quantitative defect in Hb characterized by lack of certain types of globin chains and compensatory increase in other globin chains. These changes form the basis of electrophoretic investigations and are diagnostic of respective thalassemia syndromes.

Nestroft test : Naked Eye Single Tube Red Osmotic Cell Fragility Test is used for screening of thalassemia but is not diagnostic.

HBAIC : Estimation of glycated haemoglobin is used for estimating long term Glucose control in diabetics. It has no role in thalassemia.

Target cells : May be seen in thalassemia but do not establish diagnosis of thalassemia.

- Target Cells
- Thalassemia
- Haemoglobin-C, etc.
- Liver diseases

4. Ans.— D. M3
5. Ans.— D. Hypoploidy
6. Ans.— A. α-thalassemia
7. Ans.— B. Usually are of B cell origin
8. Ans.— B. Beta thalassemia
9. Ans.— C. Sickle-cell anemia
10. Ans.— D. 0%

* As we know very well that normal HBA2 is 2%.
* It increases in case of beta thalassemia major (3.5 to 7.5%).
* It is an AR disorder.
* Genetics - If mother unaffected father affected so 100% will be carriers but no one will be affected so answer is D.

11. Ans.— D. Aspirin

Low dose aspirin is used prophylactically in cardiac patients or those with stroke to prevent coagulation.

12. Ans.— A. Cephalothin
13. Ans.— C. Erythroblastosis foetalis
14. Ans.— C. Transfusion reaction
15. Ans.— B. 35 mg bilirubin
16. Ans.— A. Packed RBC
17. Ans.— D. Hypokalaemia
18. Ans.— D. Kleihauer test
19. Ans.— D. Chronic myeloid leukaemia

ALL is the commonest malignancy of childhood.

20. Ans.— C. Great sea
21. Ans.— D. Sickle cell anemia
22. Ans.— A. Factor-VIII
23. Ans.— C. 10 gm%
24. Ans.— B. Is the same entity as Henoch-Schonlein purpura
25. Ans.— D. Infant

26. Ans.— C. Henoch-Schonlein purpura

27. Ans.— C. Peripheral smear

28. Ans.— C. Low reticulocyte count

There is reticulocytosis indicating compensatory erythropoisis. Peripheral smear shows polychromasia, burr cells, tear drop cells, spherocytes and fragmented cells.

29. Ans.— B. β chain

30. Ans.— B. Idiopathic thrombocytopenic purpura

31. Ans.— C. Oral bleeding

32. Ans.— B. Prevent CNS haemorrhage

33. Ans.— C. Blasts are peroxidase negative

34. Ans.— A. Infection

35. Ans.— C. Vit. C deficiency

36. Ans.— A. O, Rh negative

O negative is universal donor and AB positive is universal recipient.

37. Ans.— B. 2 months

38. Ans.— D. Ingestion of lead

39. Ans.— D. Iron deficiency

40. Ans.— D. Spread to the meninges unless prophylactic treatment to the central nervous system is given.

41. Ans.— A. Spontaneous haematuria

42. Ans.— C. PTT

43. Ans.— D. WBC around 10000/mm

44. Ans.— C. Breast-fed infants

45. Ans.— A. Autosomal dominant

46. Ans.— D. Phototherapy

47. Ans.— D. ↑ MCH and MCHC

MCH is normal but MCHC is high

48. Ans.— B. Thalassemia

49. Ans.— C. Idiopathic thrombocytic purpura

50. Ans.— C. Hb A2 estimation

51. Ans.— D. Splenomegaly

52. Ans.— B. Dapsone

Other drugs implicated are antimalarials, nitrofurans, Sulfas, naphthalene, Probenecid, antipyrin, PAS, nalidixic acid and fava beans etc.

53. Ans.— C. Remits of its own without any treatment in all

54. Ans.— C. Cutaneous porphyria

55. Ans.— C. Lithium

56. Ans.— A. PNH (Paroxysmal Nocturnal hemoglybinuria)

57. Ans.— C. Essential changes involving venous inflammation and subsequent thrombosis

58. Ans.— A. Intrathecal methotrexate

59. Ans.— C. Choice of Treatment-Splenectomy

60. Ans.— A. ITP

In ITP, purpura is not palpable.

61. Ans.— B. B-cell

62. Ans.— B. $\alpha_2\gamma_2$

63. Ans.— A. Mycoplasma

64. Ans.— C. Decreased iron binding capacity

65. Ans.— B. Acute myelocytic leukaemia

66. Ans.— A. Juvenile CML

67. Ans.— D. Anti Lewis

68. Ans.— D. Fanconi's anemia

69. Ans.— B. Methemoglobinemia

70. Ans.— C. Thyromboembolism

71. Ans.— B. Sickle cell anemia

72. Ans.— A. 1,2 and 3 are correct

73. Ans.— B. 7.2

74. Ans.— C. Neuroblastoma

75. Ans.— C. Packed cells

76. Ans.— B. Lead poisoning

77. Ans.— C. Liver

78. Ans.— C. Decreased bone marrow megakaryocytes

Bone marrow shows an increase in number of megakaryocytes which shows diminished budding and have intense blue cytoplasm.

79. Ans.— A. Serum iron estimation

80. Ans.— A. Staphylococcal

81. Ans.— C. HbF

82. Ans.— B. Liver

83. Ans.— C. 70%

84. Ans.— A. Goat's milk

85. Ans.— D. Prolonged bilirubinemia

86. Ans.— A. Sickle cell anaemia

87. Ans.— A. t (8; 22)

88. Ans.— D. Thalassemia and sickle cell trait occurring together

89. Ans.— C. Enteric fever

90. Ans.— D. $\beta 4$

91. Ans.— A. Idiopathic

92. Ans.— B. 250—300

93. Ans.— C. More common in formula fed infants

94. Ans.— B. CLL

95. Ans.— A. Leukopenia

96. Ans.— D. Generalised or fulminant gram negative septicaemia

97. Ans.— C. Necrotising enterocolitis

98. Ans.— C. Central nervous system involvement

99. Ans.— A. Philadelphia chromosome

Philadelphia chromosome is negative. Chemotherapy is of little help in children.

100. Ans.— D. Vitamin-E related anemia

Treatment of choice is venesection and definitive is isovolemic partial exchange with 5% albumin.

101 Ans.— A. Thrombocytopenia

102. Ans.— C. ↑ Adult Hb

There is reduced Erythrocytic count, reticulocytosis, Low MCV, MCH or MCHC, Hypercellular marrow, Erythroblasts in smear, reversed myeloid erythroid ratio and decreased fragility.

103. Ans.— D. ALL

104. Ans.— C. Cord bilirubin —5 mg%

105. Ans.— D. Acute leukaemia

106. Ans.— B. Isoimmune thrombocytopenia

107. Ans.— A. HUS

108. Ans.— A. Hemoglobin electrophoresis

In beta thalassemia, hemoglobin electrophoresis shows only fetal and α_2 hemoglobin in children with homozygous beta thalassemia.

109. Ans.— A. SLE

110. Ans.— A. Bone marrow biopsy

111. Ans.— B. 2 months

112. Ans.— D. 200 - 350

113. Ans.— A. Presence of anaemia

114. Ans.— D. pH chromosome

115. Ans.— D. Corticosteroids

116. Ans.— D. All of the above

117. Ans.— A. Serotonin

118. Ans.— D. Normal or increased number of megakaryocytes

119. Ans.— A. Chicken pox

120. Ans.— B. 2—8

Drugs e.g. antiepileptic, cotrimoxazole, PAS, rifampicin, chloromycetin can also produce thrombocytopenia.

121. Ans.— A. Usually negative

122. Ans.— D. O -ve cells suspended in AB plasma

123. Ans.— D. Bone marrow examination

124. Ans.— A. Acute leukemia

This child is suffering from acute leukaemia (Presence of spleenomegaly exclude the aplastic anaemia and ITP).

Acute Lymphatic Leukemia :

- These are the most common type of childhood malignancy.
- Peak age of onset is 3–7 years
- More common in male child
- Bone marrow is replaced by malignant lymphoblast resulting anaemia, thrombocytopenia and granulocytopenia
- Genetic disease predisposing to leukemia include Down's syndrome, Bloom syndrome Fanconi's anemia and ataxia telangiectasia.
- The symptoms in order of frequency include fever, petechiae, bleeding, anorexia, malaise and decreased activity.
- Bone pain, arthralgia, hepatosplenomegaly and rarely lymphadenopathy may occur.
- The duration of symptoms may vary from a few days to a few weeks or months at onset.
- Bone marrow aspiration or biopsy is needed to ascertain or rule out the diagnosis of acute leukaemia.

Note:

- Liver and spleen are usually not enlarged in aplastic anaemia but are often palpable in leukaemia.
- Spleen is often not palpable in ITP.
- Hypersplenism often not show thrombocytopenia (Petechial spots).

125. Ans.— C. Hemoglobin-D disease

126. Ans.— C. Blood transfusion and desferroxamine

127. Ans.— A. 14 weeks gestation

An important aspect of human globin genes is regulation of switch from fetal to adult hemoglobin. Beta globin synthesis commences early during fetal life at approximately 8-10 weeks gestation. Subsequently it continues at a low level approximately 10% of total non-alpha globin chain production, upto 36 weeks gestation after which it is considerably augmented. At the same time gamma globin chain synthesis starts to decline so that at birth there are approximately equal levels of gamma and beta chains produced.

The switch to nearly exclusive synthesis of adult hemoglobin (HbA; $\alpha_2\beta_2$) occurs at about 38 weeks. Fetuses and newborn therefore require a globin but not β-globin for normal gestation.

128. Ans.— C. Henoch Schonlein purpura

Henoch Schonlein purpura is the commonest leukocytoclastic vasculitis affecting children.

Leukocytoclastic vasculitis is characterised by a leukocytoclasis, a term that refers to the nuclear debris remaining from the neutrophils that have infiltrated in and around the vessels during the acute states.

Other causes include :

1. Subacute bacterial endocarditis
2. EBV/Infection
3. HIV infection
4. Chronic active hepatitis
5. Ulcerative colitis
6. Congenital deficiencies of various complement components
7. Retroperitoneal fibrosis
8. Primary biliary cirrhosis
9. α_1-antitrypsin deficiency
10. Intestinal bypass surgery
11. Relapsing polychondritis
12. Essential mixed cyoglobulinaemia
13. Drug induced vasculitis
14. SLE
15. Rheumatoid arthritis

C/f of leukocytoclastic vasculitis -

Hallmarks of this group of small vessel vasculitis is predominance of skin involvement.

The skin lesions appear as :

1. Palpable purpura (Mc)
2. Macules
3. Papules
4. Vesicles
5. Bullae

Other organ system may also be involved.

About other options :

1. Polyarteritis Nodosa
   - Mean age of onset is approx. 50 years.
   - It is a necrotizing inflammation of small.
2. Takayascl's disease
   - Most prevalent in adolescent girls and young women.
   - Inflammatory and stenotic disease of medium and large sized arteries characterized by a strong prediction for aortic arch and its branches.
3. Kawasaki disease
   - Acute, febrile, multisystem disease of children.
   - Immune mediated injury to blood vessel endothelium is the likely pathogenesis involved.

129. Ans.— D. Seizures

130. Ans.— B. 20

131. Ans.— C. Low complement level

132. Ans.— B. Hemarthrosis

133. Ans.— A. Echocardiography

Characteristic features such as absent thumb and thrombocytopenia suggests Fanconis anemia.

5.

MCQ's OF DISEASE & IMMUNITY

What is important in Disease & Immunity

Immune-deficiency, Immunization, Common infections (TB, Malaria, Leprosy, Diphtheria, Hepatitis, Typhoid), Fluid & Blood requirement

1. **Hypothermia is associated with all of the following in a neonate except : AIIMS 2006**
   A. Shivering
   B. Decreased peripheral resistance
   C. Cardiac arrythmias
   D. Impaired renal function
2. **A 30 years old lady delivered a healthy baby at 37 week of gestation. She was known case of chronic hepatitis-B infection. She was positive for HBsAg but negative for HBeAG. Which of the following is the most appropriate treatment for the baby : AIIMS 2005**
   A. Both active and passive immunization soon after birth.
   B. Passive immunization soon after birth and active immunization at 1 year of age.
   C. Only passive immunization soon after birth.
   D. Only active immunization soon after birth.
3. **The vaccine which is not required in the first year of life is: JIPMER 2000, 2006**
   A. Measles vaccine
   B. DPT vaccine
   C. Hepatitis-B vaccine
   D. Haemophilus influenza vaccine
4. **A child had fever and coryza for last 3 days developed maculo popular erythematous rash which lasted for 48 hours leaving behind pigmentation is most commonly due to : AIIMS 2000**
   A. Measles B. Fifth disease
   C. Roseola infantum D. Typhoid
5. **In a 6 months old baby, Floppy infant syndrome is seen commonly due to infection with : AIIMS 2000**
   A. Clostridium tetani B. Clostridium perfringens
   C. Clostridium welchii D. Clostridium botulinum
6. **Complication of chicken pox most common in children : PGI 2000**
   A. Encephalitis B. Sec. bacterial infection
   C. Pneumonia D. Otitis media
7. **Most common manifestation of HPV infection in children is : PGI 2000**
   A. Single papilloma
   B. Multiple papillomatosis
   C. Osteoma
   D. Sarcoma
8. **In a case of diphtheria, toxic cardiomyopathy usually occurs in the : TNPSC 2000**
   A. Second week of illness
   B. Fourth week of illness
   C. Sixth week of illness
   D. Eighth week of illness
9. **All of the following are toxic complications of primaquine in children, except : TNPSC 2000**
   A. Methemoglobinemia B. Ototoxicity
   C. Nephrotoxicity D. Hemolytic anemia
10. **A child is diagnosed to have acute gastroenteritis. The consulting paediatrician wants to send a stool sample to a lab which is 16-18 hrs away. Which of the following medium should be use to send this sample: AIIMS 2000**
    A. Charcol cotton bud
    B. Carry Blair medium
    C. Sterilized jar
    D. A medium with high CO_2 content
11. **A neonate suspected to have congenital syphilis, diagnostic test is : AI 2001**
    A. FTA ABS IgM B. FTA-ABS IgG
    C. TPI D. Wasserman
12. **A 6 months old infant develops high grade fever which subsided after 3 days following which there was appearance of a generalized rash which also subsided after 48 hours without any residual pigmentation. Which of the following is the most likely diagnosis : AI 2002**
    A. Fifth disease B. Roseola infantum
    C. Measles D. Rubella

Ans. 1. A 2. A 3. C 4. C 5. D 6. B 7. A 8. A 9. B 10. B 11. A 12. B

13. **All of the following methods are used for the diagnosis of HIV infection in a 2 months old child, except : AIIMS 2003**
A. DNA-PCR
B. Viral culture
C. HIV ELISA
D. p24 antigen assay

14. **The site of diphtheria include the following except : AMU 1997**
A. Larynx B. Tonsils
C. Nose D. G.I. tract

15. **Cardiovascular complications of typhoid fever include each of the following except : AP 1990**
A. Pericarditis B. Cardiomyopathy
C. Endocarditis D. Arteritis

16. **The antibiotic of choice of pertussis is : AP 1990**
A. Ampicillin B. Gentamicin
C. Erythromycin D. Penicillin

17. **Which of the following investigations is useful in the diagnosis of cystic fibrosis : BHU 1986**
A. Chest X-ray
B. ECG
C. Full blood count
D. Sweat sodium concentration

18. **Acute stage of poliomyelitis lasts for : DNB 1991**
A. 10 to 15 days B. 1 to 5 days
C. 2 to 4 weeks D. 1 to 2 years

19. **Mortality of childhood tuberculosis is highest in : AMU 1996**
A. Miliary tuberculosis
B. T.B. meningitis
C. Abdominal tuberculosis
D. Pulmonary tuberculosis

20. **Which of the following disorders is characterised by scaly lesions of the scalp, elbows, knees and buttocks : AIIMS 1995**
A. Atopic eczema B. Erythema multiforme
C. Psoriasis D. Seborrheic dermatitis

21. **Indication for use of corticosteroids in a child with meningococcemia would be presence of : AP 1991**
A. Shock
B. Petechiae
C. Meningitis
D. Temperature greater than 104°F

22. **The drug of choice for scarlet fever is : PGI 1994**
A. Penicillin B. Chloromycetin
C. Tetracycline D. Sulphadiazine

23. **True about AIDS in neonate except : Rajasthan 1998**
A. > 50% fetus involved
B. Presents as failure to grow
C. Cannot be detected by available newer methods
D. Breast feeding C/I

24. **A tuberculin test should be routinely performed prior to immunization for : Bihar 1998**
A. Pertussis B. Rubella
C. Measles D. Small pox
E. Any of the above

25. **A 3 years old is diagnosed to have H. influenza-B meningitis. The investigation to be done before discharge is : AI 1999**
A. MRI of head
B. Brainstem evoked auditory potential study
C. Physiotherapist consultation
D. Lumbar puncture

26. **Plasmodium falciparum does not grow well in red cell that contain haemoglobin : Bihar 1991**
A. HbF B. HbC
C. HbS D. Any of the above
E. Both a + b

27. **Waterhouse Friderichson syndrome is associated primarily with sepsis due to : AMU 1987; DNB 1999**
A. Pneumococci B. Meningococci
C. Streptococci D. Staphylococci

28. **The incubation period of whooping cough is : UPSC 1994**
A. 1 to 3 days B. 2 to 4 days
C. 3 to 6 days D. 7 to 14 days

29. **Infectious mononucleosis has a benign course lasting for about —— months : AIIMS 1997**
A. 2 B. 6
C. 9 D. 12

30. **The most common complication of mumps in children is : PGI 1985; AIIMS 1995**
A. Appendicitis B. Pancreatitis
C. Aseptic meningitis D. Orchitis

31. **The following are recognized complications of diphtheria except : AIIMS 1986, 99**
A. Myocarditis B. Peri-uvular-abscess
C. Polyneuritis D. Nephritis

32. **Oranism responsible for over-whelming post-splenectomy infection is : Delhi 1987; AIIMS 1997**
A. E. Coli
B. Pneumococci
C. Staphylococci
D. Pseudomonas pyocyaneu

33. **The vaccine which should be avoided in convulsive disorder is : PGI 1986; UPSC 1985, 98**
A. Diphtheria B. Measles
C. Pertusis D. Tetanus

34. **The clinical sign in measles which appears last is : UPSC 1991**
A. Koplik's spots B. Fever
C. Rash D. Coryza

Ans. 13. C 14. D 15. B 16. C 17. D 18. A 19. B 20. C 21. A 22. A
23. C 24. C 25. B 26. D 27. B 28. D 29. A 30. C 31. B 32. B
33. C 34. C

35. **Congenital passive immunity is not observed in : AIIMS 1983, 96**
A. Rubella B. Mumps
C. Poliomyelitis D. Whooping cough

36. **If a mother has measles, her newborn baby is immune to this disease for : AMU 1990; AMC 1984; AIIMS 1983, 95**
A. 4 to 6 months B. 6 to 12 months
C. 1 to 3 years D. 3 to 6 years

37. **A child with nasal regurgitation and history of pain in throat, is most likely having : AIIMS 1984, 86; UPSC 1983, 88; ESI 1999**
A. Encephalitis B. Measles
C. Chickenpox D. Palatal diphtheria

38. **The complications of measles include all of the following except : AIIMS 1993**
A. Reactivation of a tuberculous focus
B. Protein-energy malnutrition
C. Bronchiectasis
D. Bronchial asthma
E. Bronchopneumonia

39. **Dose of chloroquine at 4-6 years age-group : AI 1999**
A. 150 mg B. 300 mg
C. 450 mg D. 600 mg

40. **Most virulent form of penumococcus is : AIIMS 1986, 98**
A. Type-A B. Type-B
C. Type-C D. All are equally virulent

41. **The manifestations of disseminated tuberculosis may include : PGI 1993**
A. Anaemia B. Low grade fever
C. Splenomegaly D. All of the above
E. None of the above

42. **The schedule of universal programme of immunisation in a child begins at birth and ends at : PGI 1982; AI 1998**
A. 3rd year B. 4th year
C. 5th year D. 10th years

43. **Newborn of HBsAg +ve mother should be managed with : AI 1999**
A. Hepatitis-B active and passive (IgM) immunisation
B. Hepatitis-B active vaccination
C. No treatment
D. Stop breast feeding

44. **Thrombosis of visceral capillaries is caused by : Karnataka 1997**
A. Plasmodium vivax B. Plasmodium ovale
C. Plasmodium malariae D. Plasmodium falciparum

45. **Pick out the vaccine that give life long protection after the initial course of vaccination : Karnataka 1999**
A. TAB vaccine B. HDCV
C. Measles vaccine D. BCG vaccine

46. **Regarding typhoid in children, which of the following is true : AI 1994**
A. Encephalitis is common
B. Urine culture is positive in first few days
C. Splenomegaly
D. Tachycardia is common

47. **Alpha 1 antitrypsin deficiency is related to : AI 1994**
A. Emphysema 0B. Hepatoblastoma
C. Down's syndrome D. Cystic fibrosis

48. **Antibody related especially to GIT infection is : AI 1994**
A. IgE B. IgG
C. IgM D. IgA

49. **Alpha fetoprotein is increased in the following except : AI 1994**
A. Hepatocellular cancer
B. Seminoma testis
C. GI neoplasm
D. Inflammatory disease of liver

50. **Isolation period for mumps is : Kerala 1994**
A. Until fever subsides
B. Until pain subsides
C. Until swelling subsides
D. Until headache subsides

51. **In an infant, both IgG and IgM against syphilis are found. Which of the following is true : Delhi 1995**
A. Both mother and infant are infected
B. Mother had not passed infection in utero
C. Lab error
D. Any of the above

52. **In an infant, Hepatitis-B occur most often due to : Delhi 1995**
A. Cord Hb < 16 gm%
B. Cord bilirubin —— 3 mg %
C. Cord bilirubin — 5 mg%
D. Mother antibody titre > 1 : 64

53. **Allergic rhinitis in a 2 months old is probably due to : CMC 1995**
A. Eggs B. Milk
C. Pollens D. Dust

54. **Lymphocyte transformation is sensitive test most useful in identification of : AIIMS 1994**
A. Drug reaction B. Contact dermatitis
C. Pollen allergy D. Food allergy

Ans.										
	35. D	36. A	37. D	38. D	39. B	40. B	41. D	42. C	43. A	44. D
	45. C	46. C	47. A	48. D	49. B	50. C	51. A	52. A	53. B	54. A

55. Following scratch test is a reaction of a moderate wheal and flare, without pseudopods. The test is interpreted as : PGI 1991

A. 4 plus B. 3 plus
C. 2 plus D. 1 plus

56. False negative tuberculin reaction occurs in children of the following, except : UP 1996

A. Very severely malnourished child
B. Patient on corticosteroid therapy
C. 4-6 weeks following measles
D. Atypical mycobacteriosis

57. The dose of Engerix-B for protection of hemodialysis patients should be : Rajasthan 1995

A. 10 mg B. 20 mg
C. 40 mg D. 60 mg

58. In a child with AIDS, vaccine contraindicated is : JIPMER 1997

A. BCG B. DPT
C. Thyphoid D. Salkvaccine

59. Macular rash with red margins is seen in : Delhi 1997

A. Chicken pox B. Measles
C. Rubella D. Mumps

60. Newborns have transplacentally acquired immunity against all of the following disorders, except : UP 1997

A. Measles B. Pertussis
C. Diphtheria D. Poliomyelitis

61. Child with agammaglobinemia with respiratory tract infection and diarrhoea is most likely having infection by : TN 1997

A. Cocksackie virus B. Rota virus
C. Shigella D. None of the above

62. AIDS in children is characterised by : AIIMS 1997

A. Cryptococcus causing diarrhoea
B. Kaposi sarcoma common
C. DPT is not given
D. Recurrent candidiasis seen

63. Antisera are given in the case of : UPSC 1997

A. Tuberculosis, diphtheria and tetanus
B. Diphtheria and tetanus
C. Cholera
D. None of the above

64. Consider the following conditions : UPSC 1997

1. Phlyctenular conjunctivitis
2. Erythema nodosum
3. Positive Mantoux test

Allergy to mycobacterium tuberculosis in children may manifest as :

A. 1, 2 and 3 B. 1 and 2
C. 2 and 3 D. 1 and 3

65. The following given item consists of two statements, one labelled the 'Assertion A' and the other labelled the 'Reason R'. You are to examine these two statements carefully and decide if the Assertion A and the Reasons R are individually true and if so, whether the Reason is a correct explanation of the Assertion. Select your answer to these items using the codes given below and mark your answer sheet accordingly: UPSC 1997

Codes :

A. Both A and R are true and R is the correct explanation of A.
B. Both A and R are true but R is not a correct explanation of A.
C. A is true but R is false.
D. A is false but R is true.

Assertion (A) : Rifampicin is a useful drug in preventing H-influenzae meningitis in children

Reason (R) : Rifampicin eradicates naso-pharyngeal carrier in house-hold contacts.

66. Which of the following is not true about immunological status of the foetus : MAHE 1998

A. IgM present before birth
B. IgG in breast milk prevents against GIT & respiratory symptoms
C. IgG crosses the placenta
D. None of the above

67. Typhoid manifests in children with the following features except : Karnataka 1998

A. High grade continuous temperature
B. Manifests with Encephalopathy during the first week
C. Silent perforation may occur during first to second week
D. Constipation is common

68. Pertusis infection is characterised by the following features : Karnataka 1998

A. Subconjunctival Haemorrhage
B. Stimson's line
C. Rectal prolapse
D. Convulsions

69. A child developed bilateral blindness after getting measles. Which is the commonest cause : AIIMS 1999

A. Keratomalacia B. Viral keratitis
C. Conjunctivitis D. Encephalitis

70. In falciparum malaria, not seen in peripheral blood smear : PGI 1999

A. Crescents B. Schizonts
C. Ring forms D. Primary gametocytes

Ans.									
55. C	56. D	57. C	58. A	59. B	60. B	61. B	62. D	63. B	64. A
65. D	66. B	67. A	68. A	69. D	70. B				

71. Proper management of a 2 years old child with a positive tuberculin test and no evidence of diseases, would be to : AIIMS 1991
A. Treat with INH for three months
B. Treat with INH for one year
C. Repeat tuberculin test monthly
D. Follow the patient with serial X-ray examinations

72. Rota virus immunity in over 90% children occurs above —— years of age : AMC 1987; AIIMS 1994
A. 2 B. 5
C. 7 D. 10

73. Following is true about childhood AIDS : AIIMS 1998
A. Kaposi sarcoma
B. Recurrent candidiasis
C. Cryptococcal diarrhoea
D. Recurrent chest infection with atypical organisms

74. Which of the following cells may have an antihistaminic activity : AIIMS 1991
A. Lymphocytes B. Burr cell
C. Basophil D. Eosinophil

75. Histamine is most abundant in : Delhi 1992
A. Mast cells B. Eosinophils
C. Lymphocytes D. Paneth cells

76. Scratch tests are best read within : PGI 1992
A. 1 hour B. 4 hours
C. 5 minutes D. 15-20 minutes

77. All are considered immediate allergic reactions, except : AIIMS 1984, 85; UPSC 1996
A. Atopic dermatitis B. Contact dermatitis
C. Urticaria D. Asthma

78. What is the commonest homograft : AMC 1993
A. Heart B. Blood
C. Lung D. Kidney

79. EB virus was implicated as a cause of infectious mononucleosis by : AMC 1993
A. Koch et.al. 1962
B. Henle et.al. 1967
C. Mackinney et.al.. 1974
D. Rocchi & Ainti, 197

80. Most thermolabile vaccine is : UPSC 1983, 88; Delhi 1993
A. Measles B. OPV
C. BCG D. DP

81. The most common complication following measles is: JIPMER 1992
A. Myocarditis B. Encephalitis
C. Diarrhea D. LRI

82. Spot the true statement regarding poliomyelitis : AIIMS 1991
A. Causes a symmetrical polyneuritis
B. Is characterised by painless paralysis
C. Is diagnosed by blood culture
D. Is a viral infection affecting the anterior horn cell

83. Diphtheritic toxin affects the following system except : AMU 1994
A. Muscular system
B. Cardio vascular system
C. Central nervous system
D. Renal system

84. Which one of the following statement is not correct regarding Fifth Disease: UPSC 2004
A. It is caused by Parvovirus B 19
B. Patient has slapped cheek appearance
C. Arthritis is the most common complication
D. Incubation period varies from 2-4 days

85. Which of the following is the aetiological agent most often associated with Epiglottitis in children:
A. Streptococcus pneumoniae
B. Haemophilus influenzae type β
C. Neisseria sp.
D. Moraxella catarrhalis

86. In a completely and adequately immunized child against Diphtheria, the throat swab was collected. It showed the presence of Corynebacterium diphtheria like organisms on Albert staining. These organisms can have one of the following properties on further laboratory processing : AIIMS 2004
A. It can grow on Potassium tellurite medium.
B. It would show a positive Elek's gel precipitation test
C. It can be pathogenic to experimental guinea pigs
D. It can produce cytotoxicity in tissue cultures.

87. The antibody seen in a neonate after an intrauterine infection : Kerala 1999
A. IgG B. IgM
C. IgA D. IgD

88. A patient with fever, sore throat and +ve Paul Bunnel test : AI-2000
A. Infectious mononucleisosis
B. CMV
C. CML
D. Diphtheria

89. Vaccine with best efficacy : AI 2009
A. TT B. DPT
C. Measles D. Typhoid

Ans.									
71. B	72. B	73. B	74. D	75. A	76. D	77. B	78. B	79. B	80. B
81. D	82. D	83. A	84. D	85. B	86. A	87. B	88. A	89. A	

EXPLANATIONS OF DISEASE & IMMUNITY

1. Ans.— A. **Shivering**

Neonates are especially prone to develop hypothermia because of the increased surface to mass ratio and their lack of effective shivering and adaptive behavioural responses. In addition, the presence of malnutrition can make them more prone to the development of hypothermia.

The various physiologic changes seen in cases of hypothermia can depend on the degree of hypothermia. These changes are:

* *CNS* : It ranges from amensia, impaired judgement to increasing levels of cerebral depression.
* *CVS :* It ranges from tachycardia and increased blood pressure and CO in the milder cases to decreased BP, heart rate, CO and arrythmias in severe cases.
* *Renal :* Initial diuresis followed by decreased renal blood flow and can lead to renal failure which parallels the decline in cardiac output.

2. Ans.— A **Both active and passive immunization soon after birth**

Immunization of infants born to HbsAg positive woman.

* *These infants should receive both active and passive immunization soon after birth.*

The first dose of active immunization should be accompanied by administration of .5 ml of HBIG as soon as after delivery is possible, because the effectiveness decreases rapidly with increased time after birth.

* Subsequent doses of active immunization should be given at 1-20 months, and 6 months of age.

3. Ans.— C. **Hepatitis-B vaccine**
4. Ans.— C. **Roseola infantum**
5. Ans.— D. **Clostridium botulinum**
6. Ans.— B. **Sec. bacterial infection**
7. Ans.— A. **Single papilloma**
8. Ans.— A. **Second week of illness**

Myocarditis usually occurs towards the end of first or beginning of second week and is ushered with abdominal pain, vomiting, dypnoea, systemic venous congestion, tachycardia (or even bradycardia) extrasystoles, thready pulse and soft muffled first sound.

9. Ans.— B. **Ototoxicity**
10. Ans.— B. **Carry Blair medium**
11. Ans.— A. **FTA ABS IgM**

Passively acquired VDRL positive test from the mother, usually becomes negative within the first three months but passively transferred FTA-ABS-IgM test remains positive for over eight months.

12. Ans.— B. **Roseola infantum**

It is also called exanthem subitum. It is caused by Herpes virus-6 or Parovirus-B219 or echovirus 19. It is most common between 6 months to 3 years of age.

13. Ans.— C. **HIV ELISA**
14. Ans.— D. **G.I. tract**
15. Ans.— B. **Cardiomyopathy**
16. Ans.— C. **Erythromycin**
17. Ans.— D. **Sweat sodium concentration**
18. Ans.— A. **10 to 15 days**

Poliovirus, an RNA virus, type-I is commonest cause. It is excreted in stools of patients for 6-8 weeks after the onset of illness.

19. Ans.— B. **T.B. meningitis**
20. Ans.— C. **Psoriasis**
21. Ans.— A. **Shock**
22. Ans.— A. **Penicillin**

23. Ans.— C. **Cannot be detected by available newer methods**

24. Ans.— C. **Measles**

25. Ans.— B. **Brainstem evoked auditory potential study**

26. Ans.— D. **Any of the above**

27. Ans.— B. **Meningococci**

In meningococcomia may be associated with acute fulminating illness and adrenal insufficiency characterized by severe prostration, hypotension, shock and coma called 'Waterhouse Freiderichsen syndrome'. It is due to hemorrhage and necrosis in the adrenal glands.

28. Ans.— D. **7 to 14 days**

29. Ans.— A. **2**

30. Ans.— C. **Aseptic meningitis**

31. Ans.— B. **Peri-uvular-abscess**

32. Ans.— B. **Pneumococci**

The risk is often due to pneumococci and H. influenzae. The risk of post-splenectomy sepsis is greater in malignancies, thalasemias and reticuloendotheliosis than in children who suffer from ITP, hereditary spherocytosis or trauma.

33. Ans.— C. **Pertusis**

34. Ans.— C. **Rash**

35. Ans.— D. **Whooping cough**

36. Ans.— A. **4 to 6 months**

37. Ans.— D. **Palatal diphtheria**

38. Ans.— D. **Bronchial asthma**

39. Ans.— B. **300 mg**

40. Ans.— B. **Type-B**

41. Ans.— D. **All of the above**

42. Ans.— C. **5th year**

43. Ans.— A. **Hepatitis-B active and passive (IgM) immunisation**

Vaccine should be given within first 24 hours after birth and again at 1 and 6 months of age.

44. Ans.— D. **Plasmodium falciparum**

45. Ans.— C. **Measles vaccine**

46. Ans.— C. **Splenomegaly**

Splenomegaly is seen in about 50% cases and Tympanitis is the most useful sign.

47. Ans.— A. **Emphysema**

48. Ans.— D. **IgA**

It is present in breast milk and protects against GI infection.

49. Ans.— B. **Seminoma testis**

It is common in nonseminomatous testicular tumor (i.e. teratoma).

50. Ans.— C. **Until swelling subsides**

51. Ans.— A. **Both mother and infant are infected**

52. Ans.— A. **Cord Hb < 16 gm%**

53. Ans.— B. **Milk**

54. Ans.— A. **Drug reaction**

55. Ans.— C. **2 plus**

56. Ans.— D. **Atypical mycobacteriosis**

57. Ans.— C. **40 mg**

58. Ans.— A. **BCG**

59. Ans.— B. **Measles**

60. Ans.— B. **Pertussis**

61. Ans.— B. **Rota virus**

62. Ans.— D. **Recurrent candidiasis seen**

63. Ans.— B. **Diphtheria and tetanus**

64. Ans.— A. **1, 2 and 3**

65. Ans.— D. **A is false but R is true**

66. Ans.— B. **IgG in breast milk prevents against GIT & respiratory symptoms**

67. Ans.— A. **High grade continuous temperature**

68. Ans.— A. **Subconjunctival Haemorrhage**

69. Ans.— D. **Encephalitis**

Encephalitis is due to direct invasion of brain cells with virus or may be an allergic reaction.

70. Ans.— B. **Schizonts**

71. Ans.— B. **Treat with INH for one year**

72. Ans.— B. **5**

In rota virus diarrhoea, vomiting is an early feature and diarrhoea is more severe. Most patients have mild to moderate fever.

73. Ans.— B. **Recurrent candidiasis**

74. Ans.— D. **Eosinophil**

75. Ans.— A. **Mast cells**

76. Ans.— D. **15-20 minutes**

77. Ans.— B. **Contact dermatitis**

78. Ans.— B. **Blood**

79. Ans.— B. **Henle et.al., 1967**

80. Ans.— B. OPV

81. Ans.— D. LRI

SSPE (Subacute sclerosing panencephalitis) characterized by myoclonic jerks, mental deterioration and a fatal course within 6 months is also a complication.

82. Ans.— D. Is a viral infection affecting the anterior horn cell

83. Ans.— A. Muscular system

84. Ans.— D. Incubation period varies from 2-4 days

85. Ans.— B. Haemophilus influenzae type-β

86. Ans.— A. It can grow on Potassium tellurite medium.

87. Ans.— B. IgM

88. Ans.— A. Infectious mononucleisosis

89. Ans.— C. Measles

Among the choices mentioned above Measles Vaccine has Highest Efficacy of >95% after single vaccination.

However the book mentions the efficacy of DPT is 70% after 3 doses and this includes Tetanus Toxoid too.

Typhoid Vaccines have an efficacy range of 70-85%

6

IMPORTANT TEXT OF GIT

CAUSES OF ACUTE VOMITING

Infectious gastroenteritis
Intestinal obstruction
Infection from a non-intestinal site
- Otitis media
- Urinary tract infection
- Meningitis

Ingestion of toxic substances
Increased intracranial pressure
Encephalopathy
Pancreatitis
Self-induced

CAUSES OF CHRONIC DIARRHOEA (MORE THAN 2 WEEKS) IN CHILDREN

Dietary intolerance	Coelia disease Cow's milk protein intolerance Carbohydrate intolerance
Inborn errors	Chloridiarrhoea Acrodermatitis enteropathic Abetaliproteinaemia
Surgical	Malrotation Bind loop syndrome Stenosis
Pancreatic insufficiency	Cystic fibrosis Shwachman's syndrome
Immunodeficiency	Severe combined immunodeficiency Hypogammaglobulinaemia Opsinization defect HIV infections (AIDA)
Tumours	Ganglioneuroma Lymphoma
Others	Intestinal lymphangiectasia Addison's disease Auto-immune enteropathy Congenital microvillus atrophy

PYLORIC STENOSIS

* 1/150 males & 1/700 females & +ve family history
* Presents in 1st month - vomiting (without bile) & becomes projectile
* Failure to thrive, weight loss, but baby is hungry
* O/E - observe for peristalitic waves & palpable pyloric "tumour", after "sham" feed
* Lab: BUN (due to dehydration) & Hypochloraemic alkalosis
* Needs chlorides> 95 before surgey, NaXI & KCI are indicated & correction of alkalosis

INTUSSUSCEPTION :

* Occur 3 months to 3 years
* Child suddenly develops severe abdominal pain, which lasts a few min, then resolves (recurrent).
* May present with collapse, blood in stools, (Red current jelly) & eventually obstruction develops
* Treatment & diagnosis - Barium enema

HIRSCHPRUNG'S DISEASE	FUNCTIONAL CONSTIPATION
* Onset since birth neonatal period	* Onset 60% in 1st year
* No formed stool	* Course intermittent
* Withholding-absent	* Withholding +++
* Soiling - Nil	* Soiling++
* Delayed growth (failure to thrive)	* Normal growth
* Distended abdomean	* Variable
* Empty rectum & No dilation	* Rectum usually contains feces
* Dilated to involved Segment on X-ray	* Dilated to anus on X-ray
* Rectal biopsy reveals absence of aganglionic meyentric plexus	* —
* May develop toxic megacolon	* —

INVESTIGATION OF CHOICE

Disorder	*Investigation*
Gastro-oesophageal reflux	Barium oesophagography under fluoroscopy
Achalasia	Barium swallow
Tracheo-oesophageal fistula	Barium swallow
Ingestion of caustic agents & Benign Oesophageal structures	Endoscopy (within 24 hours and Barium swallow)
Pyloric stenosis	Radiographic evaluation - Barium study
Congenital intestinal obstruction	Flat & upright X-ray abdomen without use of contract media
Congenital deodenal obstruction	'*Double buddle*' sign on X-ray (with complete atresia- no gas is seen)
Jejunal or ileal obstruction	Plane X-ray abdomen shows 'ground glass' appearance in the right lower quadrant in meconium ileus
Differentiation of small intestinal obstruction from large intestine	Barium or Gastrogratin study of colon
Congenital megalcolon Hirschprung	Rectal biopsy by punch or suction method showing absence of ganglion disease cells in submucosa
Meckel's diverticulum	Negative 99mTc scan indicates absence of Meckel's diverticulum (Barium studies cannot demonstrate diverticulum)
Ectopic gastric tissue	99mTc scan (99m Technetium is excreted by gastric mucosa)
Intussusception	Barium enema - show filling defect or cupping in the head of barium. Coilspring sign
Colonic polyps	Sigmoidoscopy - if not visualized - a double air/barium contrast study
Foreign bodies in the stomach & intestines	Serial roentgenograms

Anorectal malformations	
Low lesions	Digital & endoscopic examination
High lesions	Lateral roentgenogram in the upside down position
Idiopathic ulcerative colitis	Colonoscopic examination
Crohn's disease	Irregular mucosa, cobblestone-like pattern, segmental distribution of lesion on barium contrast roentgenogram
Malabsorptive disorders	Per oral suction biopsy of small intestine

MCQ's OF GIT

What is important in GIT

Congenital lesions (Pyloric stenosis, Hiatus hernia, Anal atresia, Hirschsprung's disease), Cystic fibrosis, Indian Childhood Cirrhosis, Hepatosplenomegaly

1. **One of the intestinal enzymes that is generally deficient in children following an attack of severe infectious enteritis is : AI 2005**
   A. Lactase B. Trypsin
   C. Lipase D. Amylase
2. **Which of the following disease could present with history of Meconium Ileus ? Kerala 2000, 2003**
   A. Hypersensitive Pneumonitis
   B. Kartagener's Syndrome
   C. α_1 antitrypsin deficiency
   D. Cystic Fibrosis
   E. Childhood (Extrinsic) Asthma
3. **Hepatitis-B has the following characteristics except : Kerala 2000**
   A. Has the same incubation period as HBV
   B. May occur as a co-infection with HBV
   C. A biphasic illness occurs which is uncommon in other types of hepatitis
   D. It is a DNA virus
   E. May cause fulminant hepatitis
4. **In Coeliac disease, following are true except : PGI 2000, 2005**
   A. Gliadin is cause
   B. Association with HLA B_8
   C. Decreased vill to crypt ratio
   D. Increased brush border seizures
5. **Intractable diarrhoea in children is caused by following except: PGI 2000**
   A. Cystic fibrosis B. Giardiasis
   C. Secreting tumor D. Chloridorrhoea
6. **In neuroblastoma, good prognosis is indicated by : PGI 2000**
   A. myc gene amplication B. Hyperploidy
   C. Abdominal type D. Age above 1 year
7. **Ramu, 8 years old boy presents upper GI bleeding. On examination splenomegaly, no ascites, no hepatomegaly; esophageal varices present and UGIE. Diagnosis is : AI 2001, 2007**
   A. Budd chiari syndrome
   B. Non-cirrhotic portal fibrosis
   C. Cirrhosis
   D. Veno occlusive disease
8. **3 years old with hepatic failure has following complications except : Kerala 2001**
   A. Cerebral odema B. Hypoglycemia
   C. Hyponatremia D. Pancreatitis
9. **A neonate is presented to the hospital with hepatitis and clay coloured stools. Biopsy of the liver shows giant cells. The diagnosis is : AIIMS 2001**
   A. Neonatal hepatitis with extrabiliary atresia
   B. Physiological jaundice
   C. Extrabiliary atresia
   D. Neonatal hepatitis with physiological jaundice
10. **Most common age group affected by infantile colic is: UPSC 1983; JIPMER 2002**
    A. 0-3 months B. 4-6 months
    C. 6-9 months D. 9-12 months
11. **Osteogenic sarcoma is associated commonly with : Maharashtra -2000**
    A. Retinoblastoma B. Neuroblastoma
    C. Ganglioneuromas D. Ca. colon
12. **The gold standard for definitive diagnosis of extrahepatic biliary atresia is : AIIMS 2002**
    A. Perioperative cholangiography
    B. Hepatobiliary scintigraphy
    C. Alkaline phosphatase level
    D. Liver biopsy
13. **A 3-years old child develops severe dehydration following acute gastroenteritis. Investigations show blood urea 60 mg/dl, pH 7.27, base excess-10 mEq/L, sodium 134 mEq/L and potassium 3.8 mEq/L. The most appropriate fluid for initial treatment of this child is : UPSC 2002**
    A. N/3 saline in 5% dextrose
    B. N/3 saline in 10% dextrose
    C. Normal saline with 5% destrose
    D. 3% saline

Ans.									
1. A	2. D	3. D	4. B	5. B	6. B	7. B	8. D	9. A	10. A
11. A	12. D	13. C							

14. **A 2 months baby presents with history of jaundice, turmeric coloured urine, and pale stools since birth. Examination reveals liver span of 10 cms, firm in consistency and spleen of 3 cms. The most specific investigation for establishing the diagnosis would be : AI 2003**
A. Liver function tests
B. Ultrasound abdomen
C. Preoperative cholangiogram
D. Liver biopsy

15. **A 45 days old infant developed icterus and two days later symptoms and signs of acute liver failure appeared. Child was found to be positive for HBsAg. The mother was also HBsAg carrier. The mother's hepatitis-B serological profile is likely to be : AI 2003**
A. HBsAg positive only
B. HBsAg and HbeAg positivity
C. HBsAg and anti-HBe antibody positivity
D. Mother infected with mutant HBV

16. **One of the more common causes of primary peritonitis is : AP 1990**
A. Pseudomonas B. Pneumococcus
C. Staphylococcus D. E. coli

17. **Commonest cause of jaundice in a newborn within 24 hours is : Delhi 1993**
A. Septicemia B. Rh - isoimmunization
C. Physiological D. Sickle cell anemia

18. **In acute abdomen the investigation of choice is : Delhi 1992**
A. S. Amylase B. S. Alkaline phosphatase
C. SGOT D. TLC

19. **All are causes of chronic constipation in infant except: JIPMER 1992**
A. High protein diet B. High carbohydrate diet
C. Hirschsprung's disease D. Fissure-in-ano

20. **Of the following which is not an usual feature of Ascariasis : AMC 1986, AIIMS 1992**
A. Abdominal pain B. Loeffer's syndrome
C. Urticaria D. Anaemia

21. **Unconjugated hyperbilirubinemia in newborn is caused by all except : AIIMS 1986; 87, 92**
A. Breast milk jaundice B. Galactosemia
C. Spherocytosis D. Gilbert's syndrome

22. **Following are seen in Necrotizing enterocolitis except: TN 1993; Rajasthan 1998; Kerala 1999**
A. Abdominal distention
B. Exaggerated bowel sounds
C. Intestinal perforation
D. Gangrene of bowel

23. **Which of the following is not a feature of cystic fibrosis: CMC 1987**
A. Autosomal recessive inheritance
B. Offensive stools in a toddler
C. Umbilical hernia in infancy
D. Presenting as intestinal obstruction in newborn

24. **Hereditary disorder associated with cirrhosis include all except : AMU 1985**
A. Galactosemia B. Cystic fibrosis
C. Wilson's disease D. Amyloidosis

25. **Pruritus ani in childhood is usually due to : Bihar 1991**
A. Prolapsed rectum B. Polyps
C. Soap allergy D. Oxyuriasis

26. **Currant jelly stools are usually associated with : Bihar 1990**
A. Appendicitis B. Intussusception
C. Enterocolitis D. Hirschsprung's disease

27. **Gluten restricted diets are used the in treatment of : AIIMS 1983**
A. Sprue B. Galactosemia
C. Pyuria D. Epilepsy

28. **Which of the following is the most common cause of acute diarrhoea in infants and children : PGI 1986**
A. Chemical B. Bacteria
C. Parasite D. Virus

29. **Which of the following is the most common cause of constipation in infants and children : AIIMS 1981**
A. Anorectal anomaly B. Hypothyroidism
C. Hirschsprung's disease D. Functional

30. **The use of oral pancreatic enzyme replacement therapy is most helpful in patients with : DNB 1989**
A. Ulcerative colitis
B. Cystic fibrosis
C. Coeliac disease
D. Protein losing enteropathy

31. **Most likely cause of GIT haemorrhage in a newborn is: Rohtak 1984**
A. Volvulus
B. Peptic ulcer
C. Ingested maternal blood
D. Meckel's diverticulum

32. **Pathological hyperbilirubinemia due to septicemia usually occur : Rohtak 1985**
A. Within 24 hours of birth
B. Within 48 hours of birth
C. After 72 hours of age
D. Any of the above mentioned time

33. **Which of the following criteria is useful to diagnose pathological Jaundice : AMU 1986**
A. Jaundice appears within 24 hours of age
B. Serum bilirubin level less than 12 mg/dl
C. Maximum intensity of Jaundice on the 4th day
D. Jaundice persisting for 8-10 days

Ans. 14. C 15. B 16. B 17. B 18. A 19. B 20. D 21. B 22. B 23. B
24. D 25. D 26. B 27. A 28. D 29. D 30. B 31. C 32. C 33. A

34. **In a newborn, brain damage may be associated with serum bilirubin protein ratio of: AMU 1989**
A. More than 1 B. More than 2
C. More than 3 D. More than 3.5

35. **The weight of a preterm neonate is 1000g. He developed hyperbilirubinemia on day 3. The baby will need exchange transfusion at a level of : Bihar 1990**
A. More than 5 mg/dl B. More than 6 mg/dl
C. More than 8 mg/dl D. More than 10 mg/dl

36. **Phototherapy is used treat hyperbilirubinemia. Both intermittent and continuous exposure are in use. However : AIIMS 1984**
A. Intermittent exposure is as effective as continuous
B. Intermittent exposure better than continuous
C. Continuous exposure better than intermittent
D. Intermittent exposure not be used

37. **Congenital absence of spleen is suspected in the presence of the following except : AP 1989**
A. Hepatomegaly
B. Target cells in the blood
C. Increased number of spherocytes
D. Howell Jolly and Heinz bodies

38. **Unconjugated bilirubin in plasma generally does not enter the brain because off : AIIMS 1982**
A. Rapidly metabolised by C S F
B. Blood brain in impermeable to bilirubin
C. Tightly bound to albumin
D. Not soluble in lipid

39. **Major route of bilirubin excretion in foetus is probably: PGI 1980**
A. Transplacental passage
B. Reincorporation into Hb
C. Degradation to biliverdin
D. Hepatic secretion and storage in lumen of intestine

40. **Which of the following is not a factor in neonatal hyperbilirubinaemia : PGI 1982**
A. Increased portal blood flow
B. Decreased hepatic conjugation of bilirubin
C. Increased bilirubin production
D. Increased enterohepatic circulation of bilirubin

41. **Intestinal roundworms in children : AIIMS 1984**
A. Are usually asymptomatic
B. Does not produce malena
C. Cause recurrent lung infection
D. May cause convulsions

42. **Risk of kernicterus is increased in all except : PGI 1982; AIIMS 1984**
A. Low level of serum albumin
B. Prematurity
C. Acidosis
D. High levels of serum albumin

43. **Celiac disease is due to sensitivity to : UPSC 1983; AIIMS 1984**
A. Milk B. Maize
C. Wheat D. Meat

44. **In acute hepatitis-B infection, the earliest abnormality detected is : PGI 1984; AIIMS 1983**
A. Raised serum transaminases
B. Antibodies to hepatitis-B Antigen
C. Detection of surface antigen
D. Anorexia and lassitude

45. **All of the following cause splenomegaly except : AIIMS 1983**
A. Gauchers disease B. Von Gierke disease
C. Tay Sach's disease D. Niemann Pick's disease

46. **An abdominal mass palpable in an asymptomatic neonate is not likely to be : PGI 1981**
A. Polycystic kidney
B. Multicystic renal dysplasia
C. Neuroblastoma
D. Distended urinary bladder

47. **Which of the following is associated with chronic liver disease : PGI 1982; AIIMS 1983**
A. Hepatitis
B. Alpha-1 antitrypsin deficiency
C. Malaria
D. Infectious mononucleosis

48. **A faintly pea green stool indicates : PGI 1981**
A. Peptic ulcer B. Amoebic dysentery
C. Ulcerative colitis D. None of the above

49. **All are features of functional constipation, except : UPSC 1983**
A. Growth usually normal
B. Rectal biopsy normal
C. Rectum not dilated and generally empty of stool
D. Huge bowel movements at long intervals

50. **Tarry stools are usually not associated with : AMC 1982, 89**
A. Ulcerative colitis B. Peptic ulcer
C. Bleeding diathesis D. Oesophageal varices

51. **Which of the following is not usually associated with abdominal pain in infancy : AMC 1983, 91**
A. Volvulus B. Infantile colic
C. Intussusception D. Duodenal ulcer

52. **All are features of tracheo-esophageal fistula, except : UPSC 1983**
A. Laryngeal stridor
B. Pneumonia
C. Stomach distension
D. X-ray helpful in diagnosis

53. **Fissured tongue is most often associated with : UPSC 1984**
A. Herpes simplex B. Coarctation of aorta
C. Down's syndrome D. Cheilosis

Ans.									
34. D	35. D	36. A	37. A	38. C	39. A	40. A	41. A	42. D	43. C
44. C	45. B	46. B	47. B	48. D	49. C	50. A	51. D	52. A	53. C

54. Common clinical features of gluten enteropathy includes all, except : PGI 1982
A. Faecal emesis
B. Abdominal distension
C. Foul, bulky, greasy stools
D. Recurrent diarrhoea

55. Most frequent cause of paralytic ileus in infants is probably : AIIMS 1985
A. Tuberculosis B. Pneumonia
C. Peritonitis D. Cystic fibrosis

56. Clinical features of congenital megacolon include all, except : PGI 1982
A. Diarrhoea B. Vomiting
C. Enterocolitis D. Hematemesis

57. Encopresis may be associated with conditions such as : UPSC 1983
A. Emotional instability
B. Disturbed parental relationship
C. Learning disability and hyperactivity
D. All of the above

58. Commonest cause of abdominal pain in children is : PGI 1983, 87
A. Porphyria B. Worm colic
C. Lead poisoning D. Appendicitis

59. Meconium is excreted by a newborn till —— days : UPSC 1983; AIIMS 1986
A. 2 B. 3
C. 4 D. 6

60. Crigler-Najjar disease is associated with : AIIMS 1985
A. Siblings are not similarly affected
B. Hepatomegaly
C. Jaundice
D. A positive Coomb's test

61. Which of the following pairs are correctly matched : UPSC 1995
1. Physiological jaundice—Increase in indirect bilirubin
2. Erythroblastosis foetalis—Jaundice at birth
3. ABO incompatibility—Exchange transfusion
4. Cord sepsis—Increase in direct bilirubin

Select the correct answer using the codes given below:
Codes :
A. 1, 2 and 4 B. 1, 3 and 4
C. 1, 2 and 3 D. 2, 3 and 4

62. Clinical features of congenital glucose galactose malabsorption include all, except : AIIMS 1984
A. Stools contain glucose B. Refusal of feedings
C. Watery diarrhoea D. Slight glucosuria

63. Congenital sucrose isomaltose malabsorption is usually first manifested by : AIIMS 1984
A. Convulsions B. Alopecia
C. Diarrhoea D. Cataracts
E. All of the above

64. A galactosemic infant is best fed with : AMU 1986, 92
A. Alacta B. Skim milk
C. Breast milk D. Nutramigen

65. All are true about tropical splenomegaly except : AP 1994
A. Seen in superendemic
B. Increased IgM levels
C. Massive splenomegaly
D. High parasitemia is always seen

66. Which is contraindicated in treating a child with familial hypercholesterolemia ? Delhi 1980
A. Cholestyramine B. Oestrogen
C. Nicotinic acid D. Thyroxine

67. In Hypertrophic pyloric stenosis, vomitings characteristically occur after : UPSC 1980
A. 2 weeks B. 4 weeks
C. 6 weeks D. 8 weeks

68. Diarrhoea in cystic fibrosis is due to : PGI 1983
A. Deficiencies in mucosal transport
B. Abnormal intestinal secretions
C. Rapid transit time
D. Deficiency in pancreatic secretions

69. Most common aetiology of hepatic metastasis in children is : PGI 1981
A. Astrocytoma B. Neuroblastoma
C. Melanoma D. Retinoblastoma

70. Splenomegaly in the absence of hepatomegaly is most likely to be seen in : AIIMS 1980
A. Fabry's disease
B. Niemann-Pick disease
C. Infantile Gaucher's disease
D. Congenital erythropoietic porphyria

71. Classical radiological sign of duodenal atresia is the : UPSC 1984, 86
A. Anchor sign B. String sign
C. Double-bubble sign D. Reverse 3 sign

72. A narrowing and elongation of pyloric canal on X-ray, in a 12 days infant, most strongly suggests : PGI 1979
A. Annular pancreas
B. Duodenal ulcer
C. Duodenal atresia
D. Infantile hypertrophic pyloric stenosis

73. Most common cause of infantile hematemesis is : UPSC 1983
A. Duodenal ulcers
B. Stomach ulcers
C. Oesophagitis and oesophageal ulcers
D. Gastric polyps

74. Gall stones in child are frequently due to : UPSC 1984
A. Spherocytic haemolytic anaemia
B. Salmonella dysentry
C. Pyloric stenosis
D. Sickle cell anaemia

Ans.									
54. A	55. B	56. D	57. D	58. B	59. C	60. C	61. B	62. B	63. C
64. D	65. D	66. B	67. A	68. D	69. B	70. D	71. C	72. D	73. C
74. A									

75. Rapid death (kernicterus) is associated which type of congenital jaundice ? AP 1992
A. Crigler-Najjar syndrome (Type-I)
B. Crigler-Najjar syndrome (Type-II)
C. Dubin-Johnson syndrome
D. Rotor syndrome

76. Concerning Hirschsprung's disease : UPSC 1985
A. Biopsy reveals increased number of nerve fibres
B. Familial incidence
C. Diagnosis usually made in first year of life
D. All are true

77. A 3 days old infant presents with vomiting, rapidly distending abdomen and signs of shock. The vomitus is bile stained. Most likely diagnosis is : UPSC 1982
A. Meconium ileus B. Midgut volvulus
C. Achalasia D. Acute appendicitis

78. 'Lead pipe' colon is associated with : AIIMS 1983, 85; Delhi 1985, 87
A. A ganglionic megacolon
B. Enterocolitis
C. Chronic ulcerative colitis
D. All of the above

79. Radiographic 'string sign' is associated with : Delhi 1987; UPSC 1982
A. Volvulus B. Pyloric stenosis
C. Regional enteritis D. Intussusception

80. The least likely diagnosis in a 2 days old infant with bile stained vomiting would be : UPSC 1984
A. Annular pancreas
B. Duodenal atresia
C. Hypertrophic pyloric stenosis
D. Volvulus

81. Lactase deficiency in children is characterised by : UP 1996, 97
A. Dumping syndrome
B. Abdominal bloating, cramps and diarrhoea
C. High pH of the stool
D. Low lactic acid levels in blood

82. A physical sign pathognomonic of necrotizing enterocolitis is : UPSC 1986, Bihar 1988
A. Pneumoperitoneum B. Bloody stools
C. Bile stained vomitus D. Pneumatosis intestinalis

83. Dysphagia is always present when the oesophagus cannot distend beyond : AIIMS 1986
A. 1 cm B. 1.3 cm
C. 1.8 cm D. 2.5 cm
E. 4 cm

84. Which of the following conditions is associated with impaired hepatic uptake of bilirubin : Bihar 1989
A. Crigler-Najjar syndrome
B. Gilbert's syndrome
C. Rotor syndrome
D. Dubin-Johnson syndrome
E. Pregnanediol therapy

85. "Pea-soup stool" characteristically seen in : Bihar 1991
A. Cholera B. Typhoid
C. Botulism diarrhoea D. Traveller's diarrhoea

86. Splenectomy is least useful in : AI 1989
A. Congenital elliptocytosis
B. Thalassemia major
C. Congenital spherocytic anaemia
D. Hereditary non-spherocytic haemolytic anaemia

87. A case of diarrhoea with 7% blood loss, best treatment is : PGI 1995
A. ORS
B. I/V fluids
C. ORS with antibiotics
D. Antibiotics + Antidiarrhoeals

88. Which of the following is not given in meconium aspiration syndrome (MAS) : JIPMER 1997
A. I/V fluids B. IPPV
C. I/V steroids D. I/V bronchodilatation

89. Bilious vomiting in a neonate is usually due to : AI 1994
A. Hypertrophic Pyloric stenosis
B. Tetralogy of Fallot
C. Congenital atresia of III part of duodenum
D. Intussusception

90. Strongyloides stercoralis infection does not cause : AMC 1985
A. Skin eruption B. Diarrhoea
C. Bronchitis D. Severe anaemia

91. Profuse haematemesis in children is due to : PGI 1984
A. Stomach polypi B. Oesophagitis
C. Portal hypertension D. Peptic ulcer

92. What is not true of Hunter's glossitis : AIIMS 1986
A. Occurs in pernicious anemia
B. Achlorhydria
C. Sprue
D. Niacin deficiency

93. What is not true regarding pancreatic insufficiency and chronic neutropenia (Schwachman's syndrome) : AP 1988
A. Normal sweat electrolytes and normal pancreatic functions
B. Thrombocytopenia and anemia
C. Metaphyseal dysostosis
D. Response with pancreatic enzyme replacement

Ans. 75. A 76. D 77. B 78. C 79. C 80. C 81. B 82. D 83. B 84. B
85. B 86. D 87. A 88. C 89. C 90. D 91. C 92. D 93. A

94. **Following are early symptoms of analphylactoid purpura except : DNB 1993**
A. Headache B. Abdominal pain
C. Loss of appetite D. Jaundice

95. **In a 3 years old child most common cause of hepatitis-B is : PGI 1997**
A. Pin Prick B. Saliva exchange
C. Perinatal D. Water

96. **Which of the following is a characteristic sign of Oesophageal atresia in child : AIIMS 1986**
A. Dribbling of saliva B. Dyspnoea
C. Cyanosis D. Distension of abdomen

97. **Which of the following is not seen in neuroblastoma : PGI 1985; AIIMS 1986**
A. Cafe-au-lait spots
B. Proptosis
C. Mouth eaten appearance of skull
D. Hypertension rarely

98. **Commonest cause of intestinal obstruction in a child is: AIIMS 1986**
A. Gut malrotation B. Congenital bands
C. Ileal Atresia D. Meconium ileus

99. **Gilbert's syndrome is characterised by : AIIMS 1987**
A. Mild unconjugated hyperbilirubinemia
B. Normal liver function tests
C. Normal liver histology
D. Increased risk of cirrhosis

100. **Lactase deficiency is characterised by : AIIMS 1990**
A. Acidity of stools occasionally
B. ↓ S. lactic acid
C. Abd. pain and distension with diarrhoea
D. Abnormal muscle cells seen

101. **Which of the following would suggest a diagnosis of diabetes mellitus rather than appendicitis in a child : JIPMER 1998**
A. Vomiting
B. Periumbilical pain
C. Abdominal distention
D. Nocturnal enuresis over preceding four weeks

102. **Celiac disease is associated with HLA —— in more than —— % patients : AIIMS 1987**
A. A_3, 60 B. A_8, 80
C. A_3, 85 D. B_7, 90

103. **Early morning vomiting of infants is chiefly due to : UPSC 1983; PGI 1989**
A. Hypoglycaemia B. Meningitis
C. Gastroenteritis D. Intestinal obstruction

104. **In diarrhoea due to cryptosporidium, following drug may be tried : DNB 1994**
A. Furazolidone B. Vancomycin
C. Spiramycin D. Omeprazole

105. **Tracheo oesophageal fistula is associated with : Delhi 1984, 89**
A. GIT anomalies
B. CVS anomalies
C. CNS anomalies
D. Respiratory tract anomalies

106. **A 4-years old child with abdominal mass and calcification is most likely suffering from : AIIMS 1989; Delhi 1989**
A. Mesenteric cyst B. Phaeochromocytoma
C. Wilm's tumour D. Neuroblastoma

107. **Diagnosis of lactose intolerance is by : AIIMS 1987; Delhi 1982, 88**
A. Reducing substance in stool
B. Alkalinity of stool
C. Alternating constipation and diarrhoea
D. Acidotic smell of stool

108. **Gastrooesophageal reflux is usually diagnosed clinically in thriving infants under —— months of age: AIIMS 1991**
A. 2 B. 6
C. 12 D. 24

109. **Blood and mucus in stools are seen with all except : AI 1989**
A. E. histolytica B. Shigella shiga
C. E. coli D. V. cholera

110. **Pseudopancreatic cyst in a child is commonly due to : AI 1999**
A. Annular pancreatitis
B. Drug induced pancreatitis
C. Traumatic pancreatitis
D. Choledochal cyst

111. **The mechanism of diarrhoea is giardiasis is prevention of absorption of fat by : AMC 1987**
A. Mechanical coating of the wall so intensive
B. Secondary bacterial infection
C. Production of exotoxins
D. Production of endotoxins

112. **Hiatus hernia becomes symptomatic at : AMC 1991**
A. Birth B. Within 1 week
C. 2-4 weeks D. 4-6 weeks

113. **Splenic rupture in children is best diagnosed by : AIIMS 1982, 89**
A. Paracentesis B. Ultrasound
C. Plain X-ray D. Tc99 scan

114. **A 4 days old child has jaundice and serum bilirubin of 8 mg/dl. Treatment of choice is : JIPMER 1990**
A. Exchange transfusion
B. Phototherapy
C. Observation
D. Investigation for liver function

Ans.									
94. D	95. A	96. A	97. A	98. C	99. A	100. C	101. D	102. B	103. A
104. C	105. A	106. D	107. A	108. C	109. D	110. C	111. A	112. C	113. D
114. C									

115. Gastric aspiration of more than 20 ml in a child at birth suggests : AMC 1983; AI 1988
A. Tracheo esophageal fistula
B. Duodenal atresia
C. Swallowed amniotic fluid
D. Any of the above

116. Commonest cause of pathological hyperbilirubinemia in India is : AMC 1982; PGI 1986, 89
A. ABO incompatibility B. Rh incompatibility
C. Septicemia D. G-6-P-D deficiency

117. Meconium contains all except : AMC 1984; PGI 1986, 89
A. Lanugo B. Bacterial flora
C. Epithelial debris D. Bilirubin

118. Chronic persistent diarrhoea may occur in all of the following conditions except : Karnataka 1994
A. Zinc deficiency B. Niacin deficiency
C. Riley-Day syndrome D. Hypervitaminosis-D

119. Commonest cause of obstructive jaundice in a neonate is : Delhi 1994
A. Biliary atresia B. CBD stones
C. UTI D. Iatrogenic

120. The most common cause of malabsorption syndrome in Indian children is : UPSC 1994
A. Amoebiasis
B. Giardiasis
C. Escherichia coli infection
D. Malrotation of the gut

121. A 80 day old baby developed jaundice with features suggestive of non-pathological jaundice. The level of bilirubin indicative of phototherapy is : AIIMS 1999
A. 9 B. 12
C. 15 D. 18

122. 2 months old jaundice since birth, with absent urobilin, golden yellow stool, increased conjugated bilirubin in blood has : AIIMS 1999
A. Biliary atresia
B. Breast milk jaundice
C. Hypothyroidism
D. Hereditary spherocytosis

123. The investigation to be done in neonatal jaundice is : AI 2000
A. Direct bilirubin B. Total bilirubin
C. Total+direct bilirubin D. Conjugated bilirubin

124. Match List-I (Stool test) with List- II (Disease) and select the correct answer using the codes given below the Lists: UPSC 2000

List-I	List-II
A. pH less than 5.5 and reducing substances positive (more than 1+)	1. Giardiasis
B. Neutral fat more than 40 fat globules/high power field	2. Carbohydrate malabsorption
C. Occult blood positive	3. Malrotation with protein malabsorption
D. Trophozoite and cyst present	4. Enteritis or colitis
	5. Pancreatic insufficiency

Codes:

	a	b	c	d
A.	1	4	2	3
B.	2	5	4	1
C.	2	1	4	3
D.	3	5	2	1

125. Which one of the following markers increases the risk of transmission of Hepatitis-B, from mother to her newborn: UPSC 2000
A. HBs AG B. Anti HBs
C. HBe Ag D. HBc Ag

126. Protracted (or Persistent) diarrhoea is defined as : Orissa 1991; UPSC 1995
A. Diarrhoea more than 2 weeks duration.
B. Diarrhoea more than 1 week duration.
C. Diarrhoea more than 2 weeks duration with weight loss or failure to gain weight.
D. Diarrhoea more than one week duration with weight loss or failure to gain weight.

127. Which of the following parasites is not a common cause of chronic diarrhoea : UPSC 1988
A. Ent. histolytica B. Ascaris lumbricoides
C. Giardia D. H. nana

128. Jaundice in a newborn seen after 48 hours of birth, S. bilirubin not exceeding 5 mg% is : Kerala 1994
A. ABO incompatibility
B. Haemolytic disease of newborn
C. Neonatal hepatitis syndrome
D. Physiological jaundice

129. Hepatitis-C closely resembles : AIIMS 1995
A. Hepatitis-B B. Hepatitis-A
C. Hepatitis-E D. Hepatitis-D

130. Regarding congenital hypertrophic pyloric stenosis true all except : AI 1993
A. Metabolic acidosis
B. Inconstant lump
C. Regurgitation and vomiting
D. Hypochloremic alkalosis

131. Jaundice in newborn is decreased if mother is given : Delhi 1995
A. Phenobarbitone
B. Vit-K
C. Rh anti-immunoglobulins
D. Corticosteroids

Ans. 115. B 116. B 117. B 118. D 119. A 120. B 121. C 122. A 123. C 124. B
125. C 126. C 127. C 128. D 129. A 130. A 131. A

132. Turcot syndrome most commonly involves : AIIMS 1985, 89

A. Stomach B. Duodenum
C. Ileum D. Colon

133. Forceful or projectile vomiting is often found with except : Bihar 1990

A. Severe urinary tract infection
B. Adrenocortical insufficiency
C. Pyloric stenosis
D. Achalasia cardia

134. In Indian childhood cirrhosis, the most common biochemical change seen is that : UPSC 1995

A. Serum copper level is increased while serum zinc level is decreased.
B. Both serum copper level and serum zinc level are decreased.
C. Serum copper level is decreased while serum zinc level is increased.
D. Both serum copper level and serum zinc level are increased.

135. Signs and symptoms of trichobezoar include all, except: Rohtak 1987

A. Abdominal mass
B. Vague epigastric discomfort
C. Diarrhoea
D. Foul breath

136. A 3-years old male child is admitted in the casualty ward with dyspnoea, brassy type of cough and swelling in the neck which is tender on palpation. The child also complains of dysphagia. The most likely diagnosis is : UPSC 1995

A. Oesophagitis B. Achalasia
C. Hiatus hernia D. Retropharyngeal abscess

137. Which of the following complications are increased in the preterm baby : UPSC 1995

1. Hyperbilirubinaemia
2. Meconium aspiration syndrome
3. Hypothermia

Select the correct answer using the codes given below :

Codes :

A. 1 and 2 B. 1 and 3
C. 2 and 3 D. 1, 2 and 3

138. Most common manifestation of peptic ulcer in infancy is : AIIMS 1984

A. Constipation B. Diarrhoea
C. Vomiting D. Distension of abdomen

139. Each of the following observations about first stage of Indian childhood cirrhosis is true, except : Rohtak 1985

A. Jaundice is always present
B. Vague manifestations
C. Growth manifestations
D. Liver is enlarged by 3-5 cm

140. Primary symptom of hiatus hernia during the newborn period is : AMU 1984

A. Anaemia B. Anorexia
C. Vomiting D. Distended abdomen

141. Regarding congenital hypertrophic pyloric stenosis of infancy which one of the following statement is not correct : UPSC 2004

A. It is most commonly occurs in first born male child
B. It is usually presents at 3 to 4 weeks of life
C. Feeding is followed by bilious vomiting
D. Baby is hungry soon after vomiting

142. Match List-I (condition) with List-II (Timing of Surgery) and select the correct answer using the codes given below the Lists : UPSC 2004

List - I (Condition)	*List - II (Timing of Surgery)*
A. Cystic hygroma	1. Around 1 year of age
B. Undescended testes	2. Almost never needed
C. Cleft palate	3. 7 to 9 months of age
D. Umbilical hernia	4. Soon after diagnosis

Codes :

	A	B	C	D
A.	2	3	1	4
B.	4	3	1	2
C.	4	1	3	2
D.	2	1	3	4

143. One of the intestinal enzymes that is generally deficient in children following an attack of severe infectious enteritis is : AI 2005

A. Lactase B. Trypsin
C. Lipase D. Amylase

144. Which of the following is a cause for hematemesis in new born infant : MAHE 2006

A. Obstruction intestinal
B. Maternal swallowing of blood
C. Tracheoesophageal fistula
D. Pyloric stenosis

Ans. 132. D 133. D 134. A 135. C 136. D 137. B 138. C 139. A 140. C 141. C 142. C 143. A 144. B

EXPLANATIONS OF GIT

1. Ans.— A. Lactase
2. Ans.— D. Cystic Fibrosis
3. Ans.— D. It is a DNA virus
4. Ans.— B. Association with HLA B_8
5. Ans.— B. Giardiasis
6. Ans.— B. Hyperploidy

   The prognosis depends on age, location of primary tumor and degree of maturation of cells. Younger age, tumors from thorax and neck and maturation of tumor cells indicate better prognosis.
7. Ans.— B. Non cirrhotic portal fibrosis
8. Ans.— D. Pancreatitis
9. Ans.— A. Neonatal hepatitis with extrabiliary atresia
10. Ans.— A. 0-3 months
11. Ans.— A. Retinoblastoma
12. Ans.— D. Liver biopsy
13. Ans.— C. Normal saline with 5% destrose
14. Ans.— C. Preoperative cholangiogram
    * Pale stool since birth clearly suggests biliary atresia.
    * Most useful conformatory test for biliary atresia is preoperative Cholangiography.
15. Ans.— B. HBsAg and HbeAg positivity
    * Perinatal transmission occurs primarily in child born to HBsAg carrier mothers or mothers with acute Hepatitis-B during the 3rd trimester of pregnancy or during early postpartum period.
    * Likelihood of perinatal transmission of HBV corelates with the presence of HBeAg is 90% than that of mothers with Anti-HBeAg(+)ve is 10-15%.
16. Ans.— B. Pneumococcus
17. Ans.— B. Rh - isoimmunization

    Is an important cause of severe neonatal jaundice. The main danger of unconjugated hyperbilirubinemia in newborn is kernicterus or brain damage. Bilirubin protein ratio of more than 3.5 is often associated with brain damage. The antibodies involved in isosensitization are of IgG type which pass from placenta into fetus.
18. Ans.— A. S. Amylase
19. Ans.— B. High carbohydrate diet
20. Ans.— D. Anaemia
21. Ans.— B. Galactosemia
22. Ans.— B. Exaggerated bowel sounds

    The clinical picture stimulates neonatal septicemia. It is seen in premature infants especially those who are under stress during first week of life. Ileum is the most frequent site involved.
23. Ans.— B. Offensive stools in a toddler
24. Ans.— D. Amyloidosis
25. Ans.— D. Oxyuriasis
26. Ans.— B. Intussusception
27. Ans.— A. Sprue
28. Ans.— D. Virus

    Rota virus is an important cause
29. Ans.— D. Functional
30. Ans.— B. Cystic fibrosis
31. Ans.— C. Ingested maternal blood
32. Ans.— C. After 72 hours of age
33. Ans.— A. Jaundice appears within 24 hours of age
34. Ans.— D. More than 3.5
35. Ans.— D. More than 10 mg/dl
36. Ans.— A. Intermittent exposure is as effective as continuous
37. Ans.— A. Hepatomegaly

38. Ans.— C. Tightly bound to albumin

39. Ans.— A. Transplacental passage

40. Ans.— A. Increased portal blood flow

41. Ans.— A. Are usually asymptomatic

42. Ans.— D. High levels of serum albumin

43. Ans.— C. Wheat

Celiac disease is an important cause of malabsorption in childhood. Antibodies are against gliadin (a fraction of gluten). Serum levels of IgA are high and IgM are low. More than 80% have HLA A8 haplotype. All cereals containing gluten (Wheat, rye, barley, oats) should be excluded from diet.

44. Ans.— C. Detection of surface antigen

45. Ans.— B. Von Gierke disease

46. Ans.— B. Multicystic renal dysplasia

47. Ans.— B. Alpha-1 antitrypsin deficiency

48. Ans.— D. None of the above

49. Ans.— C. Rectum not dilated and generally empty of stool

50. Ans.— A. Ulcerative colitis

51. Ans.— D. Duodenal ulcer

This is not a common cause of abdominal pain in infancy.

52. Ans.— A. Laryngeal stridor

53. Ans.— C. Down's syndrome

54. Ans.— A. Faecal emesis

55. Ans.— B. Pneumonia

56. Ans.— D. Hematemesis

57. Ans.— D. All of the above

It is usually associated with enuresis and bowel and bladder training should be properly instituted.

58. Ans.— B. Worm colic

59. Ans.— C. 4

60. Ans.— C. Jaundice

In Crigler-Najjar syndrome, there is congenital absence of the enzyme UDP glucuronyl transferase. Two types are recognized Type-I (onset of jaundice at birth) and type-II-a milder disease (onset of jaundice may be delayed upto 10 years of age).

61. Ans.— B. 1, 3 and 4

62. Ans.— B. Refusal of feedings

63. Ans.— C. Diarrhoea

64. Ans.— D. Nutramigen

65. Ans.— D. High parasitemia is always seen

66. Ans.— B. Oestrogen

67. Ans.— A. 2 weeks

68. Ans.— D. Deficiency in pancreatic secretions

69. Ans.— B. Neuroblastoma

70. Ans.— D. Congenital erythropoietic porphyria

71. Ans.— C. Double-bubble sign

72. Ans.— D. Infantile hypertrophic pyloric stenosis

73. Ans.— C. Oesophagitis and oesophageal ulcers

74. Ans.— A. Spherocytic haemolytic anaemia

75. Ans.— A. Crigler-Najjar syndrome (Type-I)

76. Ans.— D. All are true

Rectosigmoid junction is most common site involved. There is absence of parasympathetic ganglion cells in Auerback and Meissner's plexuses, demonstrated on rectal biopsy.

77. Ans.— B. Midnight volvulus

78. Ans.— C. Chronic ulcerative colitis

79. Ans.— C. Regional enteritis

80. Ans.— C. Hypertrophic pyloric stenosis

81. Ans.— B. Abdominal bloating, cramps and diarrhoea

82. Ans.— D. Pneumatosis intestinalis

83. Ans.— B. 1.3 cm

84. Ans.— B. Gilbert's syndrome

85. Ans.— B. Typhoid

86. Ans.— D. Hereditary non-spherocytic haemolytic anaemia

87. Ans.— A. ORS

88. Ans.— C. I/V steroids

89. Ans.— C. Congenital atresia of III part of duodenium

Abdominal distention is minimal and constipation is present

90. Ans.— D. Severe anaemia

91. Ans.— C. Portal hypertension

92. Ans.— D. Niacin deficiency

93. Ans.— A. Normal sweat electrolytes and normal pancreatic functions

94. Ans.— D. Jaundice

95. Ans.— A. Pin Prick

96. Ans.— A. **Dribbling of saliva**
Dribbling of saliva is the characteristic sign of oesophageal atresia.

97. Ans.— A. **Cafe-au-lait spots**
Early manifestations are vague and non-specific (anorexia, fatigue, anemia and loss of weight). Cafe-au-lait spots are seen in tuberous sclerosis.

98. Ans.— C. **Ileal Atresia**

99. Ans.— A. **Mild unconjugated hyperbilirubinemia**

100. Ans.— C. **Abd. pain and distension with diarrhoea**

101. Ans.— D. **Nocturnal enuresis over preceding four weeks**

102. Ans.— B. **A_8, 80**

103. Ans.— A. **Hypoglycaemia**

104. Ans.— C. **Spiramycin**

105. Ans.— A. **GIT anomalies**

106. Ans.— D. **Neuroblastoma**

107. Ans.— A. **Reducing substance in stool**
Lactose malabsorption is common in protein energy malnutrition.

108. Ans.— C. **12**

109. Ans.— D. **V. cholera**

110. Ans.— C. **Traumatic pancreatitis**

111. Ans.— A. **Mechanical coating of the wall so intensive**

112. Ans.— C. **2-4 weeks**

113. Ans.— D. **Tc99 scan**

114. Ans.— C. **Observation**

115. Ans.— B. **Duodenal atresia**

116. Ans.— B. **Rh incompatibility**

117. Ans.— B. **Bacterial flora**

118. Ans.— D. **Hypervitaminosis-D**

119. Ans.— A. **Biliary atresia**

120. Ans.— B. **Giardiasis**

121. Ans.— C. **15**

122. Ans.— A. **Biliary atresia**

123. Ans.— C. **Total+direct bilirubin**

124. Ans.— B. **2 5 4 1**

125. Ans.— C. **HBe Ag**

126. Ans.— C. **Diarrhoea more than 2 weeks duration with weight loss or failure to gain weight.**

127. Ans.— C. **Giardia**

128. Ans.— D. **Physiological jaundice**

129. Ans.— A. **Hepatitis-B**

130. Ans.— A. **Metabolic acidosis**
It results in metabolic alkalosis.

131. Ans.— A. **Phenobarbitone**

132. Ans.— D. **Colon**

133. Ans.— D. **Achalasia cardia**

134. Ans.— A. **Serum copper level is increased while serum zinc level is decreased**

135. Ans.— C. **Diarrhoea**

136. Ans.— D. **Retropharyngeal abscess**

137. Ans.— B. **1 and 3**

138. Ans.— C. **Vomiting**

139. Ans.— A. **Jaundice is always present**
The jaundice either merges imperceptibly with cirrhosis or there is a symptom free gap of a few months to a year followed by a florid type of cirrhosis. Onset is commonly anicteric.

140. Ans.— C. **Vomiting**

141. Ans.— C. **Feeding is followed by bilious vomiting**

142. Ans.— C.

A	B	C	D
4	1	3	2

143. Ans.— A. **Lactase**

Causes of Lactase Deficiency

Congenital (very rare)	Acquired
	1. Viral gasteroenteritis
	2. Bacterial gasteroenteritis
	3. Protein energy malnutrition
	4. Prolonged use of drugs – Neomycin
	5. Celiac disease
	6. Cow's milk protein intolerance
	7 Cystic fibrosis

144. Ans.— B. **Maternal swallowing of blood**

7

IMPORTANT TEXT OF CVS

TIME OF ONSET OF CONGESTIVE HEART FAILURE IN CONGENITAL LESIONS

Age	*Lesion*
Birth to 72 hours	Pulmonary, mitral and aortic atresia
4 days to 1 week	Hypoplastic left and right heart syndromes, transposition and malposition of great arteries.
1 to 4 weeks	Transposition and malposition complexes, endocardial fibroelastosis, coarctation of aorta.
1 to 2 months	Transposition and malposition complexes, endocardial cushion defects, ventricular septal defect, patent ductus arteriosus, total anomalous pulmonary venous connection, anomalous left coronary artery from pulmonary artery.
2 to 6 months	Transposition and malposition complexes, ventricular septal defect, patent ductus arteriosus, total anomalous pulmonary venous connection, aortic stenosis, coarctation of aorta.

SYMPTOMS OF CONGESTIVE CARDIAC FAILURE

1. Poor weight gain
2. Difficulty in feeding
3. Breathes too fast
4. Breathes better when held against the shoulder.
5. Persistent cough and wheezing.
6. Irritability, excessive perspiration and restlessness.
7. Puffiness of face
8. Pedal edema

SIGNS OF CONGESTIVE FAILURE IN INFANTS

Left sided failure	*Right sided failure*	*Failure of either side*
Tachypnea	1. Hepatomegaly	1. Cardiac enlargement
Tachycardia	2. Facial edema	2. Gallop rhythm (S3)
Cough	3. Jugular venous engorgement	3. Peripheral cyanosis
Wheezing	4. Edema on feet	4. Small volume pulse
Rales in chest	5. Absence of weight gain	

NORMAL ECG VALUES IN CHILDREN

P wave	
Height<2.5mm	At any age
Duration<0.12 sec.	
PR interval	
0.06-0.12 sec	Neonate
0.08-0.14 sec	1 month-3 years
0.10-0.18 sec	3-12 years
0.12-0.21 sec	Adult
Frontal QRS axis	
60" to 180"	1 day
20" to 120"	1 month
0" to 100"	5-16 years

SIMPLE GUIDE TO MURMUR TYPE

Timing	*Likely source*
Midsystolic	Aortic or pulmonary valves, or aorta
Pansystolic	VSD or atrioventricular valve regurgitation
Diastolic	Mitral valve stenosis
	Ductus arteriosus (also systolic)

DESCRIPTION OF TYPICAL STILL'S INNOCENT MURMUR

Midsystolic
Between lower left sternal edge and apex
No redation
1/6 to 3/6, no louder
Vibratory or twanging
Louder lying down
Quieter during valsalva manoeuvre

REASONS TO DOUBT INNOCENT NATURE OF A CHILDHOOD MURMUR

Accompanied by thrill
Pansystolic
Diastolic (except venous hum)
Radiates widely
Harch character
Quieter lying down or louder with valsalva manoeuvre
Any symptoms or abnormal cardiovascular findings

CRITERIA FOR DIAGNOSIS OF RHEUMATIC FEVER

Major Criteria

1. Carditis
2. Arthritis
3. Subcutaneous nodules
4. Chorea
5. Erythema marginatum

Essential Criteria

Evidence for recent streptococcal infection as indicated by
(a) Increased antistreptolysin 'O' titer or other antistreptococcal antibody titers
(b) Positive throat culture
(c) Recent scarlet fever

Minor Criteria

A. *Clinical*
(i) Fever
(ii) Arthralgia
(iii) Previous rheumatic fever or rheumatic heart disease

B. *Laboratory*
(i) Acute phase reactants; leucocytosis, elevated sendimentation rate and C-reactive protein.
(ii) Prolonged PR interval in the electrocardiogram.

ALTERATION OF HEART SOUNDS

Loud S2	AR, SAH
Feeble S2 (A2) or absent	AA (Aortic Atresia) Calcific AS.
Late A2	AS, PDA, AR, LBB, SAH
Wide and variable	MR, VSD, CP

Splitting S2	PS, MR, VSD
Paradoxical S2	PDA. RBBB, PS
Loud P2	PAH
Febble P2 (or absent)	PS, PA
Delayed P2	PS, ASD, RBBB

NADAS'S CRITERIA OF HEART DISEASE

Major	*Minor*
(i) Systolic murmur Gr. III or more especially with a thrill	(a) Systolic murmur less than grade-III to intensity
(ii) Diastolic murmur	(b) Abnormal second sound
(iii) Cyanosis	(c) Abnormal electrocardiogram
(iv) Congestive cardiac failure	(d) Abnormal X-ray
	(e) Abnormal blood pressure

MCQ's OF CVS

What is important in CVS

Congenital lesions (Cyanotic & Acyanotic), CHF, Rheumatic fever, Hypertension, Pericarditis, Normal changes with age

1. **The most common type of total anomalous pulmonary venous connection is : AI 2005, 2008**
   A. Supracardiac B. Infracardiac
   C. Mixed D. Cardiac

2. **The following statements are true of Patent Ductus Arteriosus (PDA) except : Kerala 2000**
   A. Spontaneous closure occurs in some term infants.
   B. Pulmonary Hypertension develops.
   C. Bacterial Endocarditis is more frequent with small PDA.
   D. Recurrent chest infection and congestive failure may develop.
   E. Anatomic existence of PDA is always an indication for surgery.

3. **Eisenmenger complex common in adult is : PGI 2000, 2004**
   A. VSD B. ASD
   C. PDA D. Cushion defect

4. **A 29-days old child present with features of congestive cardiac failure and left ventricular hypertrophy. There was an associated short systolic murmur. Which of the following is the most likely cause : AIIMS 2000**
   A. Tetralogy of Fallot
   B. Ventricular septal defect
   C. Transposition of great arteries
   D. Rheumatic fever

5. **A five-years-old child presents with left ventricular hypertrophy and central cyanosis. Which of the following is the underlying cardiac lesion : AIIMS 2000**
   A. Partial anomalous pulmonary venous drainage
   B. Tricuspid atresia
   C. Eisenmenger syndrome
   D. Tetralogy of fallot

6. **A child with Ventricular septal defect developed Eisenmenger syndrome. What is the correct sequence of events which leads to this change : AIIMS 2000**
   A. Left to right shunt, Right ventricular hypertrophy, Pulmonary hypertension, Right to left shunt.
   B. Left to right shunt, Pulmonary hypertension, right ventricular hypertrophy, Right to left shunt.
   C. Left to right shunt, Right ventricular hypertrophy, Right to left shunt, Pulmonary hypertension.
   D. Pulmonary hypertension, Right to left shunt, Right ventricular hypertrophy, Left to right shunt.

7. **Neonate has recurrent abdominal pain and diaphoresis on feeding and murmur, which may lead to MI. Diagnosis is : AI 2001, 2003**
   A. ASD B. VSD
   C. TOF D. Coronary anomalous

8. **Pott's shunt is : AI 2001**
   A. Right subclavian artery to right pulmonary
   B. Descending aorta to left pulmonary
   C. Left subclavian to left pulmonary
   D. Ascending aorta to right pulmonary

9. **A neonate presents with resp. distress. On investigations, his heart was shifted towards right side : AI 2001**
   A. TOF
   B. Diaphragmatic hernia
   C. Meconium ileus
   D. Congenital bronchiectasis

10. **ECG shows biventricular hypertrophy. Examination shows systolic murmur in 4th left intercostal space. Diagnosis is : AI 2001**
    A. TOF B. TGA
    C. VS D. ASD

Ans.	1. A	2. E	3. C	4. B	5. B	6. A	7. D	8. B	9. B	10. C

11. **A blue infant was found to have oligemic lung fields with normal sized heart. The diagnosis is : AIIMS 2001**
A. Transposition of great vessels
B. Tricuspid atresia
C. TOF
D. Pulmonary stenosis

12. **A young boy had developed congestive failure and was found to have membranous VSD. He spontaneously showed improvement in his condition. This is most likely to be due to : AIIMS 2001**
A. Perimembranous closure of VSD
B. Development of AR
C. Pulmonary vascular changes
D. Infective endocarditis

13. **The fetal anomaly which can be found if a pregnant lady is on Lithium is : AIIMS 2001**
A. Renal anomalies B. Ebstein's anomaly
C. Tricuspid atresia D. VSD

14. **Sure sign of CCF in a infant is : DNB 2001**
A. Basal crepts B. JVP
C. Pedal oedema D. Liver enlargement

15. **True about pain of pericarditis : JIPMER 2002**
A. Pain increases on leaning forward
B. Pain decreases on supine position
C. Pain increases during inspiration
D. Pain increases on eating

16. **Severity of aortic stenosis is assessed by : AIIMS 2002**
A. Late peak of holosystolic murmur
B. Late carotid upstroke
C. Diastolic rumble
D. Opening snap

17. **Consider the following clinico-pathological changes in 'Rheumatic Carditis' : UPSC 2002**
1. Mitral regurgitation
2. Aortic regurgitation
3. Rise in ASLO Titre
4. Left atrial hypertrophy
The correct chronological sequence of these changes would be : UPSC 2002
A. 3,1,4,2 B. 1,2,3,4
C. 4,2,1,3 D. 3,4,1,2

18. **An 11-years old girl presents with severe hypertension. Ultrasonography shows a small sized left kidney. The DTPA radionuclide scan shows reduced function in this kidney that further declines following oral administration of enalapril. What is the most appropriate investigation that is required : UPSC 2002**
A. Renal biopsy
B. Intravenous pyelogram
C. Arterial angiography
D. Micturating cystourethrogram

19. **Which one of the following does not produce cyanosis in the first year of life : AIIMS 2003**
A. Atrial septal defect
B. Hypoplastic left heart syndrome
C. Truncus arteriosus
D. Double outlet right ventricle

20. **Management of anoxic (cyanotic) spells in a child with Fallot's tetralogy includes the following, except : UPSC 1984**
A. Knee-chest position
B. Oxygen inhalation
C. Morphia, 0.1, to 0.2 mg/kg (IM)
D. Correction of acidosis
E. Phenobarbitone, 5 mg/kg (IM)

21. **The following statement about dextrocardia with situs inversus are true, except : UPSC 1981**
A. Commonest type of dextrocardia.
B. Cardiac hemodynamics are significantly affected.
C. Incidence of cardiac defects is low.
D. Barium meal shows gastric gas bubble on right.
E. In lead 1, E.C.G. shows inverted P and T waves.

22. **Lutembacher syndrome refers to : AIIMS 1981**
A. Ostium primum defect with mitral stenosis
B. Ostium secundum defect with mitral stenosis
C. Ostium secundum defect with mitral incompetence
D. None of the above

23. **Most common cause of hypertension in a child is : PGI 1993, 98; Delhi 1992, 96**
A. Coarctation B. Aortitis
C. Chronic GN D. Chronic PN

24. **Bacterial endocarditis is very rare in : BHU 1986; UP 1999**
A. Mitral stenosis
B. Atrial septal defect
C. Ventricular septal defect
D. P.D.A

25. **Compared to the oral digitalizing dose, parenteral dose of digoxin should be : UPSC 1985**
A. 1/4 B. 1/2
C. 1/3 D. 2/3

26. **Cardiac defect in fetus is better diagnosed by : AI 1996**
A. CT scan B. X-ray chest
C. Doppler ultrasound D. Auscultation

27. **CHF in VSD usually occurs within : DNB 1992**
A. Birth to 72 hours B. 1-2 weeks
C. 3-4 weeks D. After 1 month

Ans. 11. C 12. C 13. B 14. D 15. A 16. A 17. A 18. C 19. A 20. E
21. B 22. B 23. C 24. B 25. D 26. C 27. D

28. In a patient with history of cyanotic congenital heart disease there is pericardial friction rub like murmur in left parasternal area & gallop rhythm; most probable diagnosis is : Rajasthan 1996

A. TAPVR B. Eisenmengers complex
C. TGA D. Coarctation of aorta

29. Common manifestation of Mitral Stenosis in childhood include the following except : AMU 1986

A. Palpitations B. Haemoptysis
C. Dyspnoea D. Tiredness

30. Rheumatic carditis is suspected in the presence of the following except : AMU 1988

A. Carry Coombs murmur
B. Hollow systolic murmur at the apex
C. Tachycardia disproportionate to the degree of fever
D. Loud first heart sound

31. The following findings are normal in a 5 years old child except : AIIMS 1982

A. Split second heart sound
B. A pulse rate of 100 per minute
C. A third heart sound
D. A blood pressure of 130/90

32. Cardiac failure in infancy is characterized by following except : Rohtak 1986, 92

A. Absent femoral pulse
B. Feeding difficulty
C. Enlarged palpable liver
D. A respiratory rate of more than 40 per minute

33. Which of the following congenital heart disease does not produce central cyanosis : AI 1990

A. Pulmonary stenosis
B. Transposition of great arteries
C. Fallot's tetralogy
D. Anomalous pulmonary venous drainage

34. The following may be present in a child with a normal heart except : AI 1990

A. Continuous mumur B. A thrill
C. Third heart sound D. Ventricular extrasystole

35. In rheumatic chorea the following is not true : DNB 1989

A. May be associated with carditis
B. More common in girls
C. ASO titre is usually elevated
D. The movements disappear during sleep

36. Features of pulmonary hypertension in children include all of the following except : UPSC 1996

A. Right ventricular hypertrophy
B. Complicated large ventricular septal defect
C. Diminished main pulmonary artery shadow on X-ray
D. Systolic ejection murmur in pulmonary area

37. A child with congenital heart failure, Lt. para sternal thrill & a pansystolic murmur, the probable diagnosis is : BHU 1996

A. Transposition of the great vessel
B. Ebstein's anomaly
C. Total anomalous pulmonary venous drainage
D. Eisenmenger syndrome complex

38. Most common causative organism in subacute bacterial endocarditis in children is : AP 1991

A. Streptococcus viridans
B. Haemophilus influenzae
C. Beta haemolytic streptococci
D. Neisseria catarrhalis

39. Most common cause of death from aortic stenosis in children is : AMU 1987

A. Pulmonary oedema
B. Myocardial infarction
C. Atrial flutter
D. I.H.D. with ventricular fibrillation

40. Palliative surgery for small infant with severe tetralogy, deep cyanosis and paroxysmal dyspnoea would be : Orissa 1991

A. Atrial septostomy
B. Pulmonary artery banding
C. Ductal ligation
D. Aorta to pulmonary artery anastomosis

41. Which of the following is true of hypercyanotic spell in Tetralogy of Fallot : AP 1997

A. Seen only after 4 years
B. Increased intensity of the murmur
C. Metabolic alkalosis
D. Machinary murmur

42. The best position for examination of cardiac murmurs in a child is : PGI 1985

A. Sitting B. Standing
C. Right lateral D. Recumben

43. The most important part of the treatment of rheumatic fever is : AIIMS 1985

A. Complete bed rest
B. Steroids
C. Aspirin
D. Continued prophylaxis with penicillin
E. Diuretics

44. Most common single valvular lesion result from rheumatic endocarditis is : AIIMS 1984

A. Semilunar stenosis B. Pulmonic stenosis
C. Mitral stenosis D. Aortic stenosis

45. Which of the following is present in both left sided and right sided failure : PGI 1981

A. Dependent oedema B. Pulsus alternans
C. Cardiac enlargement D. Oliguria

Ans.									
28. C	29. B	30. D	31. D	32. A	33. A	34. B	35. C	36. C	37. B
38. A	39. D	40. D	41. A	42. D	43. A	44. C	45. C		

46. **Which of the following is not characteristic of left side failure : PGI 1981**
A. Cardiac asthma
B. Pulsus alternans
C. Gallop rhythm
D. Increasing systemic venous pressure

47. **Which of the following is not a characteristic of right sided failure : PGI 1983**
A. Pulmonary oedema B. Ascites
C. Oliguria D. Dependent oedema

48. **Which of the following is not commonly observed in acute benign viral pericarditis : PGI 1982**
A. Friction rub B. No murmur
C. Cardiac tamponade D. Pleural effusion

49. **Pericardial involvement in children is most likely to occur with : PGI 1982**
A. Rheumatoid arthritis B. Rheumatic carditis
C. Acute viral infection D. Uremia

50. **Sinus bradycardia in a child is occasionally associated with all, except : PGI 1982**
A. Hypothyroidism B. Decreased systemic BP
C. Typhoid fever D. Rheumatic fever

51. **What is the universal feature of subacute bacterial endocarditis in children ? AIIMS 1986**
A. Convulsions B. Anaemia
C. Hepatomegaly D. Splenomegaly

52. **Pulmonary blood flow is increased in : Kerala 1997**
A. TS B. TOF
C. PS D. Ebstein anomaly

53. **Match List-I and List-II and select the correct answer using the codes given below the Lists : UPSC 1997**

List-I *(Radiological appearance)*	List-II *(Clinical condition)*
A. Snowman's heart	1. Down's syndrome
B. Oligemic lung fields	2. Total anomalous pulmonary venous drainage
C. Double bubble appearance	3. Transposition of great vessels
D. Egg-shaped heart	4. Pulmonary stenosis

Codes :

	A	B	C	D
A.	2	4	3	1
B.	2	4	1	3
C.	4	2	1	3
D.	4	2	3	1

54. **On radiologic examination, a patient with a large patent ductus arteriosus would not exhibit : PGI 1982**
A. Left atrial enlargement
B. Prominent pulmonary artery
C. Small aortic arch
D. Left ventricular enlargement

55. **Large ventricular septal defects are characterized by all, except : AIIMS 1983**
A. Accentuated first heart sound
B. Normal development
C. Palpable thrill in 1/2 cases
D. Dyspnoea and exercise intolerance

56. **Probably the most common cause of cor pulmonale in children is : PGI 1980**
A. Scoliosis B. Bronchopneumonia
C. Cystic fibrosis D. Pickwickian syndrome

57. **Which is not found in anaemic heart disease ? AIIMS 1980**
A. Murmur B. Distended neck veins
C. Palpitations D. Narrow pulse pressure

58. **Pure left sided failure may be seen with : PGI 1981**
A. ASD
B. Aortic atresia
C. Patent ductus arteriosus
D. Pulmonary valvular obstruction

59. **Natural course of events in untreated ventricular septal defect may include any of following, except : PGI 1981, Delhi 1985**
A. Spontaneous closure of defect
B. Development of pulmonary insufficiency
C. Subacute bacterial endocarditis
D. A normal life without symptoms

60. **The clinical picture of early onset of severe dyspnoea, minimal cardiomegaly, cyanosis and a diffuse reticular pattern of lung fields. Chest X-ray is most suggestive of : AMC 1986**
A. Total anomalous pulmonary drainage without venous obstruction.
B. Total anomalous pulmonary drainage with venous obstruction.
C. Partial anomalous pulmonary drainage.
D. Transposition of great vessels.

61. **An apical middiastolic murmur in a one year old child with acute rheumatic fever is usually : AMC 1985, 92**
A. Of no significance
B. Indicates mitral stenosis
C. Indicates carditis
D. Indicates coexisting congenital heart disease

Ans. 46. D 47. A 48. C 49. B 50. B 51. D 52. B 53. A 54. C 55. B
56. C 57. D 58. C 59. B 60. B 61. C

62. In Holt Oram syndrome, the cardiac defect is : AIIMS 1988
A. MR B. AR
C. ASD D. PDA

63. Most common type of cyanotic congenital heart disease to survive beyond infancy without surgery is : AMC 1986, 88
A. Ventricular septal defect
B. Transposition of great vessels
C. Tetralogy of Fallot
D. Tricuspid atresia

64. In Marfan's syndrome, following cardiac defects may be seen except : AIIMS 1987
A. Aortic dilatation
B. Pulm. artery dilatation
C. Mitral valve prolapse
D. None of the above

65. Large 'a' wave in IVP, LPH present and with a mid systolic murmur. Probable diagnosis is : JIPMER 1997
A. Tricuspid atresia B. PS
C. VSD D. ASD

66. A relative hypertension of arms is the pathognomonic feature of : AIIMS 1985
A. Tetralogy of Fallot
B. Coarctation of aorta
C. Pulmonary atresia
D. Large atrial septal defect

67. The great danger for a patient with patent ductus arteriosus is : PGI 1988
A. Convulsions B. Arrhythmia
C. Syncope D. Bacterial endocarditis

68. Which of the following lesions is of least clinical significance : AIIMS 1981
A. Single atrium
B. Ostium primum defect
C. Incompetent patent foramen ovale
D. Secundum atrial septal defect

69. Pulmonary plethora is seen in all except : UPSC 1982
A. VSD B. ASD
C. Fallot's tetralogy D. PDA

70. In ASD, ejection systolic murmur is :
A. Shunt murmur
B. Tricuspid flow murmur
C. Mitral flow murmur
D. Pulmonary flow murmur

71. Aortic stenosis is characterized by the following except : PGI 1996
A. Cardiac size usually normal
B. Pulse pressure indicates severity
C. Dyspnoea on exertion
D. Hypertension

72. The diagnosis of rheumatic fever is best confirmed by : AMU 1988; PGI 1988
A. Throat swab culture B. Raised ESR
C. ASLO titre D. ECG changes

73. In children with persistent hypertension where routine laboratory tests are normal what more has to be done : UPSC 1982
A. Renin activity tests
B. Rapid I.V.P's
C. Renal arteriography
D. Retrograde pyelography

74. Mustard as well as Senning's Operation are done for : AIIMS 1985
A. ASD B. VSD
C. TGA D. PDA

75. Malformation often associated with pulmonary hyperaemia include the following except : AIIMS 1982
A. Atrial septal defect
B. Ventricular septal defect
C. Patent ductus arteriosus
D. Ebsteins anomaly

76. Murmur of hypertrophic cardiomyopathy is increased by all except : AIIMS 1992
A. Valsalva manoeuvre B. Exercise
C. Squatting D. Digoxin

77. Loud and split pulmonary second sound (P2) is associated with all the following except : AIIMS 1985
A. ASD B. Pulmonary stenosis
C. VSD D. Mitral stenosis

78. The most common cause of painful pericarditis is : Bihar 1991
A. Viral B. Tuberculous
C. Uraemic D. All of these

79. The most common cause of painless percarditis is : AMU 1991
A. Neoplastic B. Uraemic only
C. Tuberculous D. Both a+c

80. Myocarditis is a recognized complication of each of the following infectious conditions, except for one : TN 1988
A. Streptococcus haemolyticus
B. Coxsackie virus
C. Rhabdovirus
D. Corynebacterium diphtheriae

81. Which is the diagnostic investigation for a suspected case of myxoma of heart ? TN 1989
A. X-ray chest (AP view) B. Conventional ECG
C. Echocardiography D. All of the above

Ans.										
	62. C	63. C	64. D	65. A	66. B	67. D	68. C	69. C	70. D	71. D
	72. C	73. C	74. C	75. D	76. C	77. B	78. A	79. B	80. C	81. C

82. **"Opening snap" a characteristic finding of mitral stenosis (MS) can be inaudible under the following circumstances, except for one : AP 1989**
A. RHD MS+MR
B. MS with prosthetic valve
C. MS postcommissurotomy
D. MS with calcified valve

83. **In rheumatic heart disease, (MS) which of the following is characteristically true about opening snap: Kerala 1988**
A. Just follows first heart sound
B. Follows second heart sound
C. Proceeds the mid-diastolic murmur
D. Both B+C above

84. **"Carey Coombs murmur" of rheumatic carditis is : Delhi 1983**
A. An apical pansystolic murmur
B. An apical mid diastolic murmur
C. An apical early diastolic murmur
D. A basal ejection systolic murmur

85. **"Pericardial Knock" is characteristically heard in which of the following heart lesion : Kerala 1988**
A. Pericardial effusion B. Rheumatic carditis
C. Cardiac myxoma only D. Toxic myocarditis

86. **The appropriate T/t for symptomatic sick sinus syndrome is : NIMHANS 1989**
A. Atropine only
B. Only bed rest
C. Pacemaker implantation
D. Propranolol only

87. **Which of the following congenital heart diseases may remain asymptomatic till adult life and is suspected/ detected after a routine X-ray chest ? JIPMER 1988**
A. ASD only
B. Tetralogy of Fallot's
C. Endocardial cushin defects
D. Transposition of great vessels

88. **In which of the following cardiac conditions, the pulmonary component of the second heart sound is soft and inaudible on cardiac auscultation : JIPMER 1988**
A. ASD secondum B. VSD only
C. COA D. Fallot's tetralogy

89. **"Constrictive pericarditis" is not a feature of : JIPMER 1989, 96**
A. Rheumatic pericarditis
B. Pyogenic pericarditis
C. Neoplastic pericarditis
D. Tuberculous pericarditis

90. **Fourth heart sound is audible in all, except : AP 1989**
A. Pulmonary hypertension
B. Pulmonary stenosis
C. Healthy young adult
D. Systemic hypertension

91. **Among the following major Jones criteria for the diagnosis of rheumatic fever, which of the following is most commonly encountered in India : Rajasthan 1990**
A. Pancarditis only B. Migratory polyarthritis
C. Subcutaneous nodules D. Chorea only

92. **Infantile hypercalcemia syndrome is most frequently associated with : AIIMS 1984**
A. ASD
B. VSD
C. Patient ductus arteriosus
D. Supravalvular aortic stenosis

93. **In tetralogy of Fallot, pulmonary stenosis is : AI 1997**
A. Infundibular B. Valvular
C. Both A+B D. Supravalvular

94. **Which of the following is not true about tricuspid atresia : Delhi 1997**
A. Cyanosis not present at birth
B. Single second heart sound
C. Left axis deviation
D. Pansystolic murmur along left sternal border

95. **At what age the muscular arteries reach the alveolar level : DNB 1989**
A. 3 months B. 5 years
C. 10 years D. 20 years

96. **Tricuspid dysmorphogenes is associated with : AIIMS 1983, 84, 86**
A. Tetralogy of Fallot B. Ebstein's anomaly
C. Marfan's syndrome D. Turner's syndrome

97. **In a pregnant female with cyanotic heart disease, foetal maturity is best assessed by : PGI 1985; AIIMS 1984**
A. Arterial O2 saturation
B. Cardiac output
C. Foetal growth
D. Foetal movements

98. **The commonest congenital heart disease is : AIIMS 1984**
A. Mitral stenosis
B. Tetralogy of Fallot
C. Pulmonary stenosis
D. Ventricular septal defect

Ans.	82. A	83. D	84. B	85. A	86. C	87. A	88. D	89. A	90. C	91. B
	92. D	93. A	94. A	95. B	96. B	97. A	98. D			

99. Systolic hypertension in children is a recognized feature of each of the following conditions except : AIIMS 1986, 89

A. Adrenogenital syndrome
B. Klinefelter's syndrome
C. Takayasu disease
D. Acute intermittent porphyria

100. 1 year old child is cyanosed with Left ventricular hypertrophy. Most common cause is : AIIMS 1987, 88

A. Tetralogy of Fallot B. Tricuspid atresia
C. Eisenmenger D. Hypertension

101. In opening snap of mitral stenosis, all are true except : AIIMS 1987

A. Present in early calcified valves
B. Best heard at diaphragm
C. Severity indicated by relation to S2
D. Lost in M.R.

102. Reverse splitting of S1 is seen in except : AIIMS 1987, 88, 91

A. ASD B. Pulmonary stenosis
C. Aortic stenosis D. Systemic hypertension

103. Least commonest complication of cardiac prosthesis is : AIIMS 1988

A. Thromboembolism
B. Bacterial endocarditis
C. Paravalvular leak
D. RBC fragmentation syndrome

104. Digitalis toxicity can be diagnosed if ECG shows : AIIMS 1983, 88

A. Prolonged PR interval
B. T-wave inversion
C. Shortening of QT interval
D. Ventricular bigeminy

105. Which of the following murmur is always abnormal: DNB 1991

A. Ejection systolic
B. Pansystolic
C. Diastolic murmur in hypertension
D. Diastolic murmur in anemia

106. Following are associated with coarctation of aorta in children except : AI 1997

A. PDA
B. Berry aneurysm rupture
C. Bicuspid aortic valve
D. Renal artery stenosis

107. Acute rheumatic fever is most commonly caused by: PGI 1989, 93

A. Beta hemolytic streptococcus, type-A
B. Beta hemolytic streptococcus, type-B
C. Staphylococcus albus
D. Pneumococcus

108. Long standing Mitral stenosis is related to : AI 1997

A. HT B. LVH
C. RVH D. Apical thrombosis

109. Commonest cardiac rhythm disturbance encountered in children is : Karnataka 1998

A. Supra ventricular tachycardia
B. Ventricular tachycardia
C. Sinus tachycardia
D. Junctional rhythm

110. 5 days old child with cyanosis around the mouth and finding similar to ASD with CCF-probable diagnosis is : Kerala 1998

A. TAGV
B. TAPV connection without obstruction
C. TAPV connection with obstruction
D. TOF

111. Congestive heart failure in chidren is best diagnosed by : PGI 1987, 88; AMC 1987, 88

A. Tachycardia and tender hepatomegaly
B. ↑ JVP
C. ↑ JVP + pedal oedema
D. Hypotension

112. A two days old baby with central cyanosis and heart failure has : Delhi 1987; AIIMS 1983, 88

A. Preductal coarctation
B. Patent ductus arteriosus
C. Transposition of great vessels
D. Tetralogy of fallot

113. Which of the following congenital cyanotic disease presents with gallop rhythm, left parasternal murmur, pericardial friction rub : Orissa 1998

A. Ebstein anomaly
B. TA PVC
C. TGA
D. Eisenmenger complex

114. The most common cause of dilated pulmonary artery in children is : UPSC 1995

A. Stenosis of pulmonary valve
B. Patent ductus arteriosus
C. Ventricular septal defect
D. Atrial septal defect

115. Congenital heart disease which causes death in the first week of life : AIIMS 1987; AI 1988

A. VSD
B. TOF
C. Ebstein's anomaly
D. Hypoplastic left ventricle

Ans.									
99. B	100. C	101. B	102. C	103. D	104. D	105. B	106. D	107. A	108. C
109. A	110. C	111. A	112. C	113. A	114. B	115. D			

116. Pick out the statement which is not true of children with ventricular septal defect : PGI 1982

A. A good proportion of small defects close spontaneously.
B. Many children remain asymptomatic.
C. Large defects never cause death in infancy.
D. Repeated respiratory infection occur with large defect.
E. Some children develop pulmonary hypertension.

117. Commonest cause of enlarged cardiac shadow in X-ray of a child is : PGI 1983

A. PDA B. Coarctation of Aorta
C. Pericarditis D. Rheumatic carditis

118. Paradoxically split second heart sound signifies severe : AIIMS 1983, 88

A. Pulmonary stenosis B. Mitral stenosis
C. Aortic stenosis D. Tricuspid stenosis

119. Among the complications in Tetralogy of Fallot is : Karnataka 1989

A. Cerebral thrombosis usually occurs in cerebral veins in the presence of extreme polycythemia.
B. Brain abscess frequently occurs in infants under one year.
C. Congestive cardiac failure frequently occurs after the age of 1 month.
D. Bacterial endocarditis never occurs in patients who have undergone palliative shunt procedure during infancy.

120. Ebstein anomaly is characterised by all of the following except : Karnataka 1994

A. Multiple heart sounds
B. Right Ventricular hypertrophy
C. Himalayan P-wave on ECG
D. Association of WPW syndrome

121. Earliest Cause of CHF in first week of life is : Delhi 1994

A. Pulmonary Atresia
B. Endocardial cushion defect
C. Transposition of great vessels
D. Hypoplastic left heart syndrome

122. Consider the following congenital heart disease: UPSC 2000

1. Patent ductus arteriosus
2. Tetralogy of fallot
3. Large ventricular septal defect
4. D-transposition of great arteries

Which of the above congenital heart disease produce congestive cardiac failure in the newborn: UPSC 2000

A. 1 and 2 B. 1 and 3
C. 1, 2 and 3 D. 3 and 4

123. The congenital heart disease commonly associated with trisomy 21 is : UPSC 1994

A. Patent ductus arteriosus
B. Fallot's tetralogy
C. Coarctation of aorta
D. Endocardial cushion defects

124. A child presents with ——— antimongoloid slant, pulmonary stenosis, short stature and undescended testis. Most likely diagnosis is : AIIMS 1994

A. Klinefelter's syndrome
B. Noonan's syndrome
C. Hypoparathyroidism
D. XYY

125. Which of the following is not a stimulus for pulmonary vasoconstriction : AIIMS 1994

A. Hypoxaemia B. PGE
C. PGIg D. Hypercapnia

126. Sustained, severe hypertension in children is commonly suggestive of : AI 1995

A. Coarctation
B. Phaeochromocytoma
C. Renal parenchymal disease
D. Aorta aortitis

127. Characteristics of VSD include all except : AI 1995

A. CHF occurs commonly in infancy
B. May close by itself
C. Vascular markings are increased in lung
D. Commonest congenital heart disease

128. Functional closure of the ductus arteriosus a normal term baby usually occurs at : UPSC 1995

A. Birth B. 15 hours
C. 3 days D. 7 days

129. Rheumatic nodules : PGI 1989

A. Are painful
B. Are attached to skin
C. Are common in adults than in children
D. Rarely occurs unless active carditis is present

130. Foetal heart starts to pump blood at : Rajasthan 1989, 93

A. 7 days B. 10 weeks
C. 3 months D. 4 months

131. Infantile myocarditis & pericarditis is due to : TN 1999

A. Coxsackie-A B. Coxsackie-B
C. Mumps D. Pox

132. Treatment for TGV : TN 1999

A. Balloon septostomy B. Oxygen
C. Ventilation D. Digoxin

Ans.										
	116. C	117. D	118. C	119. D	120. D	121. A	122. D	123. D	124. B	125. C
	126. C	127. A	128. A	129. D	130. B	131. B	132. A			

133. MC cause of heart transplantation in children is : Kerala 1999
A. Hypoplastic left heart syndrome
B. Cardiomyopathy with failure
C. Eisenmenger syndrome
D. Ebsteins anomaly

134. Loud S1 in Mitral stenosis is seen in : PGI 1999
A. Prolonged flow through mitral valve
B. 1st degree heart block
C. Calcification of the valve
D. Immobilization of the valve

135. In the newborn, artery used for palpation of pulse is: PGI 1999
A. Radial B. Carotid
C. Brachial D. Femoral

136. A 2 years old known case of RHD presents with 3 weeks history of fever, hematuria and palpitation, diagnosis is : PGI 1999
A. Streptococcal endocarditis
B. Collagen vascular disease
C. Reactivation
D. Staphylococcal endocarditis

137. A child presents with BP 190/130 with seizures, i.v. diazepam was given, next course of action is : AI 2000
A. IV. nitroprusside B. S/L nifedepine
C. S/L enalapril D. Furosemide

138. Figure of a 8 configuration is seen in : AI 2000
A. Total anomalous pulm. Venous connection
B. Partial anomalous pulm. Venous connection
C. Abnormal origin
D. VSD

139. Left heart border is abnormal in all except : AI 2000
A. Coronary art. Aneurysm
B. Azygous vein enlargement
C. Enlarged left atrial appendage
D. Left ventrical enlargement

140. Consider the following statements regarding pericardial effusion in a 10-years old boys : UPSC 2000
A. Heart sounds are distant.
B. Pericardial friction rub heard even in large effusions.
C. Bronchial breathing heard over left base.
D. Lung fields are plenthoric on chest X-ray.
Which of the above statements are correct : UPSC 2000
A. 1 and 4 B. 1 and 2
C. 1, 2 and 3 D. 2, 3 and 4

141. Spot the wrong statement concerning ASD : PGI 1981, 87, 90
A. It remains asymptomatic in most of the infants and young children.
B. Older children may have recurrent chest infection, breathlessness and bulging of the chest due to enlargement of right ventricle.
C. Growth failure may be the only manifestation in some children.
D. CCF seldon occurs.

142. Classical mumur of PDA has the following characteristics, except : AIIMS 1982
A. Begins immediately after the first heart sound and reaches its peak at the end of systole.
B. Continues in most of the diastolic phase, gradually disappearing in the later part.
C. Always accompanied by a thrill.
D. Harsh.
E. May be localized to second left intecostal space.

143. Which of the following is not a component of Fallot's tetralogy : AIIMS 1983
A. Pulmonary stenosis
B. Ventricular septal defect
C. Dextroposition of aorta
D. Left ventricular hypertrophy

144. Which of the following is not a feature of X-ray picture in Fallot's tetralogy : UPSC 1983
A. Oligemic lungs fields
B. A small boot-shaped heart
C. A small pulmonary conus
D. Right aortic arch in 50% cases

145. The following is not true of subcutaneous nodules in rheumatic fever : UPSC 1984
A. They are sometimes associated with carditis.
B. Appear on bony prominences like elbow and occiput.
C. They are nontender.
D. Subcutaneous nodules are a late manifestation and appear around 6 weeks of onset of rheumatic fever.

146. The following physical finding indicate moderate to severe VSD except : UPSC 1985
A. Onset of CCF at the age of 6 weeks of life
B. Cardiomegaly
C. Delayed diastolic murmur in mitral area
D. Pansystolic murmur in tricuspid area

147. The following cardiac lesion complicated with pulmonary hypertension and right to left shunt is associated with differential cyanosis : AIIMS 1984
A. VSD B. PDA
C. ASD D. Ebstein's anomaly

Ans.									
133. B	134. A	135. D	136. D	137. A	138. A	139. B	140. A	141. D	142. C
143. D	144. D	145. A	146. D	147. B					

148. Which of the following is incorrect in Tetralogy of Fallot : AMU 1984
A. Anoxic blue spells occur predominantly after waking up or following exertions, fever or crying on feeding.
B. Severity of cardiac lesion is directly proportional to the intensity of murmur.
C. Cardiac failure does not occur in the absence of complications.
D. All of the above.

149. Left axis deviation and left ventricular hypertrophy are characteristic of : AMU 1986
A. Transposition of great vessels
B. Tricuspid atresia
C. Total anomalous pulmonary venous drainage
D. Tetralogy of Fallot

150. In aortic regurgitation in children : Rohtak 1985
A. Females are more commonly affected than males.
B. Fatigue is an early symptom.
C. Palpitation is the main symptom.
D. A systolic pressure difference between the femoral and brachial artery of 20-40 mm of Hg indicates severe aortic incompetence.

151. Which of the following physical sign is not common in infants with heart failure : AMU 1985
A. Pulse rate greater than 180/min
B. Enlargement of liver more than 2 cms
C. Sweating
D. Loud first heart sound

152. Which of the following closes first after birth : Delhi 1984, 90
A. Ductus arteriosus B. Foramen ovale
C. Ductus venosus D. Posterior fontanella

153. In Ellis-van Creveld syndrome, following congenital defect is commonly seen in : DNB 1989
A. PS B. MR
C. ASD D. VSD

154. In Down's syndrome, following congenital defect is common : Delhi 1991, 97, 98; JIPMER 1993
A. PDA B. PS
C. ASD D. VSD

155. In which type of congenital heart disease, heart failure is not seen : PGI 1984, 91; AI 1993
A. VSD
B. TOF
C. ASD
D. Eisenmenger's syndrome

156. Congenital rubella causes which cardiac anomaly : AI 1993, 95, 97
A. PDA B. VSD
C. ASD D. Coarctation of Aorta

157. Aortic attachment of ductus arteriosus is : AIIMS 1987
A. Just proximal to right subclavian artery
B. Just distal to right subclavian artery
C. Just distal to left subclavian artery
D. Just proximal to left subclavian artery

158. Which of the following by itself need not be diagnostic of acute carditis in a patient with rheumatic heart disease : DNB 1990
A. Pericardial friction rub
B. Cardiac failure
C. Subcutaneous nodules
D. Appearance of new murmur

159. In a rheumatic heart disease patient with prolonged fever the following is diagnostic of rheumatic reactivation rather than subacute bacterial endocarditis: AIIMS 1981, 87, 91
A. Arthralgia
B. Embolic phenomena
C. Appearance of new murmur
D. Pericardial friction rub

160. Consider the following statements :
Specific features suggestive of tricuspid regurgitation consist of : UPSC 2004
1. Systolic pulsations of the liver
2. Diastolic thrill at left lower sternal border
3. Prominent V-waves in jugular venous pulse
4. Deep S-waves in V1 lead and tall R-waves in V6 lead ECG

Which of the statements given above is/are correct ?
A. 1 only
B. 1 and 3
C. 2 and 4
D. 1, 3 and 4

161. Most common type of Atrial septal defect is : UPPGME 2006
A. Endocardial hypertrophy
B. Cushion defect
C. Ostium secondum
D. Ostium primum

Ans.	148. B	149. B	150. C	151. D	152. B	153. D	154. C	155. B	156. A	157. C
	158. B	159. D	160. B	161. C						

EXPLANATIONS OF CVS

1. Ans.— A. Supracardiac
2. Ans.— E. Anatomic existence of PDA is always an indication for surgery.
3. Ans.— C. PDA
4. Ans.— B. Ventricular septal defect
5. Ans.— B. Tricuspid atresia
6. Ans.— A. Left to right shunt, Right ventricular hypertrophy, Pulmonary hypertension, Right to left shunt.
7. Ans.— D. Coronary anomalous

   Central cyanosis & CHF may be seen.
8. Ans.— B. Descending aorta to left pulmonary

   Anastomosis between subclavian artery and pulmonary artery is used in Blalock Taussig operation.
9. Ans.— B. Diaphragmatic hernia

   It is secondary to a posterolateral defect in the diaphragm (foramen of Bochdalek) or in about 5% of cases, to a retrosternal defect (foramen of Morgagni). The symptoms of mild to severe respiratory distress and cyanosis are usually present from birth, although, some patients may remain asymptomatic.
10. Ans.— C. VS

    CHF is rare in children but in adults it may develop in between 30-40 years of age.
11. Ans.— C. TOF
12. Ans.— C. Pulmonary vascular changes
13. Ans.— B. Ebstein's anomaly
14. Ans.— D. Liver enlargement
15. Ans.— A. Pain increases on leaning forward
16. Ans.— A. Late peak of holosystolic murmur
17. Ans.— A. 3,1,4,2
18. Ans.— C. Arterial angiography
19. Ans. A. Atrial septal defect
20. Ans. E. Phenobarbitone, 5 mg/kg (IM)
21. Ans.— B. Cardiac hemodynamics are significantly affected.
22. Ans.— B. Ostium secundum defect with mitral stenosis
23. Ans.— C. Chronic GN

    Renal cause contributes to about 75-80% of cases.
24. Ans.— B. Atrial septal defect
25. Ans.— D. 2/3
26. Ans.— C. Doppler ultrasound
27. Ans.— D. After 1 month
28. Ans.— C. TGA
29. Ans.— B. Haemoptysis
30. Ans.— D. Loud first heart sound
31. Ans.— D. A blood pressure of 130/90
32. Ans.— A. Absent femoral pulse
33. Ans.— A. Pulmonary stenosis

    Patients of mild to moderate pulmonary stenosis (PS) are asymptomatic, with severe PS, dysponea on effort appears.
34. Ans.— B. A thrill
35. Ans.— C. ASO titre is usually elevated
36. Ans.— C. Diminished main pulmonary artery shadow on X-ray
37. Ans.— B. Ebstein's anomaly
38. Ans.— A. Streptococcus viridans
39. Ans.— D. I.H.D. with ventricular fibrillation
40. Ans.— D. Aorta to pulmonary artery anastomosis
41. Ans.— A. Seen only after 4 years
42. Ans.— D. Recumben
43. Ans.— A. Complete bed rest
44. Ans.— C. Mitral stenosis
45. Ans.— C. Cardiac enlargement
46. Ans.— D. Increasing systemic venous pressure
47. Ans.— A. Pulmonary oedema
48. Ans.— C. Cardiac tamponade

49. Ans.— B. Rheumatic carditis

50. Ans.— B. Decreased systemic BP

51. Ans.— D. Splenomegaly

52. Ans.— B. TOF

53. Ans.— A.

A	B	C	D
2	4	3	1

54. Ans.— C. Small aortic arch

55. Ans.— B. Normal development

56. Ans.— C. Cystic fibrosis

57. Ans.— D. Narrow pulse pressure

58. Ans.— C. Patent ductus arteriosus

59. Ans.— B. Development of pulmonary insufficiency

60. Ans.— B. Total anomalous pulmonary drainage with venous obstruction.

61. Ans.— C. Indicates carditis

62. Ans.— C. ASD

63. Ans.— C. Tetralogy of Fallot

Congenital rubella may also cause congenital heart defects (PDA with or without PS), eye defects (Cataract or retinopathy) and hearing impairment. Deafness is commonest abnormality and may be the sole finding.

64. Ans.— D. None of the above

65. Ans.— A. Tricuspid atresia

66. Ans.— B. Coarctation of aorta

67. Ans.— D. Bacterial endocarditis

68. Ans.— C. Incompetent patent foramen ovale

69. Ans.— C. Fallot's tetralogy

70. Ans.— D. Pulmonary flow murmur

There are wide fixed split of S2, Pansytolic murmur, scratchy superficial murmurs are seen.

71. Ans.— D. Hypertension

72. Ans.— C. ASLO titre

73. Ans.— C. Renal arteriography

74. Ans.— C. TGA

75. Ans.— D. Ebsteins anomaly

76. Ans.— C. Squatting

77. Ans.— B. Pulmonary stenosis

78. Ans.— A. Viral

79. Ans.— B. Uraemic only

80. Ans.— C. Rhabdovirus

81. Ans.— C. Echocardiography

82. Ans.— A. RHD MS+MR

83. Ans.— D. Both B+C above

84. Ans.— B. An apical mid diastolic murmur

85. Ans.— A. Pericardial effusion

86. Ans.— C. Pacemaker implantation

87. Ans.— D. ASD only

88. Ans.— D. Fallot's tetralogy

89. Ans.— A. Rheumatic pericarditis

90. Ans.— C. Healthy young adult

91. Ans.— B. Migratory polyarthritis

92. Ans.— D. Supravalvular aortic stenosis

93. Ans.— A. Infundibular

Infundibular type is seen in 50-75%, Valvular rarely and both in 25% to 50%.

94. Ans.— A. Cyanosis not present at birth

95. Ans.— B. 5 years

96. Ans.— B. Ebstein's anomaly

97. Ans.— A. Arterial O2 saturation

98. Ans.— D. Ventricular septal defect

Rheumatic heart disease is the commonest cause in older children. Among obstructive lesions CHF is late except in PS, AS, MS (CHF within few days of life). Left-to-right shunt present with CHF in 6-8 weeks of life.

99. Ans.— B. Klinefelter's syndrome

100. Ans.— C. Eisenmenger

101. Ans.— B. Best heard at diaphragm

102. Ans.— C. Aortic stenosis

103. Ans.— D. RBC fragmentation syndrome

104. Ans.— D. Ventricular bigeminy

105. Ans.— B. Pansystolic

106. Ans.— D. Renal artery stenosis

Horse shoe kidney, double or cleft renal pelvis, perceptive hearing loss, high arched palate etc. may also be seen.

107. Ans.— A. Beta hemolytic streptococcus, type-A

108. Ans.— C. RVH

Long standing MS may cause RVH, TR, engorged neck veins and enlarged tender liver.

109. Ans.— A. Supra ventricular tachycardia

110. Ans.— C. TAPV connection with obstruction

111. Ans.— A. Tachycardia and tender hepatomegaly

112. Ans.— C. Transposition of great vessels

113. Ans.— A. Ebstein anomaly

114. Ans.— B. Patent ductus arteriosus

115. Ans.— D. Hypoplastic left ventricle

Rheumatic heart disease is the commonest cause in older children. Among obstructive lesions CHF is late except in PS, AS, MS (CHF within few days of life). Left-to-right shunt present with CHF in 6-8 weeks of life.

116. Ans.— C. Large defects never cause death in infancy.

117. Ans.— D. Rheumatic carditis

118. Ans.— C. Aortic stenosis

119. Ans.— D. Bacterial endocarditis never occurs in patients who have undergone palliative shunt procedure during infancy.

120. Ans.— D. Association of WPW syndrome

121. Ans.— A. Pulmonary Atresia

122. Ans.— D. 3 and 4

123. Ans.— D. Endocardial cushion defects

124. Ans.— B. Noonan's syndrome

125. Ans.— C. PGIg

126. Ans.— C. Renal parenchymal disease

Renal cause contributes to about 75-80% of cases.

127. Ans.— A. CHF occurs commonly in infancy

CHF is rare in children but in adults it may develop in between 30-40 years of age.

128. Ans.— A. Birth

129. Ans.— C. Are common in adults than in children

130. Ans.— B. 10 weeks

131. Ans.— B. Coxsackie-B

132. Ans.— A. Balloon septostomy

133. Ans.— B. Cardiomyopathy with failure

134. Ans.— A. Prolonged flow through mitral valve

135. Ans.— D. Femoral

136. Ans.— D. Staphylococcal endocarditis

137. Ans.— A. IV. nitroprusside

138. Ans.— A. Total anomalous pulm. Venous connection

139. Ans.— B. Azygous vein enlargement

140. Ans.— A. 1 and 4

141. Ans.— D. CCF seldon occurs

142. Ans.— C. Always accompanied by a thrill

143. Ans.— D. Left ventricular hypertrophy

TOF is the commonest cyanotic congenital heart disease in children above the age of two years. In TOF, there is right ventricular hypertrophy. The severity of cyanosis is directly proportional to severity of pulmonic stenosis, but the intensity of systolic murmur is inversely related to severity of pulmonary stenosis. The absence of main pulmonary artery segment gives heart (normal sized) the shape of Cot-en-Sabot.

144. Ans.— D. Right aortic arch in 50% cases

Right aortic arch is present in 50% cases.

145. Ans.— A. They are sometimes associated with carditis

146. Ans.— D. Pausystolic murmur in tricuspid area

147. Ans.— B. PDA

148. Ans.— B. Severity of cardiac lesion is directly proportional to the intensity of murmur.

149. Ans.— B. Tricuspid atresia

150. Ans.— C. Palpitation is the main symptom

151. Ans.— D. Loud first heart sound

In left sided failure, there is tachypnoea, tachycardia, cough wheezig and rales in chest and right sided failure, there is hepatomegaly, facial edema, jugular venous engorgement, edema on feet and in failure of either side, cardiac enlargement, Gallop rhythm (S3) peripheral cyanosis, small volume pulse and absence of weight gain.

152. Ans.— B. Foramen ovale

153. Ans.— D. VSD

154. Ans.— C. ASD

155. Ans.— B. TOF

Tetralogy of Fallot is the commonest cyanotic heart disease characterized by VSD, PS, RVH and overriding or dextroposed aorta.

156. Ans.— A. PDA

Congenital rubella may also cause congenital heart defects (PDA with or without PS), eye defects (cataract or retinopathy) and hearing impairment. Deafness is commonest abnormality and may be the sole finding.

157. Ans.— C. Just distal to left subclavian artery

158. Ans.— B. Cardiac failure

159. Ans.— D. Pericardial friction rub

160. Ans.— B. 1 and 3

161. Ans.— C. Ostium secondum

8

IMPORTANT TEXT OF RESPIRATORY SYSTEM

IATROGENIC & DRUG-INDUCED PULMONARY DISEASE

* Prolonged use of high oxygen concentration & pressure ventilation can cause ...Bronchopulmonary dysplasia.
* Overtransfusions or excessive dose of plasma expanders .. Pulmonay dysplasia.
* Prolonged intubation ... Tracheal granulomas.
* Anticoagulant therapy .. Haemoptysis.
* Radiation injury ... Inflammation followed by progressive pulmonary disease.
* Nitrofurantoin ... Acute or chronic pulmonary complication.
* Prolonged Nitrofurantoin treatement .. Chronic pulmonary fibrosis.
* Chrysotherapy (Gold therapy) .. Interstitial fibrosis.
* Aspirin intolerance ... Nasal polyps & asthma.
* Pencillamine & Methysergide ... Pulmonary fibrosis.

MCQ's OF RESPIRATORY SYSTEM

What is Important in Respiratory System

Wheezing, Stridor, Dyspnoea, Asthma, Bronchiolitis, Bronchiectasis, Common Pneumonias, Lung Function Test

1. Name an electrolyte disturbance that may follow nebulization with salbutamol : TNPSC 2000, 2005

A. Hyponatremia B. Hypernatremia
C. Hypokalemia D. Hypocalcemia

2. Child with bronchial asthma, steroid should be given as : UP 1999, 2002

A. Subcutaneous B. Aerosol
C. Intravenous D. Oral

3. A neonate delivered at 32 weeks, on ventilator, X-ray shows white shadow and reveals SpO2 of 75, ventilator settings are as, Fi O2 70, rate 50/minutes. Step to be taken : AI 2001

A. Increase rate to 60
B. Decrease rate to 60
C. Continue with the same
D. Weaning ventilator

4. A neonate presents with respiratory distress, contralateral mediastinal and multiple cystic air filled lesions in chest. Most likely diagnosis is : AI 2001

A. Congenital diaphragmatic hernia
B. Congenital lung cysts
C. Pneumonia
D. Hyaline membrane disease

5. Surfactant production in lungs starts at : AI 2001, 2004

A. 28 weeks B. 32 weeks
C. 34 weeks D. 36 weeks

6. 3 months old child presents with intermittent stridor. Most likely cause is : AI 2001

A. Laryngotracheobronchitis
B. Laryngomalacia
C. Foreign body in larynx
D. Laryngeal papilloma

7. The following are features of transient tachypnea of newborn, except : JIPMER 2002

A. Seen in early neonatal period
B. May be associated with grunting & cyanosis
C. May be associated with crepts & wheez
D. Interlobar effusion is present

8. Transient tachypnea of new born is seen in : AIIMS 2002, 2007

A. Forceps delivery
B. Elective cessarean section
C. Ventouse extraction
D. Normal vaginal delivery

9. In a newborn with respiratory distress syndrome, all the following are true except : AI 2002

A. Increased incidence in <34 weeks
B. More common in infants of diabetic mothers
C. 100% oxygen is given in treatment
D. Cyanosis is present

10. Trendelenburg test is for testing which action at hip : Maharashtra 2000

A. Flexion B. Extention
C. Abduction D. Adduction

11. Rattling sound in a child is produced due to : BHU 2002, 2004

A. Obstruction in oropharynx
B. Obstruction in trachea & larynx
C. Obstruction in bronchi & bronchioles
D. Secretions in bronchi & bronchioles

12. A 5-years old boy, a known patient of bronchial asthma, presents with cough, wheezing and breathlessness. Examination shows respiratory rate 48/ minute, pulsus oparadoxus and bilateral rhonchi. The most appropriate immediate treatment is : UPSC 2002

A. Intravenous theophylline and corticosteroids.
B. Intravenous theophylline and nebulized salbutamol.
C. Nebulized salbutamol and ipratropinm.
D. Nebulized salbutamol and intravenous corticosteroids.

Ans. 1. C 2. B 3. D 4. B 5. A 6. B 7. B 8. B 9. C 10. C
11. D 12. D

13. **Consider the following statements : UPSC 2002**
Breath holding spells in children have the following feature:
1. They are preceded by minor trauma
2. Child stops breathing and is cyanosed
3. Child becomes suddenly pale and limp
4. Frequency becomes less on zinc supplementation

Which of the above statement is correct :
A. 1, 2 and 3 B. 1 and 2
C. 2, 3 and 4 D. 1, 3 and 4

14. **A child aged 24 months was brought to the Primary health centre with complaints of cough and fever for the past 2 days. On examination, the child weighed 11 kg, respiratory rate was 38/min chest indrawing was present. The most appropriate management for this patient is : AI 2003**
A. Classify as pneumonia and refer urgently to secondary level hospital.
B. Classify as pneumonia, start antibiotics and advise to report after 2 days.
C. Classify as severe pneumonia, start antibiotics and refer urgently.
D. Classify as severe pneumonia and refer urgently.

15. **In a 7 years child, trachea would be shifted away from affected side in all, except : PGI 1980**
A. Massive atelectasis
B. Tension pneumothorax
C. Tension pleural effusion
D. Massive emphysema

16. **In a child with exercise induced asthma, true is : Delhi 1993**
A. Prophylaxis with steroids
B. Prophylaxis with β_1 agonists
C. Prophylaxis with theophyline
D. Breathing exercises

17. **Child with which of the following throat infection needs systemic antibiotic therapy : Delhi 1992**
A. Pneumococci
B. β haemolytic streptococci
C. Staph. aureus
D. All of the above

18. **Usual feature of Pneumonia in a child is : Delhi 1992**
A. Cyanosis B. Resp. rate 60/mt
C. Temp 103°F D. Gastric dilatation

19. **Primary site of T.B. in a child is : Delhi 1989, 92**
A. Ghon focus B. Intestinal
C. Skin D. Miliary

20. **Surfactant type-II deficiency leads to : Delhi 1992**
A. Hyaline Membrane Disease
B. Fine mottling
C. B/L crepts changing with coughing
D. None

21. **A child with bronchiolitis - about treatment not true is : AI 1993**
A. Humidified oxygen
B. Anti-pyretics if fever
C. Antibiotics if child is toxic and B/L rales
D. Antibiotics not required

22. **Dyspnea with unilateral translucency of Hemithorax in a 1 day old infant is suggestive of : Rohtak 1987; AIIMS 1992**
A. Pneumatocele
B. Diaphragmatic hernia
C. Multiple congenital cysts
D. Cystic fibrosis

23. **Characteristic features of pneumococcal pneumoniae include all except : PGI 1983**
A. Meningism B. Delirium
C. Petechial rash D. Hypochondrial pain

24. **Characteristics of tuberculous pleural effusion include each of the following, except : Rohtak 1985**
A. Rare before the age of 5 years.
B. Supposed to result from discharge of caseous material of a peripheral primary focus or enlarged regional lymph node.
C. Symptoms include fever, weightloss, chest pain an dyspnea.
D. Vocal fremitus is increased.

25. **Characteristics of miliary tuberculosis include each of the following, except : BHU 1986**
A. Onset is usually insidious
B. Chest signs may be absolutely absent
C. X-ray chest has show-storm appearance
D. Toxemia is frequently marked

26. **The commonest cause of haemoptysis in childhood is : UP 1992**
A. Mitral stenosis B. Bronchiectasis
C. Pertussis D. Tuberculosis

27. **In miliary tuberculosis, the method of spread is : DNB 1991**
A. Lymphatic B. Intra-bronchial
C. Contiguous D. Haematogenous

28. **Which of the following conditions is least likely to be responsible for neonatal stridor : AMU 1987; Delhi 1992**
A. Congenital goitre B. Cretinism
C. Birth trauma D. Pierre-Robin syndrome

29. **The most important drug in the treatment of primary pulmonary tuberculosis in children is : PGI 1982**
A. Rifampicin B. Isoniazide
C. Streptomycin D. PAS

Ans. 13. A 14. C 15. A 16. B 17. D 18. B 19. A 20. A 21. B 22. A
23. C 24. D 25. D 26. B 27. D 28. B 29. B

30. A newborn has signs of respiratory distress. X-ray reveals : generalised haziness of both lungs, superimposed noduloreticular pattern of increased density, the lumens of largest bronchi stand out as conspicuous air shadows. The most probable diagnosis is : UPSC 1984, 85

A. Hyaline membrane disease
B. Intrauterine pneumonia
C. Massive emphysema
D. Massive atelectasis

31. Which of the following is an indication for tonsillectomy : UPSC 1984

A. Asthma
B. Rheumatic fever
C. Glomerulonephritis
D. Persistent carrier of diphtheria bacilli

32. Pleurisy in primary tuberculosis is : AIIMS 1986

A. Never observed
B. Very common
C. Extremely rare
D. Seen only among adults

33. Chronic and recurrent pneumonia are common in all of the following, except : PGI 1981

A. Hyperglobulinaemia
B. Agammaglobulinaemia
C. Cystic fibrosis of pancreas
D. Rheumatic fever

34. Pulmonary haemosiderosis is a feature of : AIIMS 1985

A. Good pasture's syndrome
B. Thrombocytopenic purpura
C. Myocarditis, cow's milk hypersensitivity
D. All are true

35. What is the long term recognised complication of O2 therapy in newborn ? AIIMS 1986

A. Atelectasis and retrolental fibroplasia
B. Cerebral palsy
C. Bronchiectasis
D. High tone deafness

36. Croup syndrome is usually caused by : AIIMS 1983

A. Rhinoviruses
B. Coxsackie-A virus
C. Coxsackie-B virus
D. Para influenza viruses

37. A persistent, bloody, purulent nasal discharge suggests : AIIMS 1981

A. Syphilis
B. Measles
C. Poliomyelitis
D. Allergic rhinitis

38. Streptococcal pharyngitis is most frequently associated with : PGI 1980

A. Hoarseness
B. Cough
C. Rhinitis
D. Diffuse redness of tonsils

39. In staphylococcal pneumonia, acute respiratory distress is due to: AIIMS 1986; TN 1989

A. Pneumatocele formation
B. Tension pneumothorax
C. Pleural effusion
D. Spreading pneumonia

40. Respiratory syncitial virus causes all except : PGI 1982, 88; TN 1989

A. Cold in children
B. Coryza in adults
C. Pneumonia in elderly
D. Acute Resp. distress syndrome

41. Which of the following is true of bronchiolitis except: AMU 1986, PGI 1983, 88

A. Caused by RSV
B. Occurs in school age
C. Leads to asthma
D. Treatment is oxygen

42. A newborn infant is observed to be cyanotic and tachypnoeic. He is placed in 100% O2 and the cyanosis clears completely. The infant most likely has : AIIMS 1984

A. CNS disease
B. Liver disease
C. Cyanotic congenital heart disease
D. Lung disease

43. Respiratory distress syndrome type-II has the following features except : PGI 1982

A. Hypoxia & Hypocapnia
B. Tachypnoea and Cyanosis
C. Lungs show rales and rhonchi
D. Recover within 3-4 hours

44. What is true of 'Canals of Lambert' in the alveolar spaces of the lung : PGI 1980

A. Bronchio Alveolar connections
B. Prevent atelectasis
C. Delay in collapse
D. All of the above

45. A newborn infant coughs and gets cyanosed soon after ingesting fluids. There is no difficulty in swallowing, coarse rhonchi and rales are there after swallowing. There is gastric distension after crying but no symptoms after lavage feedings. The most likely diagnosis is : UPSC 1981

A. Achalasia
B. Pyloric stenosis
C. Isolated esophageal atresia
D. Tracheoesophageal fistula without esophageal atresia

46. Most important factor predisposing to respiratory distress syndrome (RDS) : AIIMS 1984

A. Cold stress
B. Prematurity
C. Hypoglycemia
D. Precipitous delivery

Ans.									
30. A	31. D	32. B	33. D	34. D	35. A	36. D	37. A	38. D	39. B
40. D	41. B	42. D	43. D	44. D	45. D	46. B			

47. Untreated infants with severe RDS usually develop: AIIMS 1985

A. Metabolic acidosis
B. Respiratory alkalosis
C. Respiratory acidosis and metabolic acidosis
D. Respiratory alkalosis and metabolic alkalosis

48. The lecithin-sphingomyelin ratio of amniotic fluid is a useful indicator of the maturity of foetal : DNB 1990

A. Liver B. Kidney
C. Lungs D. CNS

49. A lecithin-sphingomyelin ratio (greater than 2) generally indicates that the foetus : Rohtak 1986

A. Does not have intrauterine pneumonia.
B. Will be able to breath spontaneously at birth.
C. Will not develop idiopathic respiratory distress syndrome.
D. None of the above.

50. The major site of right-to-left shunting in respiratory distress syndrome is : AIIMS 1985

A. In liver B. In lungs
C. At ductus arteriosus D. At foramen ovale

51. Most important agent in therapy of RDS is : UPSC 1987

A. Lecithin B. Ampicillin
C. Digitalis D. Oxygen

52. Following are early signs of RDS in a child, except : JIPMER 1997

A. RR more than 6 of min
B. Cyanosed at ram temperature
C. Sternal regression and dropping in
D. Signs of shock grunting respiration

53. Each of the following pneumonia occurs in the basal portion of lungs (lower lobes), except for : Bihar 1990

A. Klebsiella pneumonia
B. Mycoplasma pneumonia
C. Pneumococcal pneumonia
D. Viral pneumonia

54. Which of the following organisms is most commonly associated with AIDS pneumonia : DNB 1991

A. Klebsiella
B. Streptococcus pneumonia
C. Mycoplasma pneumonia
D. Mycobacterium tuberculosis

55. Pneumatocele is commonly found in case of : AMU 1991; Bihar 1991

A. Pneumococcal pneumonia
B. Streptococcal pneumonia
C. Klebsiella pneumonia
D. H. influezae pneumonia
E. None of the above

56. The major advantage of alternate day prednisone therapy for conditions such as asthma is : AP 1989

A. There is less adrenal suppression
B. More effective
C. More convenient
D. Less expensive

57. All are true regarding Staphylococcal pneumonia, except : AI 1990

A. Uncommon below the age of 5 years
B. Pneumatoceles are pathognomonic
C. Abdomen is usually distended with ileus
D. Evidence of infection elsewhere in the body

58. What is the most efficient way to confirm pneumothorax: Kerala 1989

A. Chest X-ray
B. Chest tube insertion
C. Measuring tidal volumes
D. Aspiration in Anterior axillary line

59. Which of the following is not true about bronchiectasis : AIIMS 1984; Delhi 1984

A. Increased incidence in rheumatoid arthritis.
B. Streptococcus is the most common organism causing infection.
C. Long term antibiotic coverage required.
D. Clubbing is usually positive.

60. The commonest symptom of foreign body in child is: AIIMS 1985

A. Cough B. Wheezing
C. Vomiting D. Dyspnea

61. All of the following are associated with pulmonary hypoplasia except : Delhi 1997

A. Diaphragmatic hernia
B. Asphyxiating thoracic malformation
C. Oligohydramnios
D. Air leak syndrome

62. Postural stridor with dysphagia in an infant is usually caused by : AIIMS 1986, 87

A. Laryngomalacia
B. Abberrant vessels
C. Acute laryngotracheo-bronchitis
D. TB in upper airways

63. Inhalation of 100% oxygen results in disappearance of central cyanosis in all of the following conditions, except : AIIMS 1987

A. Tetralogy of Fallot
B. Diffuse interstitial fibrosis
C. Chronic obstructive lung disease
D. Status asthmaticus

Ans. 47. C 48. C 49. C 50. B 51. D 52. C 53. A 54. D 55. C 56. A
57. A 58. D 59. C 60. B 61. A 62. A 63. A

64. Stridor due to supraglottic obstruction differs from tracheal obstruction by following except : AIIMS 1987

A. Less serious
B. Cry muffled
C. Dyspnea more marked
D. Cough less marked

65. In children above 6 years, ASOM is most often caused by : AIIMS 1986, 87, 90

A. H. influenzae
B. Pneumococci
C. Staph. albus
D. Aspergillus

66. Regarding staph. pneumonia all are true, except : AIIMS 1988

A. Lobar in distribution
B. Hilar lymphadenopathy
C. Pneumatocole
D. Pleural involvement

67. Patient with bronchiectasis may give a past history of : AIIMS 1988

A. Chickenpox
B. Mumps
C. Whooping cough
D. Typhoid

68. Alveolar-arterial tension gradient increases in all except : AIIMS 1985, 90

A. Diffusion defects
B. Hypoventilation
C. R—> L shunt
D. Ventilation perfusion abnormality

69. A patient with blood chemistry of pH 7.3, PCO2-65 mm, PO2< 40 mm. Diagnosis is : AIIMS 1990

A. COPD
B. ARDS (Acute Resp. Distress Syndrome)
C. TOF (Tetralogy of Fallot)
D. None of the above

70. Lung abscess is caused by following except : AIIMS 1990

A. Staphylococcus
B. Pneumococci
C. Klebsiella
D. E. histolytica

71. Acute bronchiolitis is characterized by following except : PGI 1988

A. Caused by respiratory syncytial virus
B. Cough is infrequent
C. Expiratory dyspnea
D. In earlier life leads to bronchial asthma
E. Humidified oxygen is used for treatment

72. The commonest presentation of miliary tuberculosis is : AIIMS 1982, 84; AMC 1984, 88

A. Fever
B. Weight loss
C. Dyspnoea
D. Chest pain

73. Negative Mantoux test is important in : Delhi 1982, 85

A. Pulmonary Koch's
B. Sarcoidosis
C. Carcinoma bronchus
D. Lymphoma

74. Creaky or croupy cough is heard in : Delhi 1990

A. Foreign body inhalation
B. Bronchiolitis
C. Asthma
D. Tracheitis

75. Which of the following viral infection in childhood is associated with bronchiectasis : Delhi 1997

A. Mumps
B. Measles
C. Rhinovirus
D. Chicken pox

76. Which one of the following is true of Transient Tachypnoea of Newborn (TTNB) : UPSC 1997

A. It is the commonest respiratory disorder caused by absence of surfactant.
B. In premature babies, it is often fatal.
C. Onset of respiratory distress is immediately after birth and it rarely lasts beyond 48 hours.
D. It often leads to chronic lung disease.

77. Tidal volume in a 3 Kg infant with respiratory rate of 28 per min is about : AIIMS 1988

A. 10 ml
B. 16 ml
C. 25 ml
D. 50 ml

78. Hyaline membrane seen in the lung is composed of : PGI 1982; AI 1982

A. Globulin
B. Albumin
C. Mucoprotein
D. Polysaccharide

79. Surfactant precursors appear as inclusion bodies in alveolar lining cells by ——— weeks : AIIMS 1989

A. 20
B. 24
C. 28
D. 32

80. Mediastinal widening is found in : AIIMS 1987, 89

A. Histiocytic lymphoma
B. Prolymphatic leukemias
C. CML with blast crisis
D. T-cell ALL

81. Transient tachypnoea of new born, following are true except : PGI 1998

A. Mild pleural effusion
B. Air bronchogram
C. Reticular shadow
D. Prominent interlobular fissure

82. Ghon's focus is : PGI 1983

A. Primary complex of TB
B. Post-primary TB
C. Miliary TB
D. TB lymph nodes

83. Grunting respiration in the new born is suggestive of : AIIMS 1983, 90

A. Congestive cardiac failure
B. Respiratory disease
C. Acidosis
D. Choanal atresia

Ans.										
	64. C	65. B	66. B	67. C	68. B	69. A	70. D	71. B	72. A	73. A
	74. D	75. B	76. C	77. B	78. B	79. B	80. D	81. B	82. A	83. B

84. **Most common cause of Acute coryza : AIIMS 1993**
A. Rhinovirus B. RSV
C. Influenza virus D. Corona virus

W85. **Tuberculous pleural effusion is characterized by all except : AIIMS 1994**
A. Haemorrhagic B. LDH more than 60%
C. ↑ mesothelial cells D. Deaminase

86. **Low glucose in pleural effusion is seen in all except: AIIMS 1994**
A. Rheumatoid arthritis
B. Emphysema
C. Malignant pleural effusion
D. Dressler's syndrome

87. **Bronchial obstruction in children with asthma is due to : UPSC 1994**
Consider the following causes :
I. Mucosal oedema
II. Increased secretions
III. Smooth muscle spasm
IV. Mucosal necrosis
A. I, II and III B. I and III
C. II and IV D. I, II, III and IV

88. **Which is not a feature of childhood asthma : AIIMS 1994**
A. Raised IgE levels
B. History of atopic dermatitis
C. Absence of wheezing after exercise
D. Improves with age

89. **A 7-months old infant has been hospitalised with respiratory distress, fever and minimal lung signs. The X-ray chest reveals hyperlucency Blood count is normal. The most likely diagnosis is : UPSC 1995**
A. Bronchopneumonia
B. Bronchiolitis
C. Collapse of the lung
D. Foreign body

90. **In a child suffering from pneumonia with rapid deterioration of clinical conditon, pneumatoceles, and pleural effusion on roentgenogram, the causative organisms besides staphylococcus aureus would include all of the following except : UPSC 1995**
A. Klebsiella B. H. influenzae
C. E. coli D. Strept. pneumoniae

91. **The first drug for a child with evidence of severe bronchospasm in anaphylaxis is : AP 1993**
A. Oral prednisolone B. I.V. Aminophylline
C. S.C. Adrenaline D. I.M. Deriphylline

92. **All of the following occur in acute resp. distress syndrome is all except : Delhi 1996**
A. Anemia
B. Groundglass appearance on X-ray
C. L : S ratio below one associated with severe RDS
D. Cyanosis

93. **Erythromycin is the drug of choice in the treatment of childhood infection due to the following organisms, except : UP 1996**
A. Pertusis
B. Mycoplasma pneumonia
C. Pneumocystis carinii
D. Chlamydia trachomatis

94. **All of the following are beneficial in the management of acute attacks of bronchial asthma in children, except : UP 1996**
A. High concentration of humidified oxygen
B. Salbutamol nebuliser
C. Intravenous hydrocortisone
D. Sodium cromoglycate nebuliser

95. **Lung abscesses in children may be produced by all of the following organisms, except : UP 1996**
A. Pneumococcus
B. Entamoeba histolytica
C. Klebsiella pneumoniae
D. Staphylococcus aureus

96. **Unilateral blood stained nasal discharge in a 6 years old boy is commonly due to : UP 1996**
A. Enlarged adenoids
B. Chronic maxillary sinusitis
C. Foreign body in nostril
D. Choanal atresia

97. **The sequential changes in acute bronchiolitis are as follows : TNPSC 1997**
A. Dyspnoea, Resp. Acidosis, Resp. Alkalosis, Metabolic Acidosis.
B. Resp. Acidosis, Metabolic Acidosis, Resp. Alkalosis, Dyspnoea.
C. Metabolic acidosis, Dyspnoea, Resp. Alkalosis, Metabolic Acidosis.
D. Dyspnoea, Resp. Alkalosis, Resp. Acidosis, Metabolic Acidosis.

98. **In a child caesation of breathing for 20 sec. with bradycardia is : AMU 1995**
A. Apnea
B. Dyspnea
C. Cheyne Stokes respiration
D. None

99. **Break down after breath holding is due to : AIIMS 1999**
A. J-receptors
B. Increased PCO2 level
C. Fatigue of intricatory muscles
D. Elastic recoil of diaphragm/lungs

Ans.										
	84. A	85. NONE	86. D	87. A	88. C	89. B	90. C	91. C	92. A	93. C
	94. D	95. B	96. C	97. D	98. A	99. A				

100. Child's respiratory physiology differs from adult because of : PGI 1999
A. Smaller airways
B. Increased O_2 demand
C. Decreased tidal volume
D. Decreased residual volume

101. True about transient tachypnoea of the newborn is : PGI 1999
A. Air bronchogram seen
B. Common in preterm infants
C. Interlobar fissure effusion
D. Respiratory distress resolves in 6-10 days

102. An infant presents with clinical evidence of pneumonia which is confirmed with roentgenograph. The child deteriorates further and roentgenogram taken 12 hours later shows pleural effusion. The most likely cause of pneumonia is: UPSC 2000
A. H.influenzae B. Klebsiella
C. Pneumococcus D. Staphylococcus

103. In obstructive lung disease all the following pulmonary function test values are decreased except: UPSC 2000
A. Forced vital capacity (FVC)
B. Forced expiratory volume in 1 sec. as per cent of FVC
C. Forced expiratory flow from 20 to 75% of FVC
D. Residual volume

104. Match List-I (Conditions) with List-II (Findings) and select the correct answer using the codes given below the Lists: UPSC 2000

List-I	List-II
A. Transient tachypnoea of the newborn	1. Incidence is reduced by good suctioning of oropharynx after head is delivered
B. Respiratory distress syndrome	2. Often seen following cessarean section
C. Bronchopulmonary dysplasia	3. May occur following trauma to chest during delivery
D. Meconium aspiration syndrome	4. Hyperexpansion with focal hyperlucency alternating with strands of opacification in chest radiograph
	5. In preterms with surfactant deficiency

Codes:

	a	b	c	d
A.	3	4	2	1
B.	2	5	4	1
C.	5	2	4	3
D.	2	5	1	3

105. Acidemia is usually manifested clinically by : DNB 1981
A. Kussmaul's breathing B. Sunken, soft eyeballs
C. Both D. Neither

106. Digital clubbing is not found in a child with which of the following : AIIMS 1984
A. Asthma
B. Bronchiectasis
C. Cyanotic congenital heart disease
D. Lung abscess

107. The following is contraindicated in the management of bronchiolitis : AIIMS 1990
A. The child should be nursed in a humid atmosphere.
B. Adequate sedation should be given to prevent the child crying and exerting himself.
C. It is important to ensure adequate hydration.
D. There is no convincing evidence of the role of steroids in the management of bronchiolitis.

108. The most common cause of cor pulmonale in children is : UPSC 1988
A. Bronchopneumonia B. Cystic fibrosis
C. Scoliosis D. None of the above

109. Epiglottitis is commonly treated with : AMC 1986
A. Tracheostomy
B. High environmental humidity
C. Early antimicrobial therapy
D. All of the above

110. Drug of choice for a child with pneumococcal pneumonia is : AP 1991
A. Streptomycin B. Erythromycin
C. Chloromycetin D. Penicillin

111. Spasmodic croup most commonly occurs in ages of : DNB 1990
A. 1-3 months B. 6-9 months
C. 1-3 years D. 3-5 years

112. Which dose of adrenaline would be most appropriate for a 6 years old child with asthma ? AIIMS 1981
A. 0.1 ml (1 : 1000 solution)
B. 0.5 ml (1 : 1000 solution)
C. 1.5 ml (1 : 1000 solution)
D. 2.0 ml (1 : 1000 solution)

113. In case there is induction of premature labor, which of the following drug is useful in preventing hyaline membrane disease : AIIMS 1984
A. Hydrocortisone B. Indomethacin
C. Propranolol D. Salbutamol

114. A child presents with hoarseness of voice, croupy cough and asthmatic wheeze. Most probable diagnosis is : PGI 1985
A. Asthmatic bronchitis
B. Bronchopneumonia
C. Retropharyngeal abscess
D. Foreign body in larynx

Ans. 100. A 101. C 102. C 103. D 104. B 105. A 106. A 107. B 108. B 109. D
110. D 111. C 112. A 113. A 114. D

115. Intrathoracic primary tuberculosis is difficult to differentiate in X-ray from : PGI 1980

A. Carcinoma B. Sarcoidosis
C. Bronchopneumonia D. Ascariasis

116. Congenital pulmonary sequestrations are best diagnosed by : UPSC 1983

A. Tomograms B. Fluoroscopy
C. Bronchograms D. Aortography

117. Weakness and paralysis of external muscles of respiration is found most frequently in infants with: AIIMS 1985

A. Amyotonia congenial B. Pneumothorax
C. Poliomyelitis D. Bronchopneumonia

118. In a 1 year old child, during true allergic asthmatic paroxysm, the X-ray signs resemble : AIIMS 1986

A. Bilateral atelectasis
B. Bilateral obstructive emphysema
C. Bilateral pneumonia
D. Bilateral pnuemothorax

119. A 2-years old healthy child suddenly develops breath lessness while playing. What is the most likely cause: UPSC 2004

A. Status asthmaticus
B. Pneumothorax
C. Foreign body aspiration
D. Cardiac failure

120. Inhaled corticosteroid used in bronchial asthma are all except : UPPGME 2006

A. Beclomethasone B. Budesonide
C. Fluticasone D. Dexamethasone

121. A new born presented severe respiratory distress. On examination he was found to have scaphoid abdomen and absent breath sounds on left side of chest. The mots likely diagnosis is : Maharashtra 2006

A. Transient tachypnea of newborn
B. Congenital adenomatoid lung disease
C. Congenital diaphragmatic hernia
D. Sequestration of lung

Ans. 115. B 116. D 117. A 118. B 119.C 120. D 121. C

EXPLANATIONS OF RESPIRATORY SYSTEM

1. Ans.— C. Hypokalemia
2. Ans.— B. Aerosol
3. Ans.— D. Weaning ventilator
4. Ans.— B. Congenital lung cysts

   It may be a part of cystic fibrosis.
5. Ans.— A. 28 weeks

   By the 24th week of gestation, the surfactant precursors appear as inclusion bodies in the alveolar thining cells.
6. Ans.— B. Laryngomalacia

   Laryngomalacia is a benign congenital disorder in which the cartilageous support for supraglottic structures is underdeveloped. It usually presents in first six months of life and is the most common cause of persistent stridor in infants.
7. Ans.— B. May be associated with grunting & cyanosis
8. Ans.— B. Elective cessarean section
9. Ans.— C. 100% oxygen is given in treatment

   Arterial PaO2 levels with 55-80 mmHg are kept.
10. Ans.— C. Abduction
11. Ans.— D. Secretions in bronchi & bronchioles
12. Ans.— D. Nebulized salbutamol and intravenous corticosteroids.
13. Ans.— A. 1, 2 and 3
14. Ans.— C. Classify as severe pneumonia, start antibiotics and refer urgently.
15. Ans.— A. Massive atelectasis
16. Ans.— B. Prophylaxis with β_1 agonists
17. Ans.— D. All of the above
18. Ans.— B. Resp. rate 60/mt
19. Ans.— A. Ghon focus
20. Ans.— A. Hyaline Membrane Disease
21. Ans.— B. Anti-pyretics if fever

    Antihistaminics are not indicated unless nasobronchial allergy is suspected.
22. Ans.— A. Pneumatocele
23. Ans.— C. Petechial rash
24. Ans.— D. Vocal fremitus is increased
25. Ans.— D. Toxemia is frequently marked
26. Ans.— B. Bronchiectasis
27. Ans.— D. Haematogenous
28. Ans.— B. Cretinism

    Stridor indicates upper respiratory obstruction and is usually accompanied by hoarseness, brassy cough, dypnoea, retraction of chest in inspiration and restlessness. Stridor is frequently seen in infants and is often attributed to (a) small size of larynx (b) loose submucous connective tissue around glottic region and rigid cricoid cartilage encircling the subglottic zone.
29. Ans.— B. Isoniazide
30. Ans.— A. Hyaline membrane disease

    The incidence of hyaline membrane disease is higher in lower gestational age infants. Presence of maternal diabetes, asphyxia, acidosis and hypothermia are additional risk factors. Synthesis of surfactant starts at 20 weeks of fetal life when about 5% of phospholipid is produced through methyl transferase pathway. Over 90% of surfactant is however produced after 35 weeks of gestation through phosphocholine (cytidyl) transferase pathway.
31. Ans.— D. Persistent carrier of diphtheria bacilli
32. Ans.— B. Very common

    It is the one of the commonest infective cause of pleural effusion.
33. Ans.— D. Rheumatic fever
34. Ans.— D. All are true
35. Ans.— A. Atelectasis and retrolental fibroplasia
36. Ans.— D. Para influenza viruse

37. Ans.— A. Syphilis

38. Ans.— D. Diffuse redness of tonsils

39. Ans.— B. Tension pneumothorax

40. Ans.— D. Acute Resp. distress syndrome

Respiratory syncytial virus is the commonest viral cause of bronchiolitis and may cause laryngitis and laryngotracheobronchitis.

41. Ans.— B. Occurs in school age

Treatment is humidified air, oxygen therapy, maintenance of fluid and electrolytes, bronchodilators (if required) and corticosteroids (if required).

42. Ans.— D. Lung disease

43. Ans.— D. Recover within 3-4 hours

44. Ans.— D. All of the above

45. Ans.— D. Tracheoesophageal fistula without esophageal atresia

46. Ans.— B. Prematurity

47. Ans.— C. Respiratory acidosis and metabolic acidosis.

48. Ans.— C. Lungs

Prenatal diagnosis of hyaline membrane disease (HMD) can be made by L S ratio (more than 2 indicates mature lungs with no risk of HMD, Ratio between 1 to 1.49 reflects borderline maturity or mild HMD and ratio below 1 develop severe HMD. In infants of diabetic mother, phosphatidyl glycerol (PG) is important in determining pulmonary maturity.

49. Ans.— C. Will not develop idiopathic respiratory distress syndrome

50. Ans.— B. In lungs

51. Ans.— D. Oxygen

52. Ans.— C. Sternal regression and dropping in

53. Ans.— A. Klebsiella pneumonia

54. Ans.— D. Mycobacterium tuberculosis

55. Ans.— C. Klebsiella pneumonia

Hilar lymphadenopathy is common with TB.

56. Ans.— A. There is less adrenal suppression

57. Ans.— A. Uncommon below the age of 5 years

58. Ans.— D. Aspiration in Anterior axillary line

59. Ans.— C. Long term antibiotic coverage required

60. Ans.— B. Wheezing

61. Ans.— B. Diaphragmatic hernia

62. Ans.— A. Laryngomalacia

63. Ans.— A. Tetralogy of Fallot

64. Ans.— C. Dyspnea more marked

Laryngomalacia is a benign congenital disorder in which the cartilagenous support for supraglottic structures is underdeveloped. It usually presents in first six months of life and is the most common cause of persistent stridor in infants.

65. Ans.— B. Pneumococci

66. Ans.— B. Hilar lymphadenopathy

67. Ans.— C. Whooping cough

68. Ans.— B. Hypoventilation

69. Ans.— A. COPD

70. Ans.— D. E. histolytica

Lung abscess is rare in Pneumococcal infection.

71. Ans.— B. Cough is infrequent

72. Ans.— A. Fever

73. Ans.— A. Pulmonary Koch's

74. Ans.— D. Tracheitis

75. Ans.— B. Measles

76. Ans. C. Onset of respiratory distress is immediately after birth and it rarely lasts beyond 48 hours.

77. Ans.— B. 16 ml

78. Ans.— B. Albumin

79. Ans.— B. 24

80. Ans.— D. T-cell ALL

81. Ans.— B. Air bronchogram

82. Ans.— A. Primary complex of TB

83. Ans.— B. Respiratory disease

84. Ans.— A. Rhinovirus

85. Ans.— NONE

86. Ans.— D. Dressler's syndrome

87. Ans.— A. I, II and III

88. Ans.— C. Absence of wheezing after exercise

89. Ans.— B. Bronchiolitis

90. Ans.— C. E. coli

91. Ans.— C. S.C. Adrenaline

92. Ans.— A. Anemia

93. Ans.— C. Pneumocystis carinii

94. Ans.— D. Sodium cromoglycate nebuliser

95. **Ans.— B. Entamoeba histolytica**

96. **Ans.— C. Foreign body in nostril**

97. **Ans.— D. Dyspnoea, Resp. Alkalosis, Resp. Acidosis, Metabolic Acidosis.**

98. **Ans.— A. Apnea**

99. **Ans.— A. J-receptors**

100. **Ans.— A. Smaller airways**

101. **Ans.— C. Interlobar fissure effusion**

102. **Ans.— C. Pneumococcus**

103. **Ans.— D. Residual volume**

104. **Ans.— B. 2 5 4 1**

105. **Ans.— A. Kussmaul's breathing**

106. **Ans.— A. Asthma**

107. **Ans.— B. Adequate sedation should be given to prevent the child crying and exerting himself.**

108. **Ans.— B. Cystic fibrosis**

109. **Ans.— D. All of the above**

Epiglottitis is most often caused by H. influenzae type-B. Other microbes (pneumococcus, beta hemolytic strepto-coccus and staphylococcus) are not important in etiology.

110. **Ans.— D. Penicillin**

111. **Ans.— C. 1-3 years**

112. **Ans.— A. 0.1 ml (1 : 1000 solution)**

113. **Ans.— A. Hydrocortisone**

114. **Ans.— D. Foreign body in larynx**

115. **Ans.— B. Sarcoidosis**

116. **Ans.— D. Aortography**

117. **Ans.— A. Amyotonia congenital**

118. **Ans.— B. Bilateral obstructive emphysema**

119. **Ans.— C. Foreign body aspiration**

120. **Ans.— D. Dexamethasone**

121. **Ans.— C. Congenital diaphragmatic hernia**

9

IMPORTANT TEXT OF RENAL SYSTEM

CHARACTERISTIC FEATURES OF TWO-GROUPS OF NEPHROTIC SYNDROME

	Parameter	*Minimal glomerular lesions*	*Significant glomerular lesions*
1.	Age at onset	Mainly below 5 years	In order children
2.	Sex incidence	Boys predominate	Almost equal
3.	Hematuria	Rare	Usual
4.	Hypertension	Rare usual	
5.	Glomerular filtration rate	Normal	Decreased
6.	Renal biopsy: light microscopy	Normal glomeruli or mild mesangial prominence	Variety of distinct, mild to severe abnormalities.
	Immunofluorescent staining	Negative	Immunoglobulins and complement often present
7.	Serum Complement	No abnormality	Decreased in some
8.	Molecular size of urinary protein	Small (mainly albumin)	Large molecules also present
9.	Response to treatment	Abolition of proteinuria	Proteinuria persists in most
10.	Pathogenesis	Not immune complex mediated	Immune complex induced, in majority
11.	Long term prognosis	Good	Fair to poor

IMPORTANT FEATURES OF SOME FORMS OF SIGNIFICANT GLOMERULAR LESIONS

	Glomerular lesion	*Hematuria*	*B.P.*	*Serum C3*	*Response to prednisone*	*Long term Outcome*
1.	Mesangial proliferative	+	N	N	Fair	Fair
2.	Focal glomerulosclerosis	-	In late stages	N	Poor	Poor
3.	Membranoproliferative	+		↑ Decreased in some	Poor	Poor
4.	Membranous	+	N or ↑	N	Poor	variable often spontaneous improvement.

CAUSES OF HAEMATURIA

Infection
- Bacterial
- Viruses
- Tuberculosis
- Schistosomiasis

Trauma

Glomerulonephritis
- Post-streptococcal
- Mesangial IgA nephropathy (Berger's disease)

Calculus

Congenital abnormality
- Hydronephrosis due to PUJ obstruction

Tumor
- Wilms

Vascular
- Arteritis
- Infarction

Bleeding disorder

Drug induced
- Cyclophosphamide

Exercise induced

Fictitious (Munchausen by proxy)

CAUSES OF ACUTE RENAL FAILURE

(I) Pre-renal

Acute hypovolaemia
- Haemorrhage
- Gastro-enteritis
- Third space losses (burns, gut)

Peripheral vasodilatation
- Sepsis

Low cardiac output
- Cardiac failure

Bilateral renal vessel occlusion
- Renal artery/vein thrombosis

(II) Intra-renal (renal parenchymal)

Haemolytic uraemic syndrome

Acute glomerulonephritis

Acute interstitial nephritis from drug hypersensitivity

Nephrotoxins
- Antibiotics
- Anti-cancer drugs

Vasculitis
- Polyarteritis

Bilateral acute pyelonephritis

Myoglobinuria haemoglobinuria

Acute crystalline nephropathy
- Uric acid
- Oxalosis

(III) Post-renal

Posterior urethral valves

Bilateral obstruction
- Pelviureteric junction, or vesicoureteric junction obstruction

Neurogenic bladder

Stones

DIFFERENTIATION OF FUNCTIONAL OLIGURIA FROM ESTABLISHED RENAL FAILURE

Test	*Functional oliguria*	*Established renal failure*
$\frac{\text{Urine osmolality}}{\text{Plasma osmolality}}$	Above 3	Below 1.3
$\frac{\text{Urinary urea}}{\text{Plasma urea}}$	Above 15	Below 5
$\frac{\text{Urinary creatinine}}{\text{Plasma creatinine}} \times 100$	Below 1	More than 3
Urinary Sodium	Less than 20mgEq/1	More than 70 mEq/1
Urinary urea	More than 1.6 g/100 indicates good renal function.	

MCQ's OF RENAL SYSTEM

What is important in Renal System

Renal Physiology (Function Tests), GN, PN, Nephrotic syndrome, Hemolytic uremic syndrome, ARF, CRF

1. **Schwartz method of a determination of GFR in children is independent of : AIIMS 2006**
   A. Body mass
   B. Age
   C. Renal function
   D. Method of estimation of creatinine
2. **Steroid resitant Nephrotic syndrome is associated with which of the following gene : AIIMS 2006**
   A. NPHSI B. PAX
   C. HOX II D. NPHS2
3. **The juice of which of the following fruit has been found to decrease the incidence of UTI : AIIMS 2006**
   A. Grape fruit B. Cranberry
   C. Orange D. Respberry
4. **A 2-years-old boy has vitamin D refractory rickets. Investigations show serum calcium 9 mg/dl. phosphate 2.4 mg/dl, alkaline phosphatase 1040 IU, Parathyroid hormone and bicarbonate levels are normal. The most probable diagnosis is : AIIMS 2002, 2005**
   A. Distal renal tubular acidosis
   B. Hypophosphatemic rickets
   C. Vitamin-D dependent rickets
   D. Proximal renal tubular acidosis
5. **Diarrhea-related hemolytic uremic syndrome is characterized by all, except : UPSC 2002**
   A. Acute renal failure
   B. Coombs positive hemolytic anemia
   C. Thrombocytopenia
   D. Neutrophilic leukocytosis
6. **Which one of the following statements is false with regard to pyuria in children : AI 2003**
   A. Presence of more than 5 WBC/hpf for girls and more than 3 WBC/hpf for boys.
   B. Infection can occur without pyuria.
   C. Pyuria may be present without Urinary tract infection.
   D. Isolated pyuria is neither confirmatory nor diagnostic for UTI.
7. **Which one of the following statement is false with regard to Xanthogranulomatous pyelonephritis in children : AI 2003**
   A. Often affects those younger than 8 yrs of age.
   B. It affects the kidney focally more frequently than diffusely.
   C. Boys are affected more frequently.
   D. Clinical presentation in children is same as in adults.
8. **A three years old boy presents with poor urinary stream. Most likely cause is : AIIMS 2003**
   A. Stricture urethra
   B. Neurogenic bladder
   C. Urethral calculus
   D. Posterior urethral valves
9. **A 11- months old boy, weighing 3 kgs, has polyuria, polydipsia and delayed motor milestones. Blood investigations show creatinine of 0.5 mg/dl, potassium 3mEq/1, sodium 125 mEq/1, chloride 88 mEq/1, calcium 8.8 mg/dl, pH 7.46 and bicarbonate 26 mEq/1. Ultrasonography shows medullary nephrocalcinosis. The most likely diagnosis is : AIIMS 2003**
   A. Renal tubular acidosis
   B. Diabetes insipidus
   C. Bartters syndrome
   D. Pseudohypoaldosteronism
10. **The initial treatment of choice for primary grade-V vesico-ureteric reflux involving both kidneys in a 6 months old boy is : AIIMS 2003**
    A. Antibiotic prophylaxis
    B. Ureteric reimplantation
    C. Cystoscopy followed by subureteric injection of teflon
    D. Bilateral ureterostomies
11. **Urinary incontinence in children is a feature of all of the following conditions except : UPSC 1995**
    A. Ectopic ureters
    B. Chronic urinary tract infection
    C. Myelodysplasia
    D. Meningomyelocele

Ans. 1. C 2. A 3. A 4. B 5. B 6. D 7. B 8. D 9. C 10. A 11. C

12. **In nephrotic syndrome, the essential features are following except :** **PGI 1982; AIIMS 1985**
A. Proteinuria B. Hypoalbuminemia
C. Hyperlipemia D. Edema

13. **Which of the following observations concerning nephrotic syndrome is not correct :** **Rohtak 1985**
A. The so-called idiopathic cases are believed to be autoimmune.
B. Essential lesion is thickening of the foot plate of the basement membrane.
C. Congenital variety is rare.
D. Peak incidence occurs at 5-8 years.

14. **Each of the following statements concerning management of nephrotic syndrome is correct, except:** **AIIMS 1983**
A. Corticosteroids constitute the "cornerstone" of drug therapy.
B. Only justification for giving diuretics for a short period is diuresis taking unusually long time to start, and presence of gross respiratory and cardiac embarrassment as a result of much water logging.
C. Prophylactic antibiotic cover is a "must".
D. There is no justification for limiting protein intake.
E. With steroid therapy, about 80% children recover.

15. **Which of the following bacteria is most often responsible for urinary tract infection (UTI) in childhood :** **AIIMS 1983**
A. E. coli B. Proteus
C. Pseudomonas D. Aerobacter aerogens
E. Streptococcus

16. **Each of the following observation concerning acute glomerulonephritis is correct, except :** **UPSC 1983**
A. Onset is acute or insidious.
B. Result secondary to a preceding streptococcal (beta hemolyticus type 12) infection of throat or skin.
C. Responsible for 2.4% of pediatric admissions in tropical countries.
D. Kidney biopsy shows proliferation and swelling of the endothelial cells.

17. **A weak, dribbling urinary stream and the presence of a palpable distended bladder in male neonate indicates:** **Delhi 1986; UPSC 1986; AIIMS 1984, 85**
A. Hypospadias B. Posterior urethral valves
C. Polycystic kidneys D. Hydronephrosis
E. Epispadias

18. **Spot the wrong statement about haemolytic uremic syndrome :** **AMU 1985, 92**
A. Characterized by presence of haemolytic anemia, (secondary to acute renal failure) in addition to thrombocytopenia.
B. Usually occurs below the age of 6 months.
C. Consumptive coagulopathy is present in most of the cases.
D. A blood transfusion, peritoneal dialysis and heparin therapy are claimed to be of value.

19. **Lowe's syndrome is characterised by the following except :** **AIIMS 1984, 87**
A. Hypophosphatamic rickets
B. Undescended testes
C. Defect in the CNS and eyes
D. Aminoaciduria

20. **A child comes with frequency of micturition and UTI. The best method of investigation for diagnosis is :** **AP 1995**
A. Cystoscopy
B. Retrograde pylography
C. Micturating cystourethrography
D. IVP + MCU

21. **Most important cause of oedema in nephrotic syndrome is :** **CMC 1984**
A. Hypoproteinemia
B. Hyperkalaemia
C. Increased capillary permeability
D. Lymphatic obstruction

22. **The average daily urine excretion of a 4 years old child is :** **AIIMS 1983**
A. 2 litres B. 1 litre
C. 650 ml D. 200 ml

23. **Membranoproliferative glomerulonephritis is commonly associated with :** **PGI 1983**
A. Chronic liver disease
B. Nephrotic syndrome
C. A favourable outcome
D. Hypocomplementemia occasionally

24. **Chronic renal failure is seen in association with or as a sequel to all except :** **AIIMS 1980**
A. Haemolytic uremic syndrome
B. Thrombotic thrombocytopenic purpura
C. Henoch-Schonelin purpura
D. Idiopathic thrombocytopenic purpura

25. **Drooping flower kidney is associated with :** **PGI 1982**
A. Congenital megaloureter
B. Renal staghorn calculus
C. Hydronephrosis
D. Ectopic ureter
E. All of the above

26. **Diuresis in a child with nephrosis is best induced with:** **Delhi 1983**
A. Salt poor diet B. Corticosteroids
C. Blood plasma D. Mercurials

Ans.	12. C	13. D	14. C	15. A	16. A	17. B	18. B	19. B	20. B	21. A
	22. C	23. B	24. D	25. D	26. B					

27. Urinary obstruction leading to hydronephrosis is usually caused by : Delhi 1981
A. Severe phimosis
B. Urinary calculi
C. Congenital defect within urinary tract
D. Kinking of ureter secondary to prolapsed kidney
E. None of the above

28. Polycystic kidneys are most often associated with cysts in the : Delhi 1980
A. Spleen B. Liver
C. Pancreas D. Lungs
E. b or d

29. Which of the following has not been associated with thrombosis of renal veins in newborn period : AMU 1989
A. Dehydration
B. Polycythaemia
C. Cystitis
D. Babies born to diabetic mother

30. Urine production begins at : Bihar 1988
A. 2 month's gestation B. 4 month's gestation
C. At term D. Soon after birth
E. The time of adequate fluid intake

31. Causes of haematuria in children include all the following except : Bihar 1989
A. Polycystic kidneys
B. Minimal lesion nephrotic syndrome
C. SABE
D. Renal artery thrombosis
E. Wilm's tumour

32. Which of the following drugs can be injected to diagnose pheochromocytoma : PGI 1989
A. Ephedrine B. Noradrenaline
C. Adrenaline D. Phenotolamine
E. Any of the above

33. An infant with severe dehydration secondary to diarrhoea suddenly presents protein and blood in urine. The most probable diagnosis is : UPSC 1989
A. Renal vein thrombosis
B. Pyelonephritis
C. Acute glomerulonephritis
D. Lower nephrosis

34. Most often the cause of acute renal failure in childhood is : AIIMS 1989; UPSC 2000
A. Pyelonephritis
B. Renal vein thrombosis
C. Hemolytic uremic syndrome
D. Acute glomerulonephritis

35. Factors that may be associated with vesicoureteral reflux include all, except : AMU 1988, 94
A. Support of ureter
B. Ureteric diameter
C. Thickness of bladder wall
D. Length of intravesical ureter and intravesical pressure

36. Ectopic ureter may be frequently associated with : AMU 1989
A. Oliguria
B. Dysuria
C. Bilateral hydroureter
D. Paradoxical incontinence

37. In infants lower urinary tract infection is due to : AIIMS 1997
A. Parentral antibiotics given
B. Infants with septicemia
C. VUR commonly seen
D. All of the above

38. Dietary management of homocystinuria includes a diet low in : PGI 1986, 88
A. Purines B. Homogentisic acid
C. Methionine D. Cystine

39. Chromatin positive seminiferous tubule dysgenesis has been seen in association with : AIIMS 1985, 87
A. Hypothyroidism B. Hypopituitarism
C. Adrenal hyperplasia D. Down's syndrome

40. Post-streptococcal GN leads to : AI 1996
A. Nephritic syndrome B. Nephrotic syndrome
C. Haematuria D. Hypotension

41. A child passed blood in urine recently, and on examination of abdomen nothing is palpable and urine examination shows RBC, small quantities of albumin, no pus cells. The probable diagnosis is : UPSC 1985
A. Glomerulonephritis B. Pyelonephritis
C. Nephronic syndrome D. Tuberculosis of kidney

42. While giving bath to one and half year old child, mother noticed an abdominal mass (unilateral), not crossing the midline and increased hemiatrophy. He has: UPSC 1986; AIIMS 1984
A. Wilm's tumour B. Neuroblastoma
C. Carcinoma kidney D. Polycystic kidney

43. Steroids are indicated in management of nephrotic syndrome resulting from : AIIMS 1984; Delhi 1985
A. Renal vein thrombosis
B. Kimmelsteil-Wilson syndrome
C. Renal amyloidosis
D. Minimal lesion glomerulonephritis

44. Normally, about ——— % of plasma appears as filtrate in kidney : AIIMS 1989
A. 10 B. 20
C. 30 D. 40

45. In chronic renal failure, true about blood changes are: AIIMS 1985
A. ↑ Urea, ↑ K+
B. ↑ Urea, ↑ Na+
C. ↓ Creatinine
D. ↑ Creatinine, ↑ potassium

Ans.										
	27. C	28. B	29. C	30. B	31. B	32. D	33. A	34. D	35. C	36. D
	37. C	38. C	39. D	40. C	41. A	42. A	43. D	44. B	45. A	

46. Most specific urinary finding in acute glomerulonephritis is : Delhi 1988; AIIMS 1985; PGI 2000

A. Haematuria B. Red cell casts
C. Granular casts D. Proteinuria

47. A complication of diuretic phase of acute renal failure is : AIIMS 1986

A. Convulsions
B. Hypokalemia
C. Increased sodium excretion in urine
D. Metabolic acidosis

48. Acute glomerulonephritis is characterized all of the following except : AIIMS 1984, 87

A. Hematuria
B. Gross proteinuria
C. Minimal change is the commonest variety.
D. Steroids and cyclophosphamide are used for treatment in some cases.

49. All serum proteins are reduced in nephrotic syndrome except : AIIMS 1990

A. Albumin B. Transferrin
C. Ceruloplasmin D. Fibrinogen

50. Acute tubular necrosis shows all except : AIIMS 1990

A. Urine pH always < 5.5 B. Anionic gap
C. Bicarbonaturia D. Vit.-D deficiency

51. Following are seen in minimal change nephritis : AI 1996

A. Hypertension
B. Hypercholesterolemia
C. Haematuria
D. Normal serum α_2-globulin

52. In minimal change disease, correct is : PGI 1996

A. Most cases recover spontaneously
B. 20% go to CRF
C. 20% develop local glomerulosclerosis.
D. 90% of cases best respond to short course of steroid therapy.

53. Renal stones in children are seen in following except : AIIMS 1997

A. Idiopathic hypercalcemia
B. Renal tubular acidosis
C. Sarcoidosis
D. Hyperparathyroidism

54. RBC casts are seen in : PGI 1982

A. Tubular necrosis
B. Focal GN
C. Membranous GN
D. Minimal GN
E. Membranoproliferative GN

55. Tamm Horsfal protein is a component of : PGI 1985

A. Tubular protein B. Not detected by dipstik
C. Nephrotic syndrome D. Serum albumin
E. None

56. Chronic renal failure is least likely to occur in Delhi 1986, 90

A. Membranous glomerulonephritis
B. IgA nephropathy
C. Mesangioproliferative glomerulonephritis
D. Focal sclerosing glomerulonephritis

57. Following are true about Wilm's tumour except : AIIMS 1997

A. Prognosis is excellent if patient's age is less than 1 year.
B. Immediate post operative radiotherapy given.
C. Preoperatively actinomycin-D is given.
D. Commonest differential diagnosis is neuroblastoma.

58. Periorbital oedema and oliguria with hypertension in a 7-years old boy is most commonly seen in : UPSC 1982

A. Nephrotic syndrome
B. Urinary tract infection
C. Hydronephrosis
D. Acute glomerulonephritis
E. Polycstic kidney

59. A weak, dribbling urinary stream and the presence of a palpable distended bladder in male neonate indicates : Delhi 1986; UPSC 1986; AIIMS 1984, 85

A. Hypospadias B. Posterior urethral valves
C. Polycystic kidneys D. Hydronephrosis
E. Epispadias

60. A 2-years, old boy with generalised oedema, hyaline cyst, Proteinuria 3+, WBC negative, no RBC disease is : AIIMS 1999

A. Selective proteinuria
B. Focal segmental Glucosclerosis
C. Chr. GN
D. Hypocomplementemia

61. A child comes with C/o hematuria following respiratory infection, same history 5 to 9 months back, true are except : AIIMS 1999

A. Complement C_3 normal
B. Infection occurs repeatedly but condition progress
C. Biopsy show proliferative changes in 50% of patients
D. Selective proteinuria

62. Which is seen in nephrotic syndrome : PGI 1999

A. Low serum calcium B. Raised AT-III
C. Low lipid D. ↓ Platelet activation

Ans.	46. B	47. B	48. C	49. D	50. D	51. B	52. D	53. C	54. B	55. A
	56. C	57. C	58. D	59. B	60. C	61. B	62. B			

63. A 3 yr. old boy URI had been investigated. US shows dilated left ureter & left hydronephrosis, on MCU a filling defect in the bladder was found is diagnosis : AI 2000

A. Duplication of ureter
B. Grade-III VUR
C. Sacrococcygeal teratoma
D. Suspected ureterocele

64. The absolute indications for dialysis include the following except : Kerala 2000

A. Persistent or severe hyperkalaemia
B. Congestive cardiac failure
C. Pulmonary odema
D. Hyperphosphataemia
E. Severe acidosis

65. Child with B.P. 190/110, pedal edema ++; facial edema ascites - Absent. Gross hematuria diagnosis is : PGI 2000

A. Acute GN B. Nephrotic syndrome
C. Renal thrombosis D. Renal amyloidosis

66. A 5 years child is suffering from nephrotic syndrome is well responding to steroid therapy. What would be the finding on light microscopy : AI 2001

A. No finding
B. Basement membrane thickening
C. Podocyte lesions
D. Multiple fibrotic lesion

67. Proximal renal tubular acidosis is most important investigation in : AIIMS 1985, 89

A. Vitamin-D resistant rickets
B. Dehydration and fever
C. Nephrocalcinosis
D. Bicarbonate loss

68. Filtered bicarbonate absorbed in proximal tubules is ——— % DNB 1994

A. 50-60 B. 70-80
C. 80-90 D. 95-100

69. A 10-years old girl child being treated for nephrotic syndrome presents with thick, white, cheese-like vaginal discharge, intense pruritis, dysuria and frequency of urine. The most likely diagnosis is : UPSC 1994

A. Neisseria gonorrhea cervicitis
B. Trichomonas vaginalis vaginitis
C. Physiological leukorrhoea
D. Candida albicans vaginitis

70. Regarding Wilm's tumour which is correct : AIIMS 1994

A. Very commonly metastasize to lungs
B. Bone metastasis
C. Always unilateral
D. Worst prognosis among childhood tumour

71. Glomerular filtration rate in ml/min/1.73 m² in an 8 weeks old child is : AI 1995

A. 100 B. 50
C. 75 D. 10

72. Commonest presentation of Wilm's tumour is : AMU 1987

A. Acute abdominal pain B. Mass abdomen
C. Haematuria D. Hypertension

73. Recognised complications of the nephrotic syndrome include following except : Bihar 1989

A. Pyogenic infection B. Pulmonary oedema
C. Urinary tract infection D. Acute tubular necrosis
E. Thrombo-embolism

74. Commonest cause of nephrotic syndrome in children: AI 1995

A. Minimal change disease
B. Membranous GN
C. Mesangioproliferative GN
D. IgA nephropathy

75. Characteristic biochemical features of established chronic renal failure in childhood include : AP 1991

A. Hypokalaemia B. Hypouricaemia
C. Hypophosphataemia D. Hypocalcaemia
E. Hyposthenuria

76. Recognised associations with neuroblastoma include except : AMU 1984, 89, 93

A. Normal urinary VMA excretion
B. Proptosis
C. Myoclonic encephalopathy
D. Watery diarrhoea with hypokalaemic acidosis
E. Vitamin-B_1 deficiency

77. The neonatal kidney achieves concentrating ability equivalent to adult's kidney by: AI 2004

A. One year of age
B. Eighteen months of age
C. Three to six months of age
D. Just before puberty

78. The most common cause of severe obstructive uropathy in infants and children is : UPSC 2004

A. Posterior urethral valves
B. Phimosis
C. Urethral atresia
D. Bladder neck obstruction

Ans.									
63. D	64. D	65. A	66. A	67. D	68. C	69. D	70. A	71. C	72. B
73. B	74. A	75. D	76. E	77. B	78. A				

79. A 2 months old girl has failure to thrive, polyuria and medullary nephrocalcinosis affecting both kidneys. Investigations show blood pH 7.48, bicarbonate 25 mEq/l, potassium 2 mEq/1, sodium 126 mEq/1 and chloride 88 mEq/l. The most likely diagnosis is : AI 2005

A. Distal renal tubular acidosis
B. Primary hyperaldosteronism
C. Bartter syndrome
D. Psuedohypoaldosteronism

80. A 9 years old boy has steroid dependent nephrotic syndrome for the last 5 years. The patient is markedly cushingoid with blood pressure of 120/86 mm Hg and small subcapsular cataracts. The most appropriate therapy of choice is : AI 2005

A. Longterm fursemide with enalapril
B. Cyclophosphamide
C. Intravenous immunoglobulin
D. Intravenous pulse corticosteroids

81. An 8 days old breast fed baby presents with vomiting, poor feeding and loose stools. On examination the heart rate is 190/minute, blood pressure 50/30 mmHg, respiratory rate 72 breaths/minute and capillary refill time of 4 seconds. Investigations show hemoglobin level of 15 g/dl, Na 120 mEq/1, K 6.8 mEq/l, bicarbonate 15 m Eq/l urea 30 mg/dl and creatinine 0.6 mg/dL. The most likely diagnosis is : AI 2005

A. Congenital adrenal hyperplasia
B. Acute tubular necrosis
C. Congenital hypertrophic pyloric stenosis
D. Renal tubular acidosis

82. A child with recurrent urinary tract infections is most likely to show : AI 2005

A. Posterior urethral valves
B. Vesicoureteric reflux
C. Neurogenic bladder
D. Renal and ureteic calculi

83. A female child was brought with complaint of generalized swelling of her body. She was passing cast in her urine. No hematuria. The true statement is : AI 2009

A. No IgG or C3 deposition seen on renal biopsy
B. Her C3 levels could be low
C. IgA nephropathy is likely
D. Alport syndrome

Ans. 79. C 80. B 81. A 82. B 83. A

EXPLANATIONS OF RENAL SYSTEM

1. Ans.— C. Renal function

GFR is estimated in children by Schwartz formula given as :

$$GFR = \frac{X \text{ Height (in cm)}}{\text{Plasma creatinine}}$$

* Value of k depends on age
* Low birth weight infant 0.33
* Normal infants 0-18 months 0.45
* Girls 2-16 yr 0.55
* Boys 2-13 yrs 0.55
* Boys 13-16 yrs 0.70
* It can not be used in obese or malnourished children where body height does not reflext muscle mass.
* It is not of use in malnourished children as creatinine is a reflection of body mass.
* Ideally, the exact value of k should be derived from the laboratory where the plasma creatinine is measured and from inulin clearance as the reference method for estimating GFR.

2. Ans.— D NPHS2

Important facts of Genetics and Paediatric Nephrology

* Congenital Nephrotic syndrome : Gene responsible named NPHS1 (which codes for Nephrin) - AIPG2006.
* Steroid resistant nephrotic syndrome -or in FSGS-Gene responsible named as NPHS2 (which codes for Podocin).
* WT-1 gene - implicated in Wilm's tumour, Denys Drash syndrome, Frasier syndrome.

3. Ans.— D. Respberry

Cranberry juice and bacterial colonization in children – a placebo-controlled randomized trial.

The cranberry produces, antimicrobial compounds such as proanthocyanidines in response to microbial invasion. In vitro it is able to prevent growth, adhesion or biofilm formation of a large number of bacteria, whichle clinically, cranberry juice has been shown to prevent urinary tract infections (UTI) in women.

Cranberries contain two compounds with anti-adherence properties, which prevent fimbriated F. coli from adhering to uroepithelial cells in the urinary tract. Approximatley a dozen clinical trials have been performed testing the effects of cranberries on the urinary tract.

4. Ans.— B. Hypophosphatemic rickets
5. Ans.— B. Coombs positive hemolytic anemia
6. Ans.— D. Isolated pyuria is neither confirmatory nor diagnostic for UTI
7. Ans.— B. It affects the kidney focally more frequently than diffusely
8. Ans.— D. Posterior uretral valves.
9. Ans.— C. Bartters syndrome.
10. Ans.— A. Antibiotic prophylaxis.
11. Ans.— C. Myelodysplasia
12. Ans.— C. Hyperlipemia
13. Ans.— D. Peak incidence occurs at 5-8 years
14. Ans.— C. Prophylactic antibiotic cover is a "must"
15. Ans.— A. E. coli
16. Ans.— A. Onset is acute or insidious
17. Ans.— B. Posterior urethral valves
18. Ans.— B. Usually occurs below the age of 6 months
19. Ans.— B. Undescended testes
20. Ans.— B. Retrograde pylography
21. Ans.— A. Hypoproteinemia
22. Ans.— C. 650 ml
23. Ans.— B. Nephrotic syndrome
24. Ans.— D. Idiopathic thrombocytopenic purpura

25. Ans.— D. Ectopic ureter
26. Ans.— B. Corticosteroids
27. Ans.— C. Congenital defect within urinary tract
28. Ans.— B. Liver
29. Ans.— C. Cystitis
30. Ans.— B. 4 month's gestation
31. Ans.— B. Minimal lesion nephrotic syndrome
32. Ans.— D. Phenotolamine
33. Ans.— A. Renal vein thrombosis
34. Ans.— D. Acute glomerulonephritis
35. Ans.— C. Thickness of bladder wall
36. Ans.— D. Paradoxical incontinence
37. Ans.— C. VUR commonly seen
38. Ans.— C. Methionine
39. Ans.— D. Down's syndrome
40. Ans.— C. Haematuria
41. Ans.— A. Glomerulonephritis
42. Ans.— A. Wilm's turnour
43. Ans.— D. Minimal lesion glomerulonephritis
44. Ans.— B. 20
45. Ans.— A. ↑ Urea, ↑ K+
46. Ans.— B. Red cell casts
47. Ans.— B. Hypokalemia
48. Ans.— C. Minimal change is the commonest variety
49. Ans.— D. Fibrinogen
50. Ans.— D. Vit. D deficiency
51. Ans.— B. Hypercholesterolemia
52. Ans.— D. 90% of cases best respond to short course of steroid therapy.
53. Ans.— C. Sarcoidosis
54. Ans.— B. Focal GN
55. Ans.— A. Tubular protein
56. Ans.— C. Mesangioproliferative glomerulonephritis
57. Ans.— C. Preoperatively actinomycin-D is given
58. Ans.— D. Acute glomerulonephritis
59. Ans.— B. Posterior urethral valves
60. Ans.— C. Chr. GN
61. Ans.— B. Infection occurs repeatedly but condition progress
62. Ans.— B. Raised AT-III
63. Ans.— D. Suspected ureterocele
64. Ans.— D. Hyperphosphataemia
65. Ans.— A. Acute GN.
66. Ans.— A. No finding
67. Ans.— D. Bicarbonate loss
68. Ans.— C. 80-90
69. Ans.— D. Candida albicans vaginitis
70. Ans.— A. Very commonly metastasize to lungs
71. Ans.— C. 75
72. Ans.— B. Mass abdomen
73. Ans.— B. Pulmonary oedema
74. Ans.— A. Minimal change disease
75. Ans.— D. Hypocalcaemia
76. Ans.— E. Vitamin-B1 deficiency
77. Ans.— B. Eighteen months of age
78. Ans.— A. Posterior urethral valves
79. Ans.— C. Bartter syndrome
80. Ans.— B. Cyclophosphamide
81. Ans.— A. Congenital adrenal hyperplasia
82. Ans.— B. Vesicoureteric reflux
83. Ans.— A. IgG or C3 deposition seen on renal biopsy

Most likely diagnosis of this child is nephrotic syndrome due to minimal change disease. So No IgG or C3 deposition is likely to be seen in renal biopsy.

IgG nephropathy

* More common in males than females
* M/C presentation: Hematuria

Alport nephropathy

* X-linked recessive hereditary nephritis
* All patients have microscopic hematuria
* Proteinuria may be present in males but present with mild and intermittent proteinuria in females.

10

IMPORTANT TEXT OF CNS

DRUGS OF CHOICE IN VARIOUS TYPES OF EPILEPSY

	Types of Seizure	*Drugs of Choice*
Group 1	a. Generalized Tonic Clonic (grand mal) b. Tonic Clonic Partial or focal with or without secondary generalization c. Psychomotor	1. Phenytoin 2. Phenobarbitone 3. Carbamazepine/Oxcarbazepine 4. Sodium valproate 5. Primidone 6. Clonazepam
Group 2	Absences or lapses (3 per sec. wave and spike, petit mal)	1. Ethosuximide with or without 2. Sodium valproate 3. Clonazepam 4. Troxidone
Group 3	Hypsarrhythmia, infantile spasm, myoclonic attacks in infants and older children	1. ACTH 2. Nitrazepam 3. Clonazepam 4. Sodium valproate

CAUSES OF RAISED INTRACRANIAL PRESSURE

Hydrocephalus
Cerebral oedema
- Post-traumatic
- Post-hypoxic

Tumour
Intracranial haemorrhage
Cerebral abscess
Meningoencephalitis
Reye's syndrome
Status epilepticus
Benign intracranial hypertension
Hypertensive encephalopathy
Lead encephalopathy

MCQ's OF CNS

What is important in CNS

Meningitis, Reye's syndrome, SOL (Tumors, Tuberculomas), Epilepsies, Cerebral Palsy, Mental Retardation, Myopathies, Juvenile Rheumatoid Arthritis

1. **Seizure and Jitteriness can be differentiated by all except : AI 2007**
   A. Gaze
   B. Autonomic disturbance
   C. Sensitivity to stimulus
   D. Frequency of movements
2. **A neonate presents with congestive heart failure, on examination enlarging fontanellae, bruit on auscultation, on USG shows midline hypoechoeic lesion, most likely diagnosis is : AIIMS 2006**
   A. Medulloblastoma
   B. Arachnoid cyst
   C. Vein of Galen malformation
   D. Hydrocephalus
3. **Which one of the following in the characteristic feature of juvenile myoclonic epilepsy : AIIMS 2006**
   A. Myoclonic seizures frequently occur in morning.
   B. Complete remission is common.
   C. Response to anticonvulsants is poor.
   D. Associated absence seizures are present in majority of patients.
4. **A 4-years old child is hospitalised because of his inability to walk which was first noticed about two months back and worsened gradually.There is no history of fever or injury. There is a history of strees incontinence. On examination it is found that the child had paralegia and the anus is patulous. Reflexe are diminished and plantars are flexor. There is loss of sensation below the umbilicus. The segmental level of lesion is: UPSC 2000**
   A. D12 B. D 10
   C. D 8 D. D 6
5. **The deep tendon reflex present at birth is: JIPMER 2000**
   A. Knee jerk B. Ankle jerk
   C. Biceps reflex D. Triceps reflex
6. **A clinical condition which is associated with mental retardation and fits is : TNPSC 2000**
   A. Epiloia B. Gargoylism
   C. Cretinism D. None of these
7. **Persistent head tilt in children can occur in the following except : TNPSC 2000, 2005**
   A. Torticollis
   B. Visual defect
   C. Herniation of cerebellar tonsils
   D. Cervical spondylosis
8. **Ten years old boy with midline cerebral tumor. Most common diagnosis is : Kerala 2001**
   A. Astrocytoma B. Medulloblastoma
   C. Meningioma D. Glioblastoma
9. **Epileptic seizures associated with high fever can be differentiated from simple febrile seizures by which of the following : SGPGI 2002**
   A. Family history
   B. Focal lesion
   C. Associated with high rise of temperature
   D. Focal seizures
10. **Best prognosis in new born seizures is due to which of the following causes : SGPGI 2002**
    A. Hypoglycemia B. Hypocalcemia
    C. Hyponatremia D. Hypomagnesemia
11. **A neonate is born with encephalitis without any skin lesion. The most probable diagnosis is : AIIMS 2002**
    A. HSV-I
    B. Japanese encephalitis
    C. HSV-II
    D. Haemophilus influenzae
12. **Neuronal cell migration defect is present in : Delhi 2002**
    A. Neuroblastoma
    B. Dandy-Walker syndrome
    C. Meningomyelocele
    D. Lissencephaly

Ans. 1. D 2. C 3. A 4. B 5. C 6. A 7. D 8. B 9. D 10. B 11. A 12. D

13. **Floppy neonate is seen in : Delhi 2002**
A. Werding-Hoffman syndrome
B. Hypoglycemia
C. Septicemia
D. Small for date neonates

14. **Least common cause of seizure in neonates is : BHU 2002**
A. Kernicterus
B. Meningitis
C. Septicemia
D. Pertussis vaccination

15. **Neurological complications of meningitis include all of the following except : AIIMS 2002**
A. Seizures
B. Increased intra-cranial pressure
C. Cerebral hamartoma
D. Subdural effusions

16. **A 15-year old boy had 10-12 partial complex seizures per day in spite of adequate 4 drug antiepileptic regime. He had history of repeated high-grade fever in childhood. MRI for epilepsy protocol revealed normal brain scan. What should be the best non-invasive strategy to make a definite diagnosis so that he can be prepared to undergo epilepsy surgery ? AIIMS 2002**
A. Interictal scalp EEG
B. Video EEG
C. Interictal 18F-FDG PET
D. Video EEG with Ictal 99mTc-HMPAO Brain SPECT

17. **Regarding simple febrile seizure, which one of the following statement is not correct : UPSC 2002**
A. It is usually seen in children between 6 months and 6 years.
B. The seizure usually lasts for less than 15 minutes.
C. Rectal diazepam given at the onset of febrile illness can reduce the incidence of recurrent febrile seizure.
D. Oral phenobarbitone is usually prescribed after the first episode of seizure to prevent recurrences.

18. **True about Febrile convulsion : AI 1993**
A. Recurrent B. Seen from 6 yr. onwards
C. No spontaneous cure D. Follows high fever

19. **Seizure with mental retardation and sebaceous adenoma, diagnosis is : AIIMS 1986, 88; AI 1993**
A. Hypothyroidism B. Congenital syphilis
C. Toxoplasma D. Tuberous sclerosis

20. **All are true of Febrile convulsions in children except : JIPMER 1992**
A. Occurs from 6 months - 5 years
B. Temperature is more than 38°C
C. Aspirin is compulsory during spike
D. Seizures occur early during episode

21. **Dandy Walker syndrome is due to obstruction of : JIPMER 1992**
A. Foramen of Murro
B. Foramen of Morgagni
C. Foramen of Magendie and Luschka
D. Arachnoid granulations

22. **Rail road calcifications in the brain are seen in : DNB 1989; JIPMER 1992**
A. Sturge Weber syndrome B. T.B. meningitis
C. Meningioma D. Tolosa-Hunt syndrome

23. **Which is not a feature of Tuberculous meningitis : AIIMS 1992**
A. Vasculitis B. Subarachnoiditis
C. Inflammed dura D. Decreased CSF glucose

24. **Cerebral palsy which manifest after the age of 1 year is most often : JIPMER 1993**
A. Spastic B. Ataxic
C. Mixed D. Diplegia

25. **Most common cause of obstructive hydrocephalus in a child is : AMU 1988, JIPMER 1993**
A. Meningitis
B. Aqueductal stenosis
C. Arnold Chiari malformation
D. Dandy Walker syndrome

26. **Most common cause of Intracerebral calcification in a child in India is : JIPMER 1993**
A. Toxoplasmosis B. Hyperparathyroidism
C. Tuberculoma D. A-V malformation

27. **Among following, Commonest intracranial neoplasm in children is : TN 1989, 93; Delhi 1992**
A. Glioblastoma B. Meningioma
C. Medulloblastoma D. Dermoid

28. **Commonest cause of meningitis in postneonatal period is : Delhi 1993**
A. Mycobacterium tuberculosis
B. Staph. aureus
C. Str. pneumoniae
D. Klebsiella

29. **Most common cause of seizure during neonatal period : AI 1993**
A. Perinatal hypoxia B. Brain haemorrhage
C. Tetanus D. Nutrient deficiency

30. **In 'Floppy baby' the following diseases are included except : AP 1991**
A. Wardnig Hoffman disease
B. Central core disease
C. Mitochondrial myopathies
D. Little's disease

31. **Which is not diagnostic of cerebral oedema : AMU 1989**
A. Rapid pulse B. Headache
C. Vomiting D. Slow respiration

Ans.									
13. A	14. D	15. C	16. D	17. D	18. D	19. D	20. C	21. C	22. A
23. C	24. A	25. B	26. C	27. C	28. C	29. A	30. D	31. A	

32. Epidural haemorrhage usually result from a fracture involving the : BHU 1988
A. Superior sagittal sinus
B. Anterior cerebral artery
C. Middle meningeal artery
D. Vein of Galen

33. In children with cerebral oedema, which one of the following corticosteroids will be effective : UPSC 1996
A. Hydrocortisone B. Prednisolone
C. Dexamethasone D. Betamethasone

34. Neonatal seizures in the following disorders is associated with poor prognosis, except : UP 1996,97
A. Hypoglycemia
B. Intraventricular haemorrhage
C. Hypocalcemia
D. Meningitis

35. Separation of cranial sutures are not seen in : PGI 1996
A. Cranial synostosis B. Trauma
C. Intrasutural metastasis D. ↑ ICT

36. In simple partial seizure in children, treatment is : AI 1997
A. Na valproate B. Carbamazepine
C. Primidone D. Phenobarb

37. Jack in Box or Darting tongue is seen in : DNB 1992
A. Huntington's chorea B. Down's syndrome
C. Hurler's syndrome D. Rheumatic chorea

38. Chances of developing kernicterus appears to be significant when serum level of unconjugated bilirubin reaches : AIIMS 1985
A. 50 mg% B. 20 mg%
C. 10 mg% D. 5 mg%

39. The first phase of kernicterus is characterized by : AIIMS 1983
A. Paralysis
B. Diarrhoea and vomiting
C. Lethargy, poor sucking and hypotonia
D. Fever, opisthotonous and seizures

40. Maximum development of brain occurs during : AIIMS 1983
A. Infancy
B. Adolescence
C. First trimester of pregnancy
D. School going year

41. The organism that most often caused neonatal meningitis is : AIIMS 1986
A. Pneumococcus B. H. influenzae
C. Staphylococcus D. E. coli
E. Tubercle bacilli

42. Commonest complication following meningococcal meningitis is : AIIMS 1982
A. Subdural effusion
B. Hydrocephalus
C. Arthritis
D. Waterhouse Fredrickson syndrome

43. Commonest complication of hemophilus influenza meningitis is : AIIMS 1986
A. Arthritis B. Bronchopneumonia
C. Otitis media D. Subdural effusion

44. CSF glucose is markedly reduced in : UPSC 1984
A. Encephalitis B. Pyogenic meningitis
C. TB meningitis D. Viral meningitis

45. Aseptic meningitis is mostly caused by : UPSC 1985
A. Adeno virus B. Entero virus
C. Arbo virus D. Herpes virus

46. Seizures in neonates occurs when serum calcium levels fall below : Rajasthan 1996
A. 5 B. 7
C. 9 D. 11

47. Most common presentation of neonatal meningitis is : Rajasthan 1996
A. Bulging fontanelle B. Nuchal rigidity
C. Poor feeding D. Convulsions

48. Which is least common in a child with brain damage? NIMHANS 1984
A. Tics B. Hyperexcitability
C. Anxiety D. Hyperkinesis

49. What is insignificant symptom of spastic hemiplegia : AIIMS 1982
A. Leg length discrepancy
B. Raking grasp
C. Unilateral Toe walking
D. Dysarthria

50. The normal concentration of protein in CSF at 4 weeks may be as high as : Delhi 1980
A. 500 mg% B. 125 mg%
C. 50 mg% D. 25 mg%

51. Ankle clonus of 5 contractions in a 2 months old infant: PGI 1980
A. Indicates neurological disease
B. Often normal
C. Abnormal at any age
D. Normal in early years of language development

52. Chronic causes of ataxia include all, except : AMU 1984
A. Hartnup disease
B. Ataxia telangiectasia
C. Obstructive hydrocephalus
D. Multiple sclerosis

Ans.										
	32. C	33. C	34. A	35. A	36. B	37. D	38. B	39. C	40. A	41. D
	42. C	43. D	44. B	45. B	46. B	47. C	48. A	49. D	50. B	51. B
	52. D									

53. Congenital hydrocephalus most frequently results from: **UPSC 1980**

A. Atresia of foramen of Magendie
B. Atresia of aqueduct of Sylvius
C. Atresia of foramen of Luschka
D. Development failure of subarachnoid cisterns

54. Most common type of meningoencephalocele is the : **AIIMS 1981**

A. Frontal B. Temporal
C. Parietal D. Occipitation

55. 'Lacunar skull' is most frequently associated with : **AIIMS 1979**

A. Diabetes mellitus
B. Posterior fossa tumour
C. Encephalocele or meningocele
D. Arnold Chiari syndrome

56. Radioisotopic brain scans are used chiefly to localize: **Kerala 1989**

A. Hydrocephalus B. Abscesses
C. Supratentorial tumours D. Subdural haematomas

57. The disorders of movement presents in the form of chorea, athetosis and dystonia, is seen in the disease of: **PGI 1982**

A. Basal ganglia B. Pyramidal tracts
C. Sensory tracts D. Muscle involvement

58. In the C.S.F. of a new born child what is abnormal : **AIIMS 1983**

A. Xanthochromia
B. Protein more than 100 mg/dl
C. 30 leucocytes per cu. mm
D. 500 R.B.C.'s per cu. mm

59. Cephalhaematoma is best differentiated from caput succedaneum by the : **UPSC 1985**

A. Normal neurological examination
B. Sharp periosteal limitation to one bone
C. Absence of history of prolonged or difficult labour
D. None of the above

60. Birth injury to spinal roots of brachial plexus usually results in : **DNB 1987**

A. Apnoea B. Shock
C. Paralysis of arm D. None of the above

61. Which is necessary before discharge from hospital in 6-9 months old who has recovered from H. influenza meningitis : **AIIMS 1997**

A. DPT vaccine B. Chemoprophylaxis
C. CT Scan D. Immunoprophylaxis

62. Consider the following statements associated with typical febrile convulsions in children : **UPSC 1997**

1. First attack is between 6 months and 3 years of age
2. The cause of fever is extracranial in origin
3. EEG tracing must be obtained after 2 weeks

Of the statements

A. 1, 2 and 3 are correct B. 1 and 2 are correct
C. 2 and 3 are correct D. 1 and 3 are correct

63. A 9-yrs old child presents with gait disturbance and posterior fossa tumor. The cause is : **AP 1997**

A. Medulloblastoma B. Cerebellar astrocytoma
C. Craniopharyngeoma D. Ependymoma

64. Spastic hemiplegia is not usually associated with : **AP 1989**

A. Uncinate fits B. Metabolic disorders
C. Subdural hematoma D. Multiple sclerosis

65. Most common form of reflex epilepsy is produced by : **CMC 1985; AMU 1985**

A. Flashing light B. Buzzing noises
C. Monotonus sound D. Music

66. Following are true regarding petit mal epilepsy except : **AP 1990**

A. Starts in childhood between the age of 4 and 5 years.
B. It usually lasts the lifetime of the patient.
C. Hyperventilation often precipitates an attack.
D. Learning disabilities and behaviour disorders are often observed with petit mal epilepsy.

67. Which of the following is not true about neuroblastoma : **Delhi 1997**

A. Intracranial metastasis cause skull hyperostosis
B. I.V.P. shows the renal pelvicalyceal displacement
C. Calcification occurs in 50% cases
D. Usually arise in adrenal gland

68. Untrue about Acute febrile convulsions is : **PGI 1989; AMU 1995**

A. Focal in nature
B. EEG normal after 2 weeks
C. Usually occur below 6 years of age
D. None of the above

69. The following are true for cerebral palsy, except : **Bihar 1988**

A. Antigravity muscles are more commonly involved
B. 60 to 70% are mentally retarded
C. It occurs in 7 per 1000 live births
D. Associated with incidence of acute leukaemia

70. Transcient focal weakness following a convulsion is called : **AIIMS 1986**

A. Cerebral palsy B. Todd's palsy
C. Bell's palsy D. Breck's palsy

71. A child with petit mal seizures shows no response to phenobarbital. The drug of choice is : **PGI 1983**

A. Acetazolamide B. Trimethadione
C. Ethosuximide D. Phensuximide

72. Sudden flexion of body waist is called : **Rohtak 1987**

A. Focal motor seizure B. Salaam attack
C. Myoclonic seizure D. Jacksonian seizure

Ans.									
53. B	54. D	55. C	56. C	57. A	58. C	59. B	60. C	61. C	62. B
63. A	64. A	65. A	66. B	67. A	68. A	69. D	70. B	71. C	72. B

73. **Cerebral palsy is defined as a : UPSC 1987**
A. Non-progressive neuromuscular disorder of cerebral origin.
B. Progressive neuromuscular disorder of cerebral origin.
C. Non-progressive neuromuscular disorder of peripheral origin.
D. Progressive neuromuscular disorder of peripheral origin.

74. **The CSF findings in Tuberculous meningitis include all, except : DNB 1990**
A. Elevated pressure
B. Usually turbid
C. Forms cobweb coagulum
D. Increased protein content

75. **The characteristics of caput succedaneum include all of the following except : UPSC 1989**
A. Crosses midline
B. Crosses the suture line
C. It does not disappear within 2-3 days
D. It is a diffuse oedematous swelling of the soft tissues of the scalp

76. **An epileptic syndrome, manifesting by aphasia along with regression of milestones is : AIIMS 1986**
A. Dandy Walker syndrome
B. Refsum disease
C. Tuberous sclerosis
D. Klefner Landou syndrome

77. **The cause of subcutaneous calcified nodules and epilepsy in a child is : AIIMS 1984**
A. Cysticercosis B. Tuberculosis
C. Leprosy D. Ankylostoma

78. **"Milkmaid's grip" is seen in : AIIMS 1985, 88**
A. Hydrocephalus B. TBM
C. Rheumatic chorea D. Meningioma

79. **The X-ray appearance of "Brush skull" is seen in : AIIMS 1986, 87**
A. Multiple myeloma B. Haemolytic anaemia
C. Hyperparathyroidism D. Achondroplasia

80. **An 8 years old girl is admitted with low grade fever, headache, vomiting and attacks of convulsions. On local Examination no localising sign is demonstrated. The CSF Examination reveals protein 150 mg% sugar 40 mg% chloride. 520 mg% and cell count of 100/cu mm with large number of lymphocytes. The most likely diagnosis is : UPSC 1987, 97; AIIMS 1986, 87**
A. Pyogenic meningitis B. Tuberculous meningitis
C. Cerebral abscess D. Viral encephalitis

81. **Sturge-Weber syndrome is : AIIMS 1987**
A. An outcome of bilateral temporal lobes ablation
B. A tumor of pituitary with gigantism
C. A sequela of head injury
D. Multiple angiomas over face, in eyes and brain

82. **Raised ICT in 9 months infant diagnosed by all except: AIIMS 1990**
A. Bulging fontanelles B. ↑ Head size
C. Diplopia D. Papilledema

83. **A child with mental age of seven and chronological age of seven years has an I.Q. of : AIIMS 1983, 90**
A. 100 B. 120
C. 145 D. 80

84. **Symptoms of minor brain damage is : Kerala 1996**
A. Fits B. Spascity
C. Hyperactivity D. Hoarse cry

85. **The commonest anatomical type of cerebral palsy is : PGI 1990**
A. Pyramidal B. Extrapyramidal
C. Cerebellar D. Pontine
E. Spinal

86. **A typical febrile seizure is characterised by all of the following except : Karnataka 1998**
A. Age group 6 months to 6 years
B. Occurs with sudden rise of temperature
C. Manifests with generalised seizures
D. Phenobarbitone is the main drug of choice

87. **A 6 years old child has unconsciousness, rigidity, and CSF is as if pyogenic meningitis. On treatment CSF becomes clear but his condition is same. Diagnosis is : UPSC 1983; ESI 1985**
A. Aseptic meningitis
B. TB meningitis
C. Subarachnoid haemorrhage
D. Brain haemorrhage

88. **Commonest cause of intracranial calcification in a child is : PGI 1982; Delhi 1989**
A. Craniopharyngioma B. Meningioma
C. Ependymoma D. Medulloblastoma

89. **Cerebral palsy which may improve with time is : Delhi 1982, 89**
A. Ataxic type B. Spastic type
C. Athetoid type D. Cerebellar

90. **Not true about craniopharyngioma : Delhi 1982, 89**
A. Eye defects
B. Growth retardation
C. Endocrinal defects
D. Diabetes insipidus is more than 50 percent

91. **In Kernicterus, not seen in : AIIMS 1985, 86; Delhi 1986**
A. Hydrocephalus
B. Athetosis
C. Brown staining of teeth
D. Mental retardation

Ans.	73. A	74. B	75. C	76. D	77. A	78. C	79. B	80. B	81. D	82. D
	83. A	84. C	85. A	86. D	87. A	88. A	89. C	90. D	91. A	

92. Common cause of meningitis in children (above 3 years) is : AIIMS 1976; Delhi 1983, 90
A. Meningococcus
B. Pneumococcus
C. Streptococcus pyogenes
D. H. influenzae

93. Commonest cause of hydrocephalus in children in India is : AIIMS 1989
A. Perinatal trauma
B. Infections
C. Arnold Chiari syndrome
D. Brain tumours

94. In meningioma, not seen is : Delhi 1990
A. Lamellar calcification
B. ↑ diploic space
C. Bone spicule in inner table
D. Decalcification in inner table

95. Reye's syndrome may present with following except : AIIMS 1986
A. Seizures
B. Delirium
C. Rapidly developing coma
D. Characteristic meningeal signs

96. Commonest intracranial neoplasm in children is : AI 1989; DNB 1998
A. Glioma B. Meningioma
C. Medulloblastoma D. Dermoid

97. In unexplained ataxia in a child, —— poisoning is a possibility : AI 1989
A. Arsenic B. Lead
C. Salicylate D. Mercury

98. Hydrocephalus in Arnold Chiari malformation presents : Kerala 1997
A. In pregnancy B. At any time
C. Ist decade D. Ist year

99. Treatment of choice of hydrocephalus in children is : Delhi 1987, 98
A. Corticosteroids B. Antibiotics
C. Aspiration D. Shunt operation

100. The patern of petit mal epilepsy of EEG is : NIMHANS 1986; AIIMS 1981, 87
A. Spike and dome
B. Continuous shunted spikes
C. Waves at the rate of 10/sec
D. Continuous tall spikes

101. Clonazepam should be avoided alongwith : DNB 1994
A. Phenytoin B. Ethosuximide
C. Sodium valproate D. Phenobarbitone

102. CSF examination in a one day old term male infant with convulsions reveals cell count—10 RBCs/HPF, 50 cells, protein—70 mg/dl. Sugar—40 mg/dl. The child is likely to be suffering from : Karnataka 1998
A. Meningitis B. Intracranial bleed
C. Hypoglycemia D. None of the above

103. Preventable cause of mental retardation is : PGI 1986
A. Down's B. Phenylketonuria
C. Cretinism D. Cerebral palsy

104. Neonatal cause of seizures which carries the best prognosis is : Rohtak 1987
A. Birth asphyxia B. Hypoglycemia
C. Bacterial meningitis D. Late onset hypocalcemia

105. All of the following cause hydrocephalus except : Delhi 1994
A. Toxoplasma B. TBM
C. Rubella D. Arnold Chiari syndrome

106. An X-ray of the skull of an eight years old child presenting with growth failure, progressive visual loss and papilloedema showed suprasellar calcification. The most likely diagnosis is : UPSC 1994
A. Craniopharyngioma
B. Toxoplasmosis
C. Cytomegalovirus disease
D. Sturge Weber Syndrome

107. Which of the following disorders of mother may lead to microcephaly : AIIMS 1994
A. Hepatitis-A B. Phenylketonuria
C. SLE D. Rubella

108. Cause of benign intracranial hypertension in children are all except : Delhi 1995
A. Hypervitaminosis-A B. Nalidixic acid
C. Sulphonamide D. Tetracycline

109. Sequelae of TB meningitis include except : AI 1995
A. Optic atrophy B. Hydrocephalus
C. Parkinsonism D. Seizures

110. A one-year old male child is brought to the emergency room with a short history of fever and restlessness. Examination reveals temperature of 103° F (39.4°C), hypotension, bulging fontanellae and petechial rash. The most likely diagnosis is : UPSC 1995
A. Pneumococcal meningitis
B. Meningococcal meningitis
C. Tubercular meningitis
D. Aseptic meningitis

Ans.	92. C	93. B	94. D	95. D	96. A	97. B	98. D	99. D	100. A	101. C
	102. C	103. C	104. D	105. C	106. A	107. D	108. C	109. C	110. B	

111. In a standard risk case of acute lymphatic leukaemia, the preferred prophylactic treatment of the central nervous system is : UPSC 1995
A. Cranial irradiation
B. Intrathecal methotrexate
C. Intrathecal triple therapy with methotrexate, hydrocortisone and cytosine arabinoside
D. Intrathecal vincristine

112. The following EMG findings are characteristic except: AIIMS 1985
A. Reduced amplitude and duration of potentials in muscular dystrophy.
B. Polyphasic and fibrillation potentials in dermato-myositis.
C. Increased amplitude and duration of potentials in dystrophia myotonica.
D. Bursts of high frequency discharges in dystrophia myotonica.

113. Serum creatine phosphokinase is raised in all except : AIIMS 1986
A. Duchenne muscular dystrophy
B. Duchenne patients as they grow older
C. Becker type muscular dystrophy
D. Dermatomyositis
E. Viral myositis

114. Hypotonia at birth is seen in the following except : AI 1996
A. Duchenne dystrophy
B. Glycogen storage disease
C. Cerebral palsy
D. Werdning Hoffman muscular atrophy

115. Which of the following is not true regarding normal cerebrospinal fluid : AMU 1986, 91
A. Appears clear
B. Contains less than 4 lymphocytes/mm^3
C. Has a protein concentration of 0.4-1.0gm/litre
D. Contains less than 4 polymorphs/mm

116. Spasticity is associated with all except : AMU 1986
A. Clonus B. Quadriplegia
C. Clasp-knife rigidity D. LMN type paralysis

117. The highest amount of protein in CSF is seen in : AIIMS 1984
A. Acute bacterial meningitis
B. Aseptic meningitis syndrome
C. Encephalitis
D. Tuberculous meningitis

118. Subdural effusion is seen more as a complication of : JIPMER 1990
A. Pneumococcal meningitis
B. Meningococcal meningitis
C. Haemophilus influenzae meningitis
D. Staphylococcal meningitis

119. In Kernicterus, staining of brain is more intense in the : AIIMS 1981
A. Spinal cord B. Corpus callosum
C. Basal ganglion D. Cerebral cortex

120. Which of the following is true regarding petit mal epilepsy : AIIMS 1986
A. May be provoked by hyperventilation
B. Late onset
C. Confused with vasovagal attack
D. Is a sequel of breath holding of attack

121. Which of the following is not a sign of meningitis in a child : PGI 1982
A. Neck stiffness
B. Fits
C. Palpable occipital glands
D. Headache

122. An 8-years old child is hospitalised for low grade pyrexia for 21 days, headache, vomiting and generalised convulsions. Central nervous system examination does not reveal any localising sign. Fundus examination revealed early papilloedema. C.S.F. examination showed protein 150 mg%, sugar 30 mg%, chloride 520 mg% cell count 100/cu mm all lymphocytes. The most likely diagnosis is : UPSC 1996
A. Pyogenic meningitis B. Tuberculous meningitis
C. Cerebral abscess D. Viral encephalitis

123. Regarding brain tumours in children : PGI 1983
A. Metastatic tumours are more common in children.
B. Supratentorial tumours are common than infratentorial ones.
C. After leukaemias, brain tumour are the commonest malignancies in children.
D. Hydrocephalus occurs late.

124. Ventriculo-peritoneal shunt is done for : AIIMS 1983
A. Communicating hydrocephalus
B. Non-communicating hydrocephalus
C. Arrested hydrocephalus
D. In all established non-arrested hydrocephalus

125. The most reliable early cutaneous sign of tuberous sclerosis is : AP 1991
A. Erythema nodosum B. Mongolian spot
C. Erythema toxicum D. White leaf macule

126. The drug of choice for Status epilepticus in children is : UPSC 1987, 89; TN 1993
A. Hydantoin B. Phenobarbitone
C. Diazepam D. Carbamazepine

Ans. 111. B 112. D 113. B 114. A 115. C 116. D 117. D 118. C 119. C 120. A
121. C 122. B 123. C 124. D 125. D 126. C

127. **Long term neurological sequelae in children is seen in following :** **TN 1993**
A. Toxoplasmosis B. Measles
C. Mumps D. All of the above

128. **All are the features of absence seizures except:** **TN 1994**
A. Usually seen in childhood
B. 3 Hz spike wave in EEG
C. Postictal confusion
D. Precipitation by hyperventilation

129. **All of the following are neural tube defects except :** **TN 1993**
A. Myelomeningocele B. Anencephaly
C. Encephalocele D. Holoprosencephaly

130. **In a patient with Listeria meningitis who is allergic to penicillin, the antimicrobial of choice is :** **AIIMS 2004**
A. Vancomycin
B. Gentamicin
C. Trimethoprim-sulphamethoxazole
D. Ceftriaxone

131. **Which one of the following is the common cause of congenital hydrocephalus is :** **AI 2005**
A. Craniosynostosis
B. Intra-uterine meningitis
C. Aqueductal stenosis
D. Malformations of great vein of Galen

132. **The following bacteria are most often associated with acute neonatal meningitis except :** **AI 2005**
A. Escherichia coli.
B. Streptococcus agalactia
C. Nelsseria meningitis
D. Listeria monocytogenes

133. **A 8 years old girl with headache, vomiting and no localizing sign showed a normal CT study of the head. LP revealed protein 150; sugar 40; chloride 520 and lymphocytes 100/microliter. What is the diagnosis:** **AIIMS 1999**
A. Tuberculous meningitis
B. Pyogenic meningitis
C. Viral encephalitis
D. HIV

134. **False about febrile seizure :** **TN 1999**
A. > 20 mts lasting
B. Within 24 hr of fever
C. Residual palsy absent
D. Usually non-progressive

135. **True about brain tumors in children is :** **AI 2000**
A. Most of them are located infratentorially
B. They are most common childhood tumors
C. Medulloblastoma is supratentorial
D. Usually cause papilloedema

136. **Which of the following drug first choice in the treatment of neonatal seizure :** **MAHE 2006**
A. Phenobarbitone
B. Phenytoin
C. Sodium valproate
D. Ethosuximide

137. **Most common cause of seizure in newborn is :** **AIIMS 2008**
A. Hypoxia induced ischemic encephalopathy
B. Hypocalcemia
C. Metabolic abnormality
D. Sepsis

Ans. 127. B 128. C 129. D 130. C 131. C 132. C 133. A 134. A 135. A 136. A 137. A

EXPLANATIONS OF CNS

1. Ans.— D. **Frequency of movements**

Jitteriness- It usually occurs in newborns with perinatal asphyxia, that may have seizure as well. It can be distinguished from seizure by :

1. **EEG monitoring**
2. **Absence of eye movements (i.e. Gaze)**
3. **Alternation in respiratory pattern**
4. **Presence of stimulus activation**

Decrease stimulation, decreases jitteriness.

Autonomic changes such as tachycardia, increaed BP are more common with seizure not with non-epileptic events. (like Jitteriness).

2. Ans.— C. **Vein of galen malformation**

The vein of Galen is located under the cerebral hemispheres and drains the anterior and central regions of the brain into the sinuses of the posterior cerebral fossa. Aneurysmal malformations of the vein of Galen (VGAM) typically result in high-output congestive heart failure or may present with developmental delay, hydrocephalus, and seizures.

* **Direct communication between a cerebral artery and a cerebral vein results from a congenital vascular malformation. The vein of Galen abnormality is the most frequent arterior venous malformation in noenates.**

3. Ans.— A. **Myoclonic seizures frequently occur in morning**

Juvenile myoclonic epilepsy is an epilepsy syndrome. Epilepsy syndromes are disorders in which epilepsy is a predominantly feature and there is sufficient evidence to suggest a common underlying mechanism.

Juvenile Myoclonic Epilepsy

It is characterized by :

- **Appearance in early adolescence**
- **Bilateral myoclonic jerks that may be single or repetitive.**
- **Most frequent in morning after awakening.**
- **Can be provoked by sleep deprivation.**
- **Consciousness is usually preserved unless myoclonus is especially severe.**
- **Association with generalised tonic-clonic seizures and absence seizures is seen.**
- **Absence seizures occur in 1/3rd of patients**
- **Benign condition although complete remission is uncommon.**
- **Seizure responds well to appropriate anticonvulsant medication.**
- **Family history of epilepsy is common.**
- **EEG show 4-6/s irregular spike.**
- **Treatment is with valproate.**

4. Ans.— B. **D 10**
5. Ans.— C. **Biceps reflex**
6. Ans.— A. **Epiloia**
7. Ans.— D. **Cervical spondylosis**
8. Ans.— B. **Medulloblastoma**
9. Ans.— D. **Focal seizures**
10. Ans.— B. **Hypocalcemia**
11. Ans.— A. **HSV-I**
12. Ans.— D. **Lissencephaly**
13. Ans.— A. **Werding-Hoffman syndrome**

It is characterized by marked hypotonia, sluggish fetal movement and fasciculations of tongue. The child is alert. Muscle biopsy shows neurogenic atrophy. It is autosomal recessive.

14. Ans.— D. **Pertussis vaccination**
15. Ans.— C. **Cerebral hamartoma**
16. Ans.— D. **Video EEG with Ictal 99mTc-HMPAO Brain SPECT**
17. Ans.— D. **Oral phenobarbitone is usually prescribed after the first episode of seizure to prevent recurrences**

18. Ans.— D. Follows high fever

19. Ans.— D. Tuberous sclerosis

20. Ans.— C. Aspirin is compulsory during spike

21. Ans.— C. Foramen of Magendie and Luschka

22. Ans.— A. Sturge Weber syndrome

23. Ans.— C. Inflammed dura

24. Ans.— A. Spastic

25. Ans.— B. Aqueductal stenosis

26. Ans.— C. Tuberculoma

27. Ans.— C. Medulloblastoma

28. Ans.— C. Str. pneumoniae

29. Ans.— A. Perinatal hypoxia

Birth anoxia is the commonest cause of mental retardation.

30. Ans.— D. Little's disease

31. Ans.— A. Rapid pulse

32. Ans.— C. Middle meningeal artery

33. Ans.— C. Dexamethasone

34. Ans.— A. Hypoglycemia

Epileptiform attacks may occur but common is generalized spasms resulting in loss of consciousness. Pseudohypoparathyroidism is due to defect in kidney tubules making them refractory to action of PTH whereas pseudohypoparathyroidism, has features as above but without clinical or biochemical evidence of hypoparathyroidism.

35. Ans.— A. Cranial synostosis

36. Ans.— B. Carbamazepine

37. Ans.— D. Rheumatic chorea

38. Ans.— B. 20 mg%

39. Ans.— C. Lethargy, poor sucking and hypotonia

40. Ans.— A. Infancy

This is especially during first 5 years of life.

41. Ans.— D. E. coli

42. Ans.— C. Arthritis

43. Ans.— D. Subdural effusion

44. Ans.— B. Pyogenic meningitis

45. Ans.— B. Entero virus

46. Ans.— B. 7

47. Ans.— C. Poor feeding

48. Ans.— A. Tics

Tics (motor or verbal) are not commonly associated with brain damage.

49. Ans.— D. Dysarthria

50. Ans.— B. 125 mg%

51. Ans.— B. Often normal

52. Ans.— D. Multiple sclerosis

53. Ans.— B. Atresia of aqueduct of Sylvius

54. Ans.— D. Occipitation

55. Ans.— C. Encephalocele or meningocele

56. Ans.— C. Supratentorial tumours

57. Ans.— A. Basal ganglia

58. Ans.— C. 30 leucocytes per cu. mm

59. Ans.— B. Sharp periosteal limitation to one bone

60. Ans.— C. Paralysis of arm

61. Ans.— C. CT Scan

62. Ans.— B. 1 and 2 are correct

EEG is not characteristically diagnostic of febrile convulsions.

63. Ans.— A. Medulloblastoma

64. Ans.— A. Uncinate fits

65. Ans.— A. Flashing light

66. Ans.— B. It usually lasts the lifetime of the patient.

67. Ans.— A. Intracranial metastasis cause skull hyperostosis.

68. Ans.— A. Focal in nature

Febrile seizures commonly seen in age group of 5 months to 6 years, are generalized in nature.

69. Ans.— D. Associated with incidence of acute leukaemia

70. Ans.— B. Todd's palsy

71. Ans.— C. Ethosuximide

72. Ans.— B. Salaam attack

73. Ans.— A. Non-progressive neuromuscular disorder of cerebral origin.

74. Ans.— B. Usually turbid

75. Ans.— C. It does not disappear within 2-3 days

76. Ans.— D. Klefner Landou syndrome

77. Ans.— A. Cysticercosis

Albendazole or praziquantel are used for treatment. One should be careful about hypersensitivity, seizures or signs of raised intracranial pressure during its treatment.

78. Ans.— C. Rheumatic chorea

79. Ans.— B. Haemolytic anaemia

80. Ans.— B. Tuberculous meningitis

81. Ans.— D. Multiple angiomas over face, in eyes and brain.

82. Ans.— D. Papilledema

83. Ans.— A. 100

84. Ans.— C. Hyperactivity

85. Ans.— A. Pyramidal

86. Ans.— D. Phenobarbitone is the main drug of choice.

87. Ans.— A. Aseptic meningitis

88. Ans.— A. Craniopharyngioma

89. Ans.— C. Athetoid type

90. Ans.— D. Diabetes insipidus is more than 50 percent.

91. Ans.— A. Hydrocephalus

92. Ans.— C. Streptococcus pyogenes

In bacterial meningitis, 3 months to 3 years, it is H. influenzae, pneumococci and meningococci. From 3 years onwards, pneumococci. From Birth to 3 months—Esch. coli, St. pneumoniae, psuedomonas, Str. faecalis. Meningococci cause infection in all age groups.

93. Ans.— B. Infections

94. Ans.— D. Decalcification in inner table

95. Ans.— D. Characteristic meningeal signs

First clinical description of this syndrome was probably made by Najib Khan in Jamshedpur in 1956. He called it Jamshedpur fever. Its pathology was described by Reye et. al. in Australia in 1964. There is a diffuse fatty infiltration of liver and to a less extent kidney and cerebral edema. It is observed in childhood from age of 2 months to 15 years.

96. Ans.— A. Glioma

Some books (CPDT) mention astrocytoma whereas some (Ghai) mention medulloblastoma.

97. Ans.— B. Lead

98. Ans.— D. Ist year

99. Ans.— D. Shunt operation

100. Ans.— A. Spike and dome

101. Ans.— C. Sodium valproate

Because it can precipitate petit mal status.

102. Ans.— C. Hypoglycemia

103. Ans.— C. Cretinism

104. Ans.— D. Late onset hypocalcemia

105. Ans.— C. Rubella

106. Ans.— A. Craniopharyngioma

107. Ans.— D. Rubella

108. Ans.— C. Sulphonamide

109. Ans.— C. Parkinsonism

Parkinsonism is unlikely. TB meningitis is common in miliary TB.

110. Ans.— B. Meningococcal meningitis

111. Ans.— B. Intrathecal methotrexate

112. Ans .— D. Bursts of high frequency discharges in dystrophia myotonica.

113. Ans.— B. Duchenne patients as they grow older

114. Ans.— A. Duchenne dystrophy

Duchenne dystrophy develops in 2-6 years of age.

115. Ans.— C. Has a protein concentration of 0.4-1.0gm/litre

116. Ans.— D. LMN type paralysis

117. Ans.— D. Tuberculous meningitis

118. Ans.— C. Haemophilus influenzae meningitis

119. Ans.— C. Basal ganglion

Basal ganglia, hippocampus and subthalamic nuclei are involved.

120. Ans.— A. May be provoked by hyperventilation

121. Ans.— C. Palpable occipital glands

There may be separation of sutures due to raised intracranial pressure.

122. Ans.— B. Tuberculous meningitis

123. Ans.— C. After leukaemias, brain tumour are the commonest malignancies in children.

124. Ans.— D. In all established non-arrested hydrocephalus.

125. Ans.— D. White leaf macule

126. Ans.— C. Diazepam

127. Ans.— B. Measles

Febrile seizures are seen in 5 months to 6 years of age and usually remit after that.

128. Ans. C. Postictal confusion

Absence Seizures

- Start abruptly in childhood and the peak prevalence is between 6–8 years.

- The seizures last for less than 30 sec.
- No loss of posture, incontinence of urine and stools or breathing difficulty.
- Other neurological manifestations and postictal phenomena (confusion and drowsiness) are absent.
- Hyperventilation for 3 minutes often precipitates the attacks.
- EEG shows characteristic 3 per second spike and slow wave pattern.

129. Ans.— D. Holoprosencephaly

Neural tube deficit

- Anencephaly
- Encephalocele
- Myelomeningocele
- Congenital hydrocephalus

Holoprosencephaly, a developmental disorder of the brain, results from defective cleavage of the prosencephalon.

130. Ans.— C. Trimethoprim-sulphamethoxazole

The treatment of choice for listeriosis is intra-venous administration of either ampicillin or penicillin, often in combination with an aminoglycoside for synergy. Trimethoprim-sulfamethoxazoleis bactericidal against L. monocytogenes and has been used successfully in the treatment of patients with penicillin allergy.

Because L. monocytogenes is not sensitive to cephalosporins, these agents should not be used for single-agent empirical treatment of neonatal sepsis or of meningitis in newborns or immunocompromised hosts.

Penicillin-allergic patients may be treated with trimethoprim-sulfamethoxazole (15/75 mg/kg intravenously per day in three equal portions every 8 h).

131. Ans.— C. Aqueductal stenosis

Congenital Hydrocephalus

Obstructive or non-communicating
Non-obstructive or communicating

(More common)

1. Aqueductal stenosis (MC)
2. Aqueductal gliosis
3. Intrauterine viral infection
4. Vein of Galen malformation (Rare)
5. Posterior fossa brain tumour
6. Dandy walker syndrome

(Less common)

1. Subarchnoid haemorrhage in premature infant.
2. Pneumococcal and tuberculous meningitis.
3. Leukemic infiltrates.

* Craniosynostosis : Premature closure of the cranial suture, producing skull defermity.

132. Ans.— C. Nilsseria meningitis

* First 2 months of life :

- Group B and D streptococci (streptococcus agalactiae)
- Gram negative enteric bacilli (Escherichia coli)
- Listeria monocytogenes
- H. influenzae (type B and nonencapsulated strain) - Rare

* 2 months to 12 years of age

- S. penumoniae
- S. pneumoniae
- H. influenzae type B

* Subsequent to the implementation of universal immunization against the H. influenzae (beginning at 2 months of age), the incidence of H. influenzae dropped precipitously.

- Meningitis (2 months - 12 years) now is most commonly caused by S. pneumoniae and N. meningitis.
- T-lymphocyte defect (congenital or acquired by chemotherapy, AIDS or malignancy) : ↑ risk of L. monocytogenes infection.
- Peak incidence of H. influenzae type B : 6-9 months of age.

133. Ans.— A. Tuberculous meningitis

134. Ans.— A. > 20 mts lasting

135. Ans.— A. Most of them are located infratentorially

Repeat Ques and Answer is controversial. Some books (Ghai's) mention that one third to half are medulloblastoma and one third are astrocytoma of cerebellum (pp 330), Other books (Current Paediatric Diagnosis) mention Astrocytoma as the commonest brain tumor (pp 1108).

136. Ans.— A. Phenobarbitone

137. Ans.— A. Hypoxia induced ischemic encephalopathy

11

IMPORTANT TEXT OF ENDOCRINOLOGY

DIFFERENTIAL DIAGNOSIS OF SHORT STATURE

		Constitutional delay in growth	*Familial short stature*	*Pituitary dwarfism*	*Hypothyroidism*	*Turner's syndrome*
1.	Family history	+ve	+ve	usually -ve	-ve	usually -ve
2.	Birth weight & height	N	↓	N	N	Slightly reduced
3.	Pattern of growth birth	Slow from birth	Slow from	Slow from a few months after birth	Slow from birth	Slow from birth
4.	Epiphyseal development	moderate but not progressive	almost normal	progressive retardation	marked retardation	within normal with variation
5.	Clinical features	immature, later normal	mature	immature	infantile	characteristic facies
	Puberty	delayed	normal	delayed	delayed	usually no signs
	Serum cholesterol	N	N	↑	↑	N
	hGH cholesterol	N	N	↓	N	N
	Gonadotrophin levels (after puberty)	N	N	↓ except in isolated hGH deficiency	N (or ↑)	↑

CAUSES OF TRUE PRECOCIOUS PUBERTY AND PSEUDO-PUBERTY.

True precocious puberty (central or complete)	*Pseudo-puberty (peripheral or incomplete)*
* Constitutional/idiopathic	Congenital adrenal hyperplasia
* Intracranial lesions with hypothalamic activation	Sex steroid administration (e.g. contraceptive pill)
* Associated with syndromes such as	Tumours
* Silver-Russell, Albright	Oestrogen producing
* Hypothyroidism	Androgen producing (arising from ovary, adrenal, testicle or interstitial cell)

BIOCHEMICAL AND CLINICAL ABNORMALITIES IN THE VARIETIES OF CONGENITAL ADRENAL HYPERPLASIA

	Hormone status				*Genitalia*			
Enzyme defect	*ACTH*	*17-OH prog.*	*Cortisol*	*Aldo.*	*Male*	*Female*	*Salt balance*	*BP*
20-22	↑	↓	↓	↓	Amb	N	Loss ++	↓
3	↑	↓	↓	↓	Amb	± Viril	Loss +	↓
17	↑	↓	N or ↓	↓	Amb	N	Retention	↑
21	↑	↑	N or ↓	N or ↓	N	Viril	N or Loss ++	N or ↓
11	↑	↑	↓	↓	N	Viril	Retention	↑
18	N	N	N	↓	N	N	Loss +	↑

MCQ's OF ENDOCRINOLOGY

What is important in Endocrinology

Cretinism, Hypothyroidism, Diabetes mellitus, Hypoglycemia, Short stature, Congenital adrenal hyperplasia, Delayed puberty

1. Commonest feature of hypoparathyroidism in children is : AI 1989

A. CataracT B. Recurrent seizures
C. Cold extremities D. Laryngospasm

2. True about children with diabetes mellitus : PGI 1982

A. Usually have an abrupt onset compared to adult onset.
B. Should not be treated with oral hypoglycemic agents.
C. Need not be concerned about developing renal eye complications at any time.
D. Have marked variations in insulin response.

3. A newborn 7 days old with vomiting and dehydration. Clinical examination was normal except for hyperpigmentation of nipple. Serum electrolytes Na—120 meq/L, K+ - 9 meq/L. Most likely diagnosis is : Mahe 1998

A. Primary hypothyroidism
B. Congenital adr. hyperplasia
C. Panhypopituitarism
D. Pyloric stenosis

4. In primary adrenal hyperplasia, incorrect is : AIIMS 1994, 96

A. Hyponatremia B. Hypokalemia
C. Hypernatremia D. Water retention

5. Which is not a feature of hypothyroid : AIIMS 1994

A. Delayed bone age
B. Delayed puberty
C. Altered upper-lower segment ratio
D. Short metacarpals in hand

6. Which of the following statement regarding sex steroid metabolism is not correct : UPSC 1995

A. All steroid hormones are synthesised from cholesterol.
B. Progesterone can be converted into estradiol.
C. Estradiol can be converted into progesterone.
D. Testosterone can be converted into estradiol.

7. Which of the following are true of congenital hypothyroidism : UPSC 1995

1. The child has stunted growth
2. Constipation is common
3. Mental development is subnormal
4. Bone age sometimes corresponds to chronological age

Select the correct answer using the codes given below:

A. 1 and 3 B. 2,3 and 4
C. 1, 2 and 4 D. 1, 2 and 3

8. Foetal distress in diabetic mother is caused by all except : Rajasthan 1993, 94

A. Oral hypoglycemic agents
B. Insulin
C. Analgesics
D. Sedatives

9. An infant with an enlarged clitoris may have been born to a mother who received the following except: AIIMS 1983

A. Progesterone B. Adrenocortical steroids
C. Testosterone D. Stilbestrol

10. ACTH secretion is highest during : PGI 1999

A. Noon B. Evening
C. Morning D. Night

11. Acromegaly is due to excess of : PGI 1999

A. ICAM-3 B. GH
C. Somatomedian-C D. ILGF

12. MC enzyme defect in congenital Adr. hyperplasia : PGI 2000

A. 21-hydroxylase B. 17 hydroxylase
C. 17 Desmolase D. 11-beta hyperoxylase

W13. A male pseudohermaphrodite child of 46 XY karyotype presents with B.P. 110/80 mmHg. Most likely enzyme deficiency is : AI 2001

A. 21 hydroxylase
B. 17 alpha hydroxylase
C. 11 hydroxylase
D. 3-beta hydroxylase

Ans. 1. C 2. C 3. B 4. A 5. D 6. C 7. D 8. B 9. D 10. B
11. B 12. A 13. B,D

14. An 11-years-old child, who is mentally and physically retarded with delayed bone age had wormian calcifications in the epiphysis on X-ray. The probable diagnosis is : AIIMS 2001

A. Hypopituitarism B. Hypothyroidism
C. Malnutrition D. Hypoadrenalism

15. In neonatal screening programme for detection of congenital hypothyroidism, the ideal place and time to collect the blood sample for TSH estimation is : AIIMS 2003

A. Cord blood at time of birth.
B. Heal pad blood at the time of birth.
C. Heal pad blood on 4th day of birth.
D. Peripheral venous blood on 28th day.

16. Child with recurrent hypoglycemic attacks and hepatomegaly is likely to have : JIPMER 1993

A. von Gierke disease B. Tetralogy of Fallot
C. Neonatal hepatitis D. Neonatal diabetes

17. Disproportionate dwarfism occurs in : TN 1993, 98,99

A. Hypothyroidism
B. Growth hormone deficiency
C. Achondroplasia
D. Laron dwarf

18. Following is not a true feature of short stature following hypopituitarism : Kerala 1981

A. Children are short at birth
B. Proportional dwarfism
C. Bone age is significantly delayed
D. Intelligence is usually normal

19. The following is not true regarding Laron's syndrome : AIIMS 1985, 92, 97

A. HGH levels are decreased
B. Somatomedin levels are decreased
C. Autosomal recessive inheritance
D. Shows clinical features of pituitary dwarfism

20. Symptoms seen in infants with hypoglycaemia include all except : AMC 1980, 88

A. Cyanosis B. Apnoea
C. Convulsions D. Persistent hunger

21. Major cause of death in diabetics having onset in early childhood is : AMC 1982, 85, 94

A. Cardiac lesions
B. Renal microangiopathy
C. Pneumonia
D. Hypertensive encephalopathy

22. Which of the following X-ray finding in a newborn infant would be most suggestive of hypothyroidism: AIIMS 1980

A. Osteoporosis
B. Epiphyseal dysgenesis
C. Prominent thymic shadow
D. Absence of ossification of hamate bone

23. Which of the following is associated with increased sweat electrolytes : PGI 1980

A. Glycogen storage disease
B. Adrenal insufficiency
C. Diabetes insipidus
D. All of the above

24. Precocious puberty is seen in : PGI 1995, 97

A. Hyperthyroidism
B. Addison's disease
C. McCune Albright syndrome
D. Neuroblastoma

25. Which is not associated with tetany : TN 1989

A. Seizures B. Carpopedal spasm
C. Fixed pupils D. Laryngospasm

26. Hyperthyroid children excrete increased amounts of all, except : DNB 1990

A. Tryptamine B. Tyramine
C. Phenylalanine D. Catecholamines

27. A primary manifestation of vasopresin deficiency results from : DNB 1990

A. Loss of phosphate in urine
B. Loss of potassium in urine
C. Loss of sodium in urine
D. Loss of solute free water

28. Water tolerance test is useful in differentiating the short stature as a result of : DNB 1989

A. Hypopituitarism B. Gonadal dysgenesis
C. Primordial dwarfism D. Mild hypothyroidism

29. In evaluating a child with short stature, birth weight is often low in a patient with : TN 1987

A. Gonadal dysgenesis B. Hypopituitarism
C. Hypothyroidism D. Constitutional delay

30. The chief presenting complaint of infants with idiopathic hypopituitarism is : AIIMS 1988

A. Short stature B. Headache
C. Convulsion D. Visual disturbance

31. Treatment of thyrotoxicosis is : AIIMS 1983

A. Subtotal thyroidectomy
B. Subtotal ablation with radioactive iodine
C. Blocking thyroid hormone production by drugs
D. Any of the above

32. All are characteristics of Hashimoto's strauma, except: AIIMS 1989

A. Variable uptake of I^{131}
B. Marked exophthalmos
C. May be preceded by viral infection
D. 95% patients have circulating antithyroid antibodies

Ans.										
	14. B	15. A	16. A	17. C	18. A	19. A	20. D	21. B	22. B	23. D
	24. C	25. C	26. C	27. D	28. A	29. A	30. A	31. D	32. B	

33. A newborn with goitre large enough to cause dyspnoea is best treated with : AIIMS 1984

A. Thyroidectomy
B. Tracheostomy
C. T3
D. Iodides

34. Goitrogenic substances associated with neonatal goitres include all, except : AMU 1987, 91

A. Sulfonamides
B. Iron containing preparation
C. Thioureas
D. Asthma medications containing iodides

35. Metabolic defects shown by hypothyroid infant are all, except : AMU 1987

A. Carotenemia
B. Sensitivity to barbiturates
C. Polycythemia
D. Impaired GFR

36. Suspicious signs of hypothyroidism in a newborn are all, except : Kerala 1988

A. Respiratory distress with feeding
B. Subnormal temperatures
C. Persistent diarrhoea
D. Failure to nurse properly

37. In Pendred's syndrome, there is an association between familial goiter and : Kerala 1988

A. Harelip
B. Deaf mutism
C. Cataracts
D. Hypospadias

38. Pendred's syndrome associated with cretinism is due to : UPSC 1986

A. Peroxidase defect
B. Failure to concentrate iodine
C. Failure to deiodinate iodotyrosines
D. Failure to form iodotyronines

39. Growth hormone does not effect : AMU 1986

A. Carbohydrate metabolism
B. Phosphorus levels
C. Potassium levels
D. Skeletal maturation

40. Adrenocortical insufficiency in infancy usually does not exhibit : DNB 1989; AMC 1992

A. Metabolic acidosis
B. Hyperkalemia
C. Hypernatrémia
D. Poor feeding

41. Biochemical finding associated with deficiency of 21-hydroxylase in congenital adrenal hyperplasia usually include : AIIMS 1990

A. Increase in oestrogens
B. Decrease in ACTH
C. Decrease in testosterone
D. Decreased total 17-ketosteroids

42. The Commonest cause of congenital hypothyroidism is : AP 1997

A. Thyroid dysgenesis
B. Pendred's syndrome
C. Defective release
D. Deficiency of deiodinase

43. Changes associated with adrenocortical tumours include all, except : UPSC 1985

A. Clitoral atrophy
B. Pubic hair development
C. Rugation of labia majora
D. Stippling and pigmentation of scrotum

44. Hypercorticalism of the adrenal gland is characterised by all of the following except : Rohtak 1988

A. Sodium retention
B. Hypertension
C. Gluconeogenesis
D. Hypotension

45. Peripheral utilization of glucose is increased in the following : AMC 1984

A. Pancreatic tumours
B. Tumours of mesothelial origin
C. Prediabetic state
D. All the above

46. What is the best line of therapy for Cushing's disease : AP 1988

A. ACTH
B. Cortisone
C. Adrenalectomy
D. Hypophysectomy

47. Virilisation of females is present in all of the following except : AIIMS 1987, 88

A. 21 β-hydroxylase deficiency
B. 11 β-hydroxylase deficiency
C. 12 β-hydroxylase deficiency
D. 17 α-hydroxylase deficiency

48. In cretinism all of the following are seen except : AIIMS 1987

A. Mental retardation
B. Obesity
C. Sexual infantilism
D. Hypoglycemia

49. Congenital hypothyroidism is diagnosed most early by : AIIMS 1986, 90; UPSC 1985

A. ↑ RAIU
B. ↑ TSH
C. T3 levels
D. PBI

50. For Cushing's syndrome in children, best test is : AIIMS 1990

A. Dexamethasone suppression test
B. ACTH levels
C. CT Scan
D. Steroid assays

51. In the case of male infertility under which one of the following conditions is hormonal therapy indicated: UPSC 1995

A. Hypopituitary hypogonadism
B. Aspermia
C. Retrograde ejaculation
D. Impotency

Ans.									
33. C	34. B	35. B	36. C	37. B	38. A	39. D	40. C	41. A	42. A
43. A	44. D	45. D	46. C	47. D	48. C	49. B	50. D	51. C	

52. Tetany may be seen with all except : **Delhi 1986; AIIMS 1988; PGI 1986, 89**
A. Hypocalcaemia B. Hypomagnesemia
C. Acidosis D. Alkalosis

53. Differentiation between Down's syndrome and Cretinism is : **JIPMER 1997**
A. Wide set eyes
B. Eyebrows elevated
C. Short neck and fatty appearance
D. Hair growth line recessed

54. In Hyperparathyroidism seen in : **PGI 1990; UPSC 1986**

	Ca^+	PO_4^-
A.	↑	↓
B.	↑	↑
C.	↓	↓
D.	↓	↑

55. Features of congenital hypothyroidism are following except : **AIIMS 1997**
A. Delayed puberty
B. Disproportionate upper-lower segment ratio
C. Normal bone age in comparison to height age
D. Short metacarpals

56. Not seen in Reye's syndrome is : **Delhi 1980; AIIMS 1988**
A. Bilirubin more than 3 mg%
B. Aminoaciduria
C. Hypoglycemia
D. Seizures

57. Diabetes insipidus in children may result from all except : **AMC 1986**
A. A sex-linked dominant genetic disease of the kidneys
B. Hand-Schuller-Christian disease
C. Head injuries
D. Hyperinsulinemia

58. Hypoglycemia in children may result from following except : **AIIMS 1984**
A. Glucose-6-phosphatase deficiency
B. Hypersensitivity to an amino acid leucine
C. Adrenal insufficiency
D. Islet cell insufficiency

59. Deficiency of growth hormone leads to : **AI 1989**
A. Delayed fusion of epiphysis
B. Proportionate dwarfism
C. Acromegally
D. Mental retardation

60. Suppression of lactation is indicated in all except : **AI 1989**
A. Neonatal death
B. Mid-trimester abortion
C. IDDM
D. Lithium administration

61. Milk let down reflex is initiated by ——— hormone : **Delhi 1993, 95**
A. Oxytocin B. Oestrogen
C. Prolactin D. Progesterone

62. Consider the following features : **UPSC 1996**
1. Infantile external genitalia
2. Chromosomal defect
3. Primary amenorrhea
4. Decreased urinary gonadotropins

Features of Turner's syndrome include :
A. 1,2,3 B. 1,3,4
C. 1,2,4 D. 2,3,4

63. Dietary treatment of galactosaemia : **Delhi 1986**
A. Must be continued life long.
B. Can be relaxed after puberty.
C. Involves delayed weaning.
D. Ensures normal intellectual development if started in the first week of life.
E. Is best monitored by liver fuction test.

64. Pelvis showing a characteristic appearance acetabular roof is a feature of : **UPSC 1996**
A. Down's syndrome B. Cretinism
C. Gargoylism D. Morquio disease

65. True about Klinefelter's syndrome is : **AI 1996**
A. Mental retardation B. Short stature
C. Chromosomal pattern XO D. Cubitus valgus

66. Side effects of corticosteroids include all, except : **Kerala 1990**
A. Cataracts B. Hypoglycaemia
C. Growth retardation D. Pseudotumour cerebri

67. Endocrine status of the newborn exhibits : **PGI 1982**
A. High calcium and low phosphorus
B. High PBI and BEI in first weeks
C. High production of ADH
D. All of the above

68. Diabetes mellitus in children most often requires and can be controlled by : **PGI 1984**
A. Restricted carbohydrate in the diet.
B. Oral hypoglycaemic drugs.
C. Dietary restriction and oral hypoglycaemic drugs.
D. Insulin without dietary restrictions.
E. Insulin and some restriction of dietary sugars.

69. Infants of diabetic mothers may exhibit the following except : **PGI 1986**
A. Low blood sugar
B. Low blood calcium
C. Low insulin blood levels
D. Increased proportion of body fat

Ans.	52. C	53. A	54. A	55. D	56. A	57. D	58. D	59. B	60. C	61. A
	62. A	63. A	64. D	65. A	66. B	67. B	68. E	69. C		

70. Obesity is associated with : AMU 1983, 90

A. Frolich's syndrome
B. Prader Willi syndrome
C. Laurence-Moon-Biedl syndrome
D. All of the above

71. Upper and lower portion of body disproportion with growth retardation is characteristically seen in: AIIMS 1989; AI 1993

A. Down's syndrome
B. Turner's syndrome
C. Congenital hypothyroidism
D. Cerebral palsy

72. Familial polyostosis, precocious puberty and pigmentation, the diagnosis is : AI 1993

A. Cretinism
B. Tuberous sclerosis
C. McCune Albright syndrome
D. Toxoplasma infection

73. Nutritional dwarfism is due to : JIPMER 1992

A. Acute undernutrition
B. Past and persistent malnutrition
C. Chronic malnutrition
D. Kwashiorkor

74. Which of the following is a feature of Hypothyroid certinism: UPSC 1986; AIIMS 1992

A. Deafness with facial palsy
B. Goitre with focal seizures
C. Blindness with mental retardation
D. Goitre with facial palsy

75. Treatment of choice in childhood thyrotoxicosis is : UPSC 1984, AIIMS 1992

A. Surgery B. Lugol's iodine
C. Carbimazole D. Radio iodine

76. Consider the following : UPSC 2004

1. Small for date baby
2. Large for date baby
3. Erythroblastosis fetalis
4. Birth asphyxia

Which of these clinical settings predispose(s) to neonatal hypoglycemia :

A. 1 only B. 1 and 3
C. 2, 3 and 4 D. 1,2 3 and 4

77. A 13 years old boy has bilateral gynaecomastia. His height is 1.48 cm, weight 58 kg; the sexual maturity rating is stage 2. The gynaecomastia is most likely due to : AIIMS 2004

A. Prolactinoma
B. Testicular tumor
C. Pubertal gynaecomastia
D. Chronic liver disease

78. A 9 years old boy presents with growth retardation and propensity to hypoglycemia. Physical examination reveals short stature, micropenia, increased fat and high-pitched voice. The skeletal survey reveals bone age of 5 years. Which of the following is most appropriate diagnosis: AIIMS 2004

A. Malabsorption
B. Growth hormone deficiency
C. Adrenal tumor
D. Thyroxin deficiency

79. Hypothalmopituitary axis becomes active and functional at : Maharashtra-2006

A. 5th month of life
B. 5th week of life
C. 5th year of life
D. 20th week of gestation

80. Mental retardation is associated with deficiency of : MAHE 2006

A. Triiodothyronine B. TSH
C. GH D. Testosterone

Ans. 70. D 71. C 72. C 73. C 74. A 75. A 76. A 77. C 78. B 79. D 80. A

EXPLANATIONS OF ENDOCRINOLOGY

1. Ans.— C. Cold extremities
2. Ans.— C. Need not be concerned about developing renal eye complications at any time.
3. Ans.— B. Congenital adr. hyperplasia
4. Ans.— A. Hyponatremia
5. Ans.— D. Short metacarpals in hand
6. Ans.— C. Estradiol can be converted into progesterone.
7. Ans.— C. 1, 2 and 4
8. Ans.— B. Insulin
9. Ans.— D. Stilbestrol
10. Ans.— B. Evening
11. Ans.— B. GH
12. Ans.— A. 21-hydroxylase

    It most often results due to 21 hydroxylase deficiency.
13. Ans.— B. 17 alpha hydroxylase
    & D. 3-beta hydroxylase

    Pseudohermaphroditism is also seen in 3 beta hydroxylase deficiency but hypertension is not seen.
14. Ans.— B. Hypothyroidism
15. Ans.— A. Cord blood at time of birth.
16. Ans.— A. von Gierke disease
17. Ans.— C. Achondroplasia
18. Ans.— A. Children are short at birth
19. Ans.— A. HGH levels are decreased
20. Ans.— D. Persistent hunger
21. Ans.— B. Renal microangiopathy
22. Ans.— B. Epiphyseal dysgenesis
23. Ans.— D. All of the above
24. Ans.— C. McCune Albright syndrome.

    Puberty before age of 8 years in girls or 9 years in boys is considered precocious puberty. It is central (true) or peripheral (pseudo type).
25. Ans.— C. Fixed pupils
26. Ans.— C. Phenylalanine
27. Ans.— D. Loss of solute free water
28. Ans.— A. Hypopituitarism
29. Ans.— A. Gonadal dysgenesis
30. Ans.— A. Short stature

    In hypopituitarism, birth weight and height are normal and there is slow growth from a few months after birth (progressive retardation), puberty is delayed and GH levels are low.
31. Ans.— D. Any of the above
32. Ans.— B. Marked exophthalmos
33. Ans.— C. T3
34. Ans.— B. Iron containing preparation
35. Ans.— B. Sensitivity to barbiturates
36. Ans.— C. Persistent diarrhoea
37. Ans.— B. Deaf mutism

    Pendred's syndrome is autosomal recessive and there is congenital deafness and goitre. Hearing loss is usually present at birth and goitre appears at puberty.
38. Ans.— A. Peroxidase defect
39. Ans.— D. Skeletal maturation
40. Ans.— C. Hypernatremia
41. Ans.— A. Increase in oestrogens
42. Ans.— A. Thyroid dysgenesis

    Goitrous hypothyroidism can result due to dyshormonogenesis, iodine deficiency antithyroid drugs and Hashimoto's disease.
43. Ans.— A. Clitoral atrophy
44. Ans.— D. Hypotension
45. Ans.— D. All the above
46. Ans.— C. Adrenalectomy
47. Ans.— D. 17 α-hydroxylase deficiency
48. Ans.— C. Sexual infantilism
49. Ans.— B. $\uparrow$ TSH

50. Ans.— D. Steroid assays

51. Ans.— C. Retrograde ejaculation

52. Ans.— C. Acidosis

53. Ans.— A. Wide set eyes

54. Ans.— A. ↑ ca+ ↓ PO_4^-

Alkaline phosphatase is also raised.

55. Ans.— D. Short metacarpals

56. Ans.— A. Bilirubin more than 3 mg%

57. Ans.— D. Hyperinsulinemia

58. Ans.— D. Islet cell insufficiency

59. Ans.— B. Proportionate dwarfism

60. Ans.— C. IDDM

It is due to increase in dopamine levels, stimulating prolactin Inhibiting factor.

61. Ans.— A. Oxytocin

62. Ans.— A. 1, 2, 3

63. Ans.— A. Must be continued life long

64. Ans.— D. Morquio disease

65. Ans.— A. Mental retardation

Chromosomal pattern is XXY. Cubitus valgus, XO patternn and short stature are seen in Turner's syndrome.

66. Ans.— B. Hypoglycaemia

67. Ans.— B. High PBI and BEI in first week

68. Ans.— E. Insulin and some restriction of dietary sugars.

69. Ans.— C. Low insulin blood levels

70. Ans.— D. All of the above

71. Ans.— C. Congenital hypothyroidism

Ratio between upper and lower segment is increased. Child appears short and stocky.

72. Ans.— C. McCune Albright syndrome

It is a diaphyseal disorder like Englemann and Caffey's diseases.

73. Ans.— C. Chronic malnutrition

74. Ans.— A. Deafness with facial palsy

75. Ans.— A. Surgery

76. Ans.— A. 1 only

77. Ans.— C. Pubertal gynaecomastia

During early to mid puberty, approximately two-thirds of boys develop various degrees of subareolar hyperplasia of the breasts. *Physiologic pubertal gynecomastia* may involve only one breast, and it is not unusual for both breasts to enlarge at disproportionate rates or at different times. Tenderness of the breast is common but transitory. Spontaneous regression may occur within a few months; it rarely persists longer than 2 yr.

Several boys with the *Peutz-Jeghers syndrome* and gynaecomastia had sex-cord tumors with annular tubules of the testes. The testes may not be enlarged; the tumor is usually multifocal and bilateral. Excessive aromatase production accounts for the gynaecomastia.

78. Ans.— B. Growth hormone deficiency

Congenital Hypopituitarism

The head is round, and the face is short and broad. The frontal bone is prominent, and the bridge of the nose is depressed and saddle-shaped. The nose is small, and the nasolabial folds are well developed. The eyes are somewhat bulging. The mandible and the chin are underdeveloped and infantile, and the teeth, which erupt late, are frequently crowded. The neck is short and the larynx is small. The voice is high-pitched and remains high after puberty. The extremities are well proportioned, with small hands and feet. The genitals are usually underdeveloped for the child's age, and sexual maturation may be delayed or absent. Facial, axillary, and pubic hair usually is lacking, and the scalp hair is fine. Length is mainly affected, giving todders a pudgy apearance.

Acquired Hypopituitarism :

Sexual maturation fails to take place or regresses if already present. There may be atrophy of the gonads and genital tract with amenorrhea and loss of pubic and axillary hair. There is a tendency to hypoglycemia. Growth shows dramatically.

79. Ans.— D. 20th week of gestation

80. Ans.— A. Triiodothyronine

81. Ans.— B. Coarctation of aorta

- **Turner's syndrome is commonly associated with congenital heart diseases.**
- **The most common anomaly associated is bicuspid Aortic valves in one third to one half of the patients (50%)**

Other congenital anomalies associated with Turner's syndrome

- **Aortic coarctation (30%)**
- **Aortic stenosis**
- **Mitral valve prolapse**
- **Anomalous pulmonary venous drainage**

ALL INDIA MD ENTRANCE EXAMINATION
(Conducted by AIIMS)
(By Dr. M.S. Bhatia & Kaur)

- First bok with **explanatory** answer to MCQ's of PG Entrance Examination.
- Contains original solved uptodate papers from 1988 onwards.
- Book is **subjectwise** and **year-wise** arranged.
- Each answer is **referenced** to the pages of standard textbook of each subject which also indicates the usefulness fo the book for this examination.
- **Explanation to each MCQ** contains very important information of a particular subject around a MCQ.
- **Important tips** for preparing and useful **references,** examination wise are also indicated in the beginning and also at the start of each chapter
- **Errata** in question bank is given in the beginning of each chapter.
- Always read this book along with papers of **AIIMS MD Entrance Exam** (given in a separate book by Dr. M.S. Bhatia) because the question bank for these two exams are the same.
- Suited for **Quick** revision after reading a particular subject.
- All suggestions are welcome and write to **Dr. M.S. Bhatia,** D-1, Naraina Vihar, New Delhi-110 028.

12

IMPORTANT TEXT OF MISCELLANEOUS

TUMORS COMMON IN CHILDHOOD

0—4 years	*5—9 years*	*10—14 years*
Leukemia	Leukemia	
Retinoblastoma	Retinoblastoma	
Neuroblastoma	Neuroblastoma	
Wilm's tumour	Hepatoblastoma	Hepatocarcinoma
Hepatoblastoma		
Soft tissue sarcoma (esp. rhabdomyosarcoma)	Soft tissue sarcoma	Soft tissue sarcoma
Teratomas	CNS tumors	Osteogenic sarcoma
CNS tumors	Ewing's tumor	Thyroid carcinoma
	Lymphoma	Hodgkin's disease Carcinoma of colon

EXAMPLES OF AUTOSOMAL DOMINANT DISORDERS

System	*Principle clinical features*
Skeletal and connective tissue	
Achondroplasia	Large head, short stature and short limbs
Marfan's syndrome	Tall stature, lens dislocation and aortic aneurysm
Osteogenesis imperfecta	Brittle bones, blue sclerac and deafness
Malformations	
Apert's syndrome	Craniosynostosis and syndactyly
Holt-Oram syndrome	Atrial septal defect and thumb abnormality
Noonan's syndrome	Pulmonary stenosis, ptosis and neck webbing
Phakomatosis	
Neurofibromatosis	Cafe-au-lait patches and neurofibromata
Tuberous sclerosis	Adenoma sebaceum and depigmented naevi
Neurological	
Huntington's chorea	Adult onset chorea and dementia
Myotonic dystrophy	Myotonia, muscle weakness and wasting
Peroneal muscular atrophy	Distal muscle weakness and wasting
Gastrointestinal	
Peutz-Jeghers syndrome	Oral freckling and intestinal polyps
Polyposis coli.	Intestinal polyps, and high risk of malignancy
Haematological and metabolic	
Familial hypercholesterolaemia	Xanthomata and coronary artery disease
Spherocytosis	Mild haemolysis
Von Willebrand's disease	Haemorrhage and factor-VIII deficiency
Renal	
Adult polycystic kidney disease	Renal cysts and renal failure
Alport's syndrome (some forms)	Nephritis and deafness

INBORN ERRORS OF METABOLISM

Disease Enzyme deficiency

Aminoacidurias :

	Disease		Enzyme deficiency
*	Phenylketonuria	—	Phenylalanine hydroxylase
*	Variant of phenylketonuria	—	Dihydropteridine
*	Hereditary tyrosinemia	—	p-hydroxyphenylpyruvic acid oxidase
*	Homocystinuria	—	Cystathione synthetase
*	Cystathioninemia	—	Cystathionase
*	Maple syrup urine disease	—	Not known
*	Histidinemia	—	Histidase
*	Oatshouse urine disease	—	Methionine malabsorption
*	Hartnup disease	—	Tryptophan

Carbohydrate Metabolism :

	Disease		Enzyme deficiency
*	von Gierke's disease	—	Glucose-6-phosphatase
*	Pompe's disease	—	Acid maltase
*	Cori or Forbe's disease	—	Amylo-1,6-glycosidase (debranching enzyme)
*	Andersen disease	—	Amylo (1,4,1,6) transglucosidase (branching enzyme)
*	McArdle's disease	—	Muscle phosphorylase
*	Hers' disease	—	Liver phosphorylase
*	Tarui's disease	—	Phosphofructokinase
*	Fabry's disease	—	a-galactosidase
*	Gaucher's disease	—	Glucocebrosidase
*	Niemann-Pick's disease	—	Sphingomylinase
*	Tay-Sach's disease	—	Hexosaminidase-A
*	Sandhoff disease	—	Hexosaminidase-A & B
*	Metachromatic leukodystrophy	—	Arylsulfatase-A
*	Kraffe leukodystrophy	—	Galactocerebroidase

Mucopolysaccharide Disorders :

	Disease		Enzyme deficiency
*	Hurler's syndrome	—	α-L-Iduronidase
*	Scheie's syndrome	—	α-L-Iduronidase
*	Hunter's syndrome	—	Iduronate-sulfate sulfatase
*	Sanfilippo-A	—	Heparan-N-sulfaminidase
*	Sanfilippo-B	—	N-Acetyl-α-Dglucosaminidase
*	Sanfilippo-C	—	Acetyl-CoA-Glucosaminide-N-acetyltransferase
*	Sanfilippo-D	—	N-Acetyl-glucosamine-6-sulfatase
*	Morquio-A	—	Galactosamine-6-sulfatesulfatase
*	Maroteaux-Lamy	—	Arylsulfatase B
*	Sly syndrome	—	β-gluuronidase

Lipoproteinemias :

	Type		Raised levels of
*	Type-I	—	Chylomicrons
*	Type-IIa	—	LDL (β type)
*	Type-IIb	—	LDL (β) & VLDL (pre-β)
*	Type-III	—	Mostly LDL & some VLDL
*	Type-IV	—	VLDL (pre-β)
*	Type-V	—	Chylomicrons & VLDL

Miscellaneous Metabolic Disorders :

* Galactosemia	—	Galactose-1-phosphate Uridyl transferase
* Albinism	—	Tyrosinase
* Lesh-Nyhan syndrome	—	Hypoxanthine Guanine phosphoribosyl transferase
* Refsum's disease	—	Phytic acid malabsorption
* Orotic aciduria	—	Pyrimidine metabolism
* Gout	—	Purine metabolism

NORMAL ODOUR OF URINE IN AMINO ACID METABOLIC DISORDER

* Mousy or musty odour	—	Phenylketonuria
* Maple syrup odour	—	Maple syrup urine disease
* Tomcat urine odour	—	β-Methylcrotomyl-glycinuria
* Rotten fish odour	—	Trimethylaminuria
* Cabbage odour	—	Methionine malabsorption
* Rancid, fishy or cabbage	—	Tyrosinemia
* Hoplike odour	—	Oatshouse disease
* Swimming pool odour	—	Hawkinsinuria
* Sweaty feet odour	—	Glutaric acidemia (type-II) & Isovaleric acidemia

MCQ's OF MISCELLANEOUS

What is Important in Miscellaneous

Leukemias, Lymphomas, Syndromes (Down's Klinefelter's, Turner's), Neuroblastoma, Phenylketonuria, Maple Syrup Disease, Homocystinuria, Common Poisonings, Drugs (uses, side effects, teratogenicity)

1. A 3 years old child is poor in language development and has poor concentration, no friends, plays only with himself, and has some delay in milestones. The likely diagnosis is: AIIMS 2007
A. ADHD
B. Autism
C. Specific learning disorder
D. Normal for age

2. The karyotype of a patient with Androgen Insensitivity Syndrome is : AI 2005
A. 46 XX B. 46 XY
C. 47 XXY D. 45 XO

3. Enzyme replacement therapy is available for which of the following disorders : AIIMS 2006
A. Gaucher's disease
B. Niemann Pick disease
C. Mucolipidosis
D. Metachromatic leukodystrophy

4. At what gestation does the switchover from fetal to adult hemoglobin synthesis begin : AIIMS 2005
A. 30 weeks B. 36 weeks
C. 7 days postnatal D. 3 weeks postnatal

5. A 5 years old child is rushed to casualty reportedly electrocuted while playing in a park. The child is apneic and is ventilated with bag and mask. There are burns on each hand. What will be the next step in the management: AIIMS 2005
A. Check pulses
B. Start chest compressions
C. Intubate
D. Check oxygen saturation

6. Characteristic clinical picture of Maple syrup urine disease is : AMC 1983
A. Choreoathetosis B. Flaccid paralysis
C. Petitmal disorder D. Decerebrate rigidity

7. Abetalipoproteinemia is first manifested clinically by : PGI 1980
A. Hypohydrosis B. Tremors
C. Steatorrhoea D. Convulsions

8. Episodic coma and vomiting are most frequently identified with : AIIMS 1980
A. Histidinemia B. Hyperammonemia
C. Homocystinuria D. Hyperlysinemia

9. Skin manifestations of Hartnup disease most closely resemble withthose of : UPSC 1983
A. Psoriasis B. Pityriasis rosea
C. Pellagra D. Rubella

10. Scalded skin syndrome (Ritter's disease) of newborn is associated with : PGI 1980
A. Riboflavin deficiency
B. Maternal diabetes
C. Staphylococcal infection
D. None of the above

11. Children with squints need to be referred to eye specialists if they persist : AMC 1982
A. Beyond 3 months of age
B. Beyond 6 months of age
C. No need to refer
D. It is a normal phenomenon

12. Acrodermatitis enteropathica has the following features except : AIIMS 1980
A. Alopecia and Diarrhoea
B. Occurs in new born children
C. Bullous lesions
D. Skin biopsy is diagnostic

13. Enamel hypoplasia is not associated with : AIIMS 1981
A. Cerebral palsy B. Nephrosis
C. Rubella D. Gardner's syndrome

14. A non-neural cause of scoliosis and kyphoscoliosis : CMC 1983
A. Arthrogryposis B. Klippel-Feil syndrome
C. Neurofibromatosis D. Syringomyelia

Ans.										
	1. B	2. B	3. A	4. B	5. A	6. D	7. C	8. B	9. C	10. C
	11. B	12. C	13. D	14. B						

15. What is not true of classical Niemann Pick's disease : AIIMS 1981
A. Infantile convulsions
B. Mascular degeneration
C. Hepatosplenomegaly
D. Partial blindness

16. Commonest cause of chronic arthritis in children is: Delhi 1992
A. Rheumatic fever
B. Rheumatic arthritis
C. Gout
D. Juvenile rheumatoid arthritis

17. The blast cell of acute lymphocytic leukemia in childhood contain : AIIMS 1986; AI 1993
A. Surface antigen
B. CALLA Ag +ve
C. Antibodies on WBCs
D. Excessive mitochondria

18. Which is not a complication of varicella infection in childhood : AIIMS 1987; AI 1993
A. Enteritis B. Encephalitis
C. Bronchopneumonia D. Herpes

19. In a child to examine the fundus, used is : AI 1993
A. 1% Atropinc ointment B. Homatropine
C. Atropine drops D. Phenyl epherine

20. Following are Tumors of first decade of life except : AIIMS 1992
A. Retinoblastoma B. Neuroblastoma
C. Rhabdomyosarcoma D. Amyloblastoma

21. Semipurposive movements in a boy is seen in : Delhi 1986; AIIMS 1992
A. SLE B. Rheumatic fever
C. Brain abscess D. Encephalitis

22. Serum alpha feto protein is decreased in : AIIMS 1990, 92
A. Down's syndrome B. Spina bifida
C. Intra-Uterine death D. Exomphalos

23. Recovery in T.B. Spine is delayed in children because of : AIIMS 1992
A. Increased vascularity B. Fragile bone
C. Cartilage is more D. Inadequate rest

24. Normal height with decreased bone age is seen in : PGI 1993
A. Cushing's syndrome B. Hypothyroidism
C. Thanatotrophic dwarfs D. Down's syndrome

25. The most common complication of long term-IV fluids in a comatose child is : JIPMER 1993
A. Overhydration B. Hyponatremia.
C. Hyperkalaemia D. Hypothermia

26. Bone age is normal in : AIIMS 1992
A. Genetic short stature B. Hypopituitarism
C. Hypothyroidism D. Emotional deprivation

27. Which of the following is not a feature of lead poisoning : AMU 1986
A. Convulsions
B. Renal Colic
C. Abdominal pain
D. Weariness and irritability

28. Which of the following childhood malignancies has highest cure rate : AMU 1986
A. Wilm's tumour B. Neuroblastoma
C. Retinoblastoma D. Rhabdomyosarcoma

29. Hereditary disorders associated with cirrhosis include all except : AMU 1986
A. Amyloidosis B. Galactosemia
C. Cystic fibrosis D. Wilson's disease

30. Treatment of choice for salicylate intoxications is intravenous : AMU 1984
A. BAL B. Calcium gluconate
C. Sodium bicarbonate D. Sodium chloride

31. Specific antidote for opiate poisoning is : DNB 1990
A. Atropine B. Nalorphine
C. Versenate D. BAL

32. Antidote for muscarine poisoning is : DNB 1991
A. Sodium benzoat B. Thiocynate
C. Atropine D. BAL

33. If the odour of bitter almonds is noted in breath, the following is suspected : AIIMS 1981
A. Plumbism
B. Arsenic poisoning
C. Atropine poisoning
D. Cyanide poisoning

34. Poisoning with antihistaminic may resemble : BHU 1986
A. Plumbism B. Atropine poisoning
C. Salicylate intoxication D. Flavism

35. Atropine poisoning may cause all, except : Kerala 1991
A. Fever B. Flushing
C. Strabismus D. Visual disturbances

36. A 15-months old child with erythematous rash, diagnosed as otitis media and prescribed ampicillin 6 hours later, child became irritable and uncooperative and developed diffuse erythematous rash, some of which do not blanch on pressure. Ear showed dull tympanic membranes. Next treatment is: MAHE 1998
A. Continue I/V ampicillin
B. Substitute ampicillin with cotrimoxazole
C. Order LP
D. Prescribe diphenylhydantoin

37. Common manifestations of Reye's Syndrome include each of the following except : AIIMS 1987
A. Hepatomegaly B. Vomiting
C. Convulsions D. Marked jaundice

Ans.									
15. A	16. D	17. B	18. A	19. A	20. D	21. B	22. A	23. D	24. B
25. D	26. A	27. B	28. A	29. A	30. C	31. B	32. C	33. D	34. B
35. C	36. B	37. D							

38. In infants, eczema generally starts on the : **AIIMS 1987**

A. Face B. Trunk
C. Arms D. Scalp

39. In chronic lead poisoning there is an increased urinary excretion of : **AMU 1988**

A. Bile B. Coproporphyrin-III
C. Urobilinogen D. Porphobilinogen

40. A useful agent in treatment of methanol poisoning would be : **Delhi 1982**

A. Ethanol B. KMnO4
C. Na citrate D. Vit. B_{12}

41. Permanent joint damage may result from at except : **CMC 1987**

A. Hemophilia
B. Still's disease
C. Tuberculosis
D. Henoch-Schonlein syndrome

42. Henoch-Schonlein Syndrome is associated with : **AIIMS 1986**

A. Mitral stenosis
B. Glomerulonephritis
C. Tuberculosis
D. Thrombocytopenic purpura

43. The following karyotypes are appropriate except : **DNB 1989**

A. 45, XO 46, XX—Turner mosaic
B. 47, XX—13—Patau's syndrome
C. 46, XY—Noonan's syndrome
D. 47, XYY—Klinefelter's syndrome
E. 45, XX, t (14q21q)—normal female phenotype

44. Aspirin is to be avoided in a child for fear of : **Bihar 1998**

A. Duodenal ulceration
B. Hypothermia
C. Electrolyte abnormalities
D. Possible association with Reye's syndrome

45. Drugs secreted in breast milk is clinically significant levels include all, except : **AIIMS 1981**

A. Cascara B. Metronidazole
C. Bromides D. Codeine

46. Acute potassium deficits may produce all, except : **Rohtak 1984**

A. Abdominal distension
B. Muscle paresis and ileus
C. Flattened and inverted T-waves
D. Nystagmus

47. Acute hyponatremia in 8 months infant may produce all, except : **Rohtak 1985**

A. Diarrhoea
B. Convulsions
C. Muscle cramps and weakness
D. Vascular collapse

48. The major toxicity of acetaminophen overdose involves : **AIIMS 1984**

A. CNS B. Heart
C. Liver D. Acid-base metabolism

49. In infants, the cause of blindness arising out of oxygen toxicity is : **UPSC 1997**

A. Degeneration of cystaline lens
B. Growth of blood vessels into vitreous followed by fibrosis
C. Damage to cornea
D. Enzymic defect in lens

50. The nicotinic effects of anticholinesterase (insecticide) would be diminished or reversed by prompt administration of : **DNB 1989**

A. PAM (Pyridine aldoxime methiodide)
B. Bicarbonate
C. Atropine
D. Acetylcysteine

51. The following is most diagnostic of Wilson's disease: **BHU 1986**

A. Kayser-Fleischer ring
B. Low level serum copper
C. Low serum ceruloplasmin
D. Raised SGPT

52. Wilson's disease is characterised by the accumulation of copper in : **AMC 1986**

A. Brain B. Kidney
C. Lung D. All of the above

53. William's syndrome includes all the following except: **AMU 1987**

A. Small mandible
B. Sharp upturned nose
C. Prominent maxilla
D. Upward slanting of eyes

54. Commonest malignancy in a child is : **UPSC 1987; Delhi 1993**

A. Retinoblastoma B. Renal cell carcinoma
C. Neuroblastoma D. Leukemias

55. Commonest congenital disease in a child is : **DNB 1990; Delhi 1993**

A. Down's syndrome B. Klinefelter's syndrome
C. Turner's syndrome D. Cri du chat disease

56. "Radius Hypoplasia" comes under the terminology of : **UPSC 1980**

A. Phocomelia B. Amelia
C. Hemimelia D. Poromelia

57. Discoloured teeth may result from the use of : **Delhi 1983**

A. Streptomycin B. Penicillin
C. Tetracycline D. Sulfonamide

Ans.										
	38. A	39. B	40. A	41. D	42. B	43. D	44. D	45. D	46. D	47. A
	48. C	49. B	50. A	51. A	52. D	53. D	54. D	55. A	56. A	57. C

58. Congenital laxity of ligaments is : PGI 1982, 89, 99

A. Linked with birth trauma
B. Extremely common
C. Transmitted as dominant trait
D. Not treated with steroids

59. Cloidocranial dysostosis is characterized by all, except : PGI 1986, 99

A. Absence of clavicles
B. Huge fontanelles
C. Death by time of puberty
D. Transmitted as a dominant

60. Bone most commonly involved in tuberculous lesions of the : Delhi 1984, 87, 94

A. Humerus B. Femur
C. Sternum D. Vertebra

61. Marfan's syndrome includes : DNB 1989

A. Anophthalmia B. Luxation of lens
C. Spastic muscles D. Congenital dwarfism

62. A hypertensive child presents with hypokalemia, hypernatremia, metabolic acidosis. The hypokalemia is unaffected by potassium therapy but responding to salt restriction should be suspected of having : UPSC 1984

A. Hyperparathyroidism B. Hyperaldosteronism
C. Cushing's syndrome D. Adrenal adenoma

63. Which one of the following is not a common finding in juvenile rheumatoid arthritis: CSE 1997

A. Subcutaneous nodules
B. Fever
C. Symmetrical involvement of joints
D. Splenomegaly

64. In foetus, HbA first appears at ——weeks : Rajasthan 1998

A. 16 B. 24
C. 28 D. 32

65. The APT test is : Bihar 1988

A. Crude test for carbon monoxide
B. Semiquantitative test for foetal haemoglobin
C. Semiquantitative test for lead poisoning
D. Screening test for haemoglobin 'S'
E. None of these

66. Which is not a characteristic of lead poisoning ? UPSC 1983

A. Anaemia B. Jaundice
C. Paraesthesia D. Ataxia

67. Mongolian spots in a neonate are most common over : AIIMS 1987

A. Chest B. Face
C. Back D. Upper extremities
E. Lower extremities

68. Which one of the following is usually associated with trisomy 18 syndrome: AIIMS 1985, 86

A. Polydactyly
B. Prominent occiput
C. Micrognathia
D. Cleft palate and hare lip
E. Low set ears

69. In a 70 kg human the amount of sodium (Na+) present in human body is 105 gm, then what should be the level/quantity of potassium (K+)? Bihar 1990

A. 105 gms B. 105 mgs
C. 245 gms D. 5 mg only

70. Sweaty feet syndrome is associated with : DNB 1989

A. Isovaleric acidemia
B. Hypophosphatasia
C. Phenylalanine deficiency
D. Branched chain ketonuria

71. Which of the following skin disorders is usually associated with neurofibromatosis: DNB 1989

A. Cafe-au-lait spots B. Pellagra rash
C. Eczema D. Areas of vitiligo

72. Treatment of Type-1 glycogen storage disease should include all, except : AIIMS 1984, 85

A. Routine immunizations
B. Oral bicarbonate
C. Atleast one quart of milk of a day
D. Feeding every 3-4 hours around the clock

73. Which of the following does not belong to trisomy : AIIMS 1986

A. Down's syndrome
B. Patau's syndrome
C. Edward's syndrome
D. Pendred's syndrome

74. Infantile body proportions are seen in each of the following conditions except : AIIMS 1985, 86

A. Cretinism B. Achondroplasia
C. Bowed legs D. Malnutrition

75. All of the following are the causes of hypokalemia except : AIIMS 1987

A. Diarrhoea B. Sweating
C. Duodenal fistula D. Essential hypertension

76. Lowe's syndrome is characterized by all the following except : AIIMS 1987

A. Aminoaciduria B. Phosphaturia
C. Mild jaundice D. Undescended testis

77. Sodium excretion of Rota virus diarrhoea is over : AIIMS 1987, 88

A. 20 meq/L B. 60 meq/L
C. 120 meq/L D. 150 meq/L

Ans. 58. D 59. C 60. D 61. B 62. B 63. D 64. C 65. B 66. B 67. C
68. D 69. C 70. A 71. A 72. C 73. D 74. B 75. D 76. D 77. B
78. B

78. In Mc Ardle's disease (Type-V glycogenesis), enzyme deficient is : PGI 1988

A. Liver phosphorylase
B. Muscle phosphorylase
C. Glucose-6-phosphatase
D. Glucose, 1,6 phosphatase
E. 2, 3 DPG

79. Nuchal mass is seen in : Rajasthan 1998

A. Klinefelter's syndrome
B. Trisomy 21
C. Cri du chat syndrome
D. Fregoli syndrome

80. Surfactant synthesis starts at ———weeks : Rajasthan 1998

A. 24 B. 28
C. 32 D. 36

81. In Galactosemia-enzyme deficiency seen is : PGI 1990

A. Galactokinase B. Epimerase
C. GALT D. Phosphoglycomutase
E. All of the above

82. Following are features of Turner's syndrome except: Delhi 1998

A. Tall stature
B. Cubitus valgus
C. Gonadal dysgenesis
D. Broad chest with wide spaced nipples

83. The intake of steroids during pregnancy is associated with : AIIMS 1989; ESI 1989, 90

A. Cardiovascular anomalies
B. Cleft palate
C. GIT abnormalities
D. Anencephaly

84. Respiratory acidosis is more common in : Delhi 1989

A. Asthma B. Hyperventillation
C. Aspirin poisoning D. Pyloric stenosis

85. Maximum fluid requirement per body area is in : Delhi 1981, 88

A. First week B. 1-4 weeks
C. 4-12 weeks D. 24 weeks

86. The fall in calcium concentration is seen in : Delhi 1988

A. Respiratory acidosis B. Respiratory alkalosis
C. Metabolic alkalosis D. Metabolic acidosis

87. Anabolic steroids are not prescribed in a child because it causes : PGI 1986; Delhi 1990

A. Hirsutism
B. Precocious puberty
C. Delay in Growth
D. Premature closure of epiphysis

88. The malignancies of childhood include following except : PGI 1987, 89

A. ALL B. Wilm's tumour
C. Retinoblastoma D. AML

89. Visceromegaly, microcephaly with blood sugar below 20 mg/dl with sinusitis is : Orissa 1998

A. Prader Willi syndrome
B. Beckwith Wiedemann syndrome
C. Alport syndrome
D. Cockyne syndrome

90. Streptococcal vaginitis in a child is treated with : AIIMS 1984; Kerala 1986, 87

A. Systemic penicillin B. Local gentian violet
C. Estrogens D. Penicillin and estrogens

91. The commonest causative organism in osteomyelitis is : UPSC 1989

A. Streptococcus B. Staphylococcus
C. Tubercular bacillus D. Spirochete of aphilis
E. Pseudomonas

92. All of the following are associated with increased bone age except : Kerala 1998

A. Congenital adrenal hyperplasia
B. Gonadal tumours
C. Turner's syndrome
D. Polyostotic dysplasia

93. Phenylketonuria is diagnosed by : AMC 1986; AI 1988

A. Guthrie test B. Ferric chloride test
C. Gerhard's test D. VMA in urine

94. A child comes with migratory polyarthritis, the investigation of choice to confirm the diagnosis would be : AIIMS 1986, 87

A. Pharyngeal swab for culture and sensitivity
B. ASLO titre
C. ESR
D. ECG

95. Children under five years of age with joint pain may have following except : AIIMS 1983, 98

A. Growing pains B. Leukemia
C. Neuroblastoma D. Rheumatoid arthritis

96. Fructose is not used for IV infusion as it causes : AIIMS 1989, 90

A. Thrombosis
B. Reactive hyperglycemia
C. Hyperosmolarity
D. Lactic acidosis

97. Serum cholesterol is high in all except : AIIMS 1982

A. Kwashiorkar
B. Diabetes mellitus
C. Primary biliary cirrhosis
D. Nephrotic syndrome

Ans.										
	79. B	80. A	81. A	82. A	83. B	84. A	85. B	86. B	87. D	88. D
	89. B	90. D	91. B	92. C	93. A	94. B	95. A	96. D	97. A	

98. Epiphyseal dysgenesis is a pathognomonic feature of: **AMU 1984; AIIMS 1982, 86**

A. Hypoparathyroidism B. Hyperparathyroidism
C. Hypothyroidism D. All of the above

99. In the management of a child unconscious from poisoning, the first thing to do is to : **AIIMS 1983, 87**

A. Establish airways
B. Take detailed history
C. Blood for chemical analysis
D. Gastric washout

100. Rickets with hearing loss occur in all except : **WB 1994**

A. Engleman disease B. Jeune syndrome
C. Marfan syndrome D. Marble bone disease

101. Pamityl Lecithin is a component of : **AIIMS 1993**

A. Surfactant B. Sweat
C. Meconium D. Conjunctival secretion

102. A 2-years old child comes with loose motions and vomiting. On examination, he is found to have severe dehydration with peripheral circulatory failure. As an emergency treatment, the child should be given : **UPSC 1994**

A. Ringer's lactage B. Whole blood
C. Normal saline D. 5% dextrose-saline

103. The presence of alpha-fetoprotein in the amniotic fluid without neural or intestinal defects is diagnostic of : **UPSC 1994**

A. Congenital idiopathic nephrotic syndrome
B. Down's syndrome
C. Hyaline membrane disease
D. Congenital rubella syndrome

104. High-arched palate, micrognathia and glossoptosis are features of : **UPSC 1994**

A. Pierre Robin syndrome
B. Treacher Collin's syndrome
C. Laurence-Moon-Biedl syndrome
D. McCune-Albright syndrome

105. Retinopathy of prematurity is caused by : **UPSC 1994**

A. Hypoxia B. Neonatal conjunctivitis
C. Oxygen therapy D. Hypoglycaemia

106. A female child aged 3 years is brought in well past mid-night with a history of not sleeping and crying continuously. No other symptom is given by the mother. On examination, the child is of average build with no systemic symptoms like fever, vomiting, cough or breathlessness or fits. No other systemic signs like neck rigidity or dehydration except scratch marks in and around congenital area with redness around without any generalised rash. What is the most probable diagnosis : **UPSC 1994**

A. Insect bites
B. Enterobious vermicularis infestation
C. Allergic rash
D. Napkin rash

107. Mucopolysaccharidosis (Hurler's Syndrome) is characterised by all of the following except : **UPSC 1994**

A. Hepatosplenomegaly B. Corneal clouding
C. Skin lesions D. Mental retardation

108. A child with uveitis and joint pain should be investigated for : **AI 1994**

A. Rheumatoid arthritis B. SLE
C. Systemic sclerosis D. Cretinism

109. Which is not used in ORS : **Kerala 1994**

A. Na+ B. K+
C. Glucose with salt D. Glucose without salt

110. A child usually gets atropine poisoning from : **PGI 1993**

A. Atropine eye drops
B. Ingestion of belladonna
C. Atropic inject. induced accidentally
D. Overdose & Atropine in organosphosphorus poisoning

111. The cause of osteomalacia is : **PGI 1994**

A. Phenytoin B. Malabsorption
C. Cushing's syndrome D. Vincristine

112. Bilateral edema of legs in children is seen in : **PGI 1994**

A. Turner's syndrome
B. Meig's syndrome
C. Haemorrhagic diathesis
D. Down's syndrome

113. Marfan's syndrome is characterised by : **AI 1993**

A. Tortuous aorta B. Venous thrombosis
C. Mitral incompetence D. Aortic root dilatation

114. Uric acid levels estimation in children is required in: **AP 1994**

A. Pica B. Self-mutilation
C. Episodic vomiting D. Hepatosplenomegaly

115. In Laurence Moon Biedl syndrome, not true is : **PGI 1996**

A. Pigmentary degeneration
B. Obesity
C. Mental retardation
D. Retinal detachment

Ans. 98. C 99. A 100. A 101. A 102. A 103. A 104. A 105. C 106. B 107. C
108. A 109. D 110. B 111. A 112. D 113. D 114. B 115. A

116. Osteogenesis imperfecta is : **PGI 1996**

A. Autosomal dominant B. Autosomal recessive
C. Both A & B D. None of the above

117. True about Still's disease is all except : **AIIMS 1996**

A. Evanescent rash
B. Rheumatoid factor '+' ve
C. Kidney
D. Sacroilitis rare in monopauciarticular onset

118. A child is advised admission to a hospital in following condition, except : **AI 1997**

A. Fever 39°C B. Cyanosis
C. Refusal to feed D. Indrawing chest wall

119. Interstitial keratitis in an 8 years old girl can occur in all of the following conditions except : **UPSC 1996**

A. Tuberculosis B. Leprosy
C. Filaria D. Syphilis

120. An infant is crying excessively even after being given good feed. He is passing a large quantitiy of urine and repeatedly getting dehydrated. Urine examination shows no proteinuria and a specific gravity of 1004. The most likely diagnosis is: **UPSC 1996**

A. Diabetes mellitus
B. Diabetes insipidus
C. Congenital nephrotic syndrome
D. Protein losing enteropathy

121. Match List-I (Poisoning) with List-II (Anti-dotes in paediatric practice) and select the correct answer using the codes given below the lists : **UPSC 1996**

List -I	List-II
A. Morphine	1. Diphenhydramine
B. Cyanide	2. Pralidoxime
C. Organophosphorus compounds	3. Desferoxamine
D. Atropine	4. Amylnitrate
	5. Narcan
	6. Physostigmine

Codes :

	A	B	C	D
A.	5	4	1	3
B.	4	1	2	6
C.	5	4	2	6
D.	4	2	5	3

122. A six-months old infant fed totally on cow's milk has been brought with bleeding spots, anaemia, fever and generalised tenderness. On examination, there were swellings in both the lower extremities and the blood count was normal. The most likely diagnosis is : **UPSC 1996**

A. Arthritis B. Poliomyelitis
C. Osteomyelitis D. Scurvy

123. Match List-I with List-II and select the correct answer using the codes given below the lists : **UPSC 1996**

List-I	List-II
A. Craniopharyngioma	1. Kidney
B. Wilm's tumour	2. Adrenal medulla
C. Neuroblastoma	3. Pituitary
D. Ewing's tumour	4. Bone

Codes :

	A	B	C	D
A.	2	1	3	4
B.	2	4	3	1
C.	3	4	2	1
D.	3	1	2	4

124. Corrigan line is seen in : **Delhi 1996**

A. Measles B. Rubella
C. Lead poisoning D. Copper poisoning

125. In pica, the deficiency of ----------- is implicated : **Delhi 1996**

A. Zinc B. Iron
C. Calcium D. Selenium

126. In CMV infection, drug of choice is : **Delhi 1996**

A. Acyclovir B. Ribavarine
C. Ganciclovir D. Amantadine

127. Death in malnourished children can be due to any one of the following codes : **TNPSC 1997**

I. Hyperglycemia
II. Infections
III. Hypothermia
IV. Dyselectrolytemia

Codes :

A. I alone is correct
B. I and III are correct
C. II, III and IV are correct
D. All are correct

128. Long term complication of steroids in child would be : **JIPMER 1998**

A. Arthralgia
B. Posterior subcapsular cataract
C. Pigmentation
D. Osteoarthritis

129. Earliest manifestation of Alport's disease is : **AIIMS 1997**

A. Microscopic haematuria
B. Proteinuria
C. Oliguria
D. Sensori neural deafness

Ans. 116. C 117. A 118. A 119. C 120. D 121. C 122. D 123. D 124. D 125. B
126. C 127. C 128. B 129. A

130. A neonate normal till 5 days of age suddenly threw a seizure and developed irritability with refusal to feed, recurrent hypoglycemia, ketonuria, metabolic acidosis. He could be suffering from : AIIMS 1999

A. Organic aciduria B. Metabolic acidosis
C. Phenylketonuria D. Alkaptonuria

131. The child of a mother having phenylketonuria with uncontrolled phenylalanine in blood can develop : AIIMS 1999

A. Phenylketonuria
B. Blond hair with MR
C. MR with cataract
D. Microcephaly, mental retardation and cardiac defects

132. 31 weeks pregnant lady delivered, within 4 hours baby developed dyspnoea. X-ray shows ground glass appearance and cyanosis, disease is : AIIMS 1999

A. HMD
B. Esophageal atresia
C. Muconium aspiration
D. Tracheoesophageal fistula

133. 3 years old girl's parents complains of her not eating anything. Weight 11 Kg (50 percentile), height 88 cm (75 percentile). What should be done : AIIMS 1999

A. Vitamin Tablets
B. Nothing should be done
C. Forceful eating
D. Complete investigation for UTI

134. HIV mother delivers a baby, all are true except : AIIMS 1999

A. Risk of HIV upto 90%.
B. Not able to diagnose in new born by routine investigation.
C. Maximum chance of transmission in perinatal period.
D. None of the above.

135. A boy comes with c/o vomiting, bloated abd, pain abd, H/o attended ice cream eating competition, H/o similar episodes in past is due to deficiency of : AIIMS 1999

A. Lactase B. Maltase
C. Salivary amylase D. Saccharidase

136. About Down's syndrome, following are true except : AIIMS 1999

A. Decreased Nuchal fold thickness
B. Decreased femur length
C. Decreased humerus length
D. Duodenal atresia

137. Commonest tumor of face in children is : PGI 1999

A. Rhabdomyosarcoma B. Sq. cell carcinoma
C. Basal cell carcinoma D. Mixed parotid tumor

138. Most common cause of dwarfism in children is : PGI 1999

A. Familial B. Hypothyroidism
C. Hypopituitarism D. Constitutional

139. Taste perception of baby develops at : TN 1999

A. Birth B. 4 months
C. 6 months D. 8 months

140. Deafness is a complication of : Kerala 1999

A. Congenital syphilis
B. Late tertiary syphilis
C. Both a & b
D. None of above

141. The age of onset of Juvenile RA is before : Kerala 1999

A. 8 yrs B. 12 yrs
C. 13 yrs D. 16 yrs

142. Lazy left colon syndrome is seen in neonate with maternal : Kerala 1999

A. DM
B. Rubella
C. Hirchsprung's disease
D. All of the above

143. Best location for intradural instillation of medication in a child is between : Kerala 1999

A. L1, L2 B. L2, L3
C. L3, L4 D. L4, L5

144. Juvenile rheumatoid arthritis is arthritis before the age of —— years : Kerala 1999

A. 8 B. 12
C. 15 D. 16

145. Seen in systemic onset JRA except : AI 2000

A. Rheumatoid factor positive
B. Hepatosplenomegaly
C. Fever
D. HLA B27

146. An infant of phenylketonuria presents at 3 weeks, all are true except : AI 2000

A. Start diet therapy immediately with complete restriction of phenylalanine.
B. There will be increased blood phenylalanine and urine phenylacetate levels.
C. Tyrosine is an essential amino acid.
D. It is diagnosed after institution of protein diet.

Ans. 130. A 131. B 132. A 133. B 134. A 135. A 136. A 137. A 138. D 139. A
140. C 141. D 142. A 143. D 144. D 145. A 146. A

147. Match List-I (Maternal medication) with List-II (Fetal effect) and select the correct answer using the codes given below the Lists: UPSC 2000

List-I	List-II
A. Vit. D	1. Supravalvular aortic stenosis
B. Steroids	2. Cleft palate
C. Imipramine	3. Limb deformities
D. Thiazide diuretic	4. Skeletal defect
	5. Neonatal bleeding

Codes:

	A	B	C	D
A.	2	1	3	4
B.	1	4	2	5
C.	3	2	4	1
D.	1	2	3	5

148. Ochronosis, Arthritis, Darkening of urine on standing and high incidence of heart disease are features of : UPSC 2000

A. Alkaptonuria B. Hartnup disease
C. Homocystinuria D. Phenyl Ketonuria

149. In Ringer lactate, which is not present : JIPMER 2000

A. Na+ B. K+
C. HCO3- D. Cl-

150. Maternal antenatal exposure to which of the following drugs can cause neural tube defects in the child : Kerala 2000

A. Corticosteroids B. Clomiphene
C. Vitamin-D D. Quinine
E. Propranolol

151. The following does not occur with Duchenne and Becker Muscular Dystrophy except : Kerala 2000

A. Poor head control in infancy may be the first sign of weakness.
B. The disease of rarely symptomatic at birth or in early infancy.
C. It is inherited as an X-linked recessive trait.
D. Cardiomyopathy is a constant feature of the disease
E. Death occurs usually in infancy.

152. Commonest cause of intestinal obstruction in Down's syndrome is : AIIMS 2000

A. Duodenal atresia B. Colonic atresia
C. Intestinal atresia D. Oesophageal atresia

153. A child with fever & sore throat developed acute cervical lymphadenopathy, most likely investigation to be done is : AIIMS 2000

A. Open biopsy of node
B. Neck X-ray
C. Radical neck dissection
D. Complete hemogram

154. A girl of 8 years suffering from vomiting and diarrhoea for last two days when punched on abdomen, skin goes back with seconds, is most likely to be suffering from : AIIMS 2000

A. Skin turgor cannot be commented
B. Some dehydration
C. Severe dehydration
D. No dehydration

155. Triple test for Down syndrome include all except : UP 1999, 2002

A. Oestriol estimation
B. Human placental lactogen
C. Karyotyping
D. Ultrasound

156. Iron poisoning in 4 years child, Rx includes : PGI 2000

A. Stomach lavage
B. Desferroxamine IV 100 mg
C. X-ray abdomen
D. Blood transfusion

157. A child presents with complaints of oliguria, abdominal distension and diarrhoea. On examination there is deep jaundice. Hepatomegaly was present measuring 4 cm below the costal margin. Conjugated bilirubin in blood was 38 mg/dL, and there was urine urobilinogen and bile pigments. Hemoglobin was 4 mg/dL and serum creatinine was 3 mg/dL. Which of the following tests is of least importance to diagnose in this case : AIIMS 2000

A. G-6-P-D level in blood
B. Serum ceruloplasmin
C. Reticulocyte count
D. Leptospiral antibody level

158. A child presents with complaints of abdominal colic and hematuria. USG showed a renal stone 2.5 cm in diameter in the renal pelvis. The next step in management of this case is : AIIMS 2000

A. ESWL
B. Pyelolithotomy
C. Nephroureterostomy
D. Conservative

Ans. 147. C 148. A 149. C 150. B 151. E 152. A 153. B 154. D 155. D 156. A 157. B 158. A

159. A five-years-old child of normal intelligence presents with features of hypotonia. On examination there was tongue fasciculations and he keeps his body in a frog like position. What is the most probable diagnosis : AIIMS 2000

A. Down's syndrome
B. Guillain Barre syndrome
C. Spinal muscular atrophy
D. Limb girdle atrophy

160. A five-years-old male child presents with complaints of fever and abdominal destension. He is having vomiting for the last five days. On examination there are 6—8 pus cell/hpf in urine. WBC count shows 78% neutrophils. What is the best line of management : AIIMS 2000

A. Send urine for culture and sensitivity and wait for results.
B. Send urine for culture and sensitivity and start I.V antibiotics immediately.
C. Send urine for culture, do an USG and start chloroquine.
D. Radio nucleotide studies.

161. A breast fed child presents with hypernatremia (serum, sodium > 170m Eq/L). His urine sodium is 70mEq/L. Which of the following is the most likely cause : AIIMS 2000

A. Diabetes insipidus
B. Acute necrosis
C. Severe dehydration
D. Excessive intake of sodium

162. Which of the following congenital malformation is seen in a child of a mother who is on treatment with oral anticoagulants : AIIMS 2000

A. Craniofacial malformations
B. Renal agenesis
C. Long bone defects
D. Chondrodysplasia punctata

163. A child presents with seborrheic dermatitis, lytic skull lesions, ear problem, hepatosplenomegaly, likely diagnosis is : AI 2001

A. Leukemia B. Lymphoma
C. Histioxytosis-X D. Porphyria

164. Treatment of kawasaki disease in children is : AI 2001

A. Oral steroids
B. IV steroids
C. IV Ig
D. Mycophenolate mefentil

165. A baby with refusal to feed, skin lesions, seizures, organic acids, lactic acidosis with normal ammonia. Diagnosis is : AI 2001

A. Isovoleric acidemia
B. Multiple carboxylase deficiency
C. Pripionic acidemia
D. Glutaric acidemia type-I

166. Which of the following is true about Ankylosing Spondylitis in children : Kerala 2001

A. Involvement of hip, ankles
B. Asymtric involvement
C. Uveitis & conduction defects
D. Incidence in infants

167. In the laboratory, for amplification of a single DNA chain, polymerase chain reaction was allowed to continue for 3 cycles. At the end of this, the number of DNA chains would be : AIIMS 2001

A. 4 B. 8
C. 16 D. 3

168. A 2-years boy with coarse facial features and hepatosplenomegaly showed tall QRS waves in the ECG. The diagnosis is most likely to be : AIIMS 2001

A. Glycogen storage disease type-II
B. Hurler's disease
C. Hunter's disease
D. Hemochromatosis

169. A neonate was born with cleft lip, cleft palate and cardiac anomalies. There is a history of drugs, which the mother was on. The drug most likely to be implicated: AIIMS 2001

A. Isotretinoin B. Lithium
C. Valproate D. Phenytoin

170. A six years old girl child presents with spotting, no secondary sexual characteristic present, cause can be: DNB 2001

A. Menarch
B. Foreign body
C. Gonococcal infection
D. Haemorrhagic disease

171. Metabolic acidosis is accompanied with : DNB 2001

A. Acetazolamide B. Phenformin
C. Verapamil D. Triamterene

172. Combination of retinitis pigmentosa icthyosis is seen in : JIPMER 2002

A. Netherton syndrome B. Refsum's disease
C. Down's syndrome D. Mob's syndrome

173. The following are features of cerebral palsy except : JIPMER 2002

A. Hypotonia B. Spasticity
C. Erbs palsy D. Epilepsy

Ans. 159. C 160. B 161. D 162. D 163. C 164. C 165. B 166. A 167. B 168. B
169. A 170. B 171. A 172. B 173. C

174. A baby born with hypotinia, and a reflexia. Mother antenatally had oligohydramnios and decreased fetal movements. The most probable cause is : AIIMS 2002

A. Congenital myopathy
B. Congenital myasthenia
C. Congenital muscular dystrophy
D. Spinal muscular dystrophy

175. A child presents with recurrent fever and failure to thrive. Most likely diagnosis is : AIIMS 2002

A. Recurrent urinary tract infection
B. Malaria
C. Protein malabsorption
D. Typhoid fever

176. A newborn was brought with persistent crying and was found to have rashes. On laboratory examination, it was found to have lactic acidosis. The diagnosis is likely to be : AI 2002

A. Organic aciduria
B. Urea cycle defect
C. MELAS with lactic acidosis
D. Aminoacidopathy

177. A child was brought 6 hours after a snake bite. On examination a localized edema of less than two inches was present at the site of the bite. There were no systemic signs and symptoms. The most correct management would be : AI 2002

A. Incision and suction
B. Inject antivenom locally
C. Polyvalent antivenom should be given i.v.
D. Observe for progression of symptoms

178. A 2 years old child weighing 6.7 kg and with a history of diarrhea and vomiting for 2 days is brought to the hospital. On examination, the skin, when pinched-up took few seconds to return to normal. Which of the following is the most likely diagnosis : AI 2002

A. No dehydration
B. Some dehydration
C. Severe dehydration
D. Skin pinching is not reliable in making a diagnosis

179. Most common cause of Metabolic Acidosis in Indian children is : Maharashtra 2000

A. Diarrhoea B. Starvation
C. DKA D. Septicemia

180. The length of the feeding tube to be inserted for transpyloric feeding is measured from the tip of : AIIMS 2002

A. Nose to umbilicus
B. Ear lobe to the umbilicus
C. Nose to the knee joint
D. Ear lobe to the knee joint

181. In pediatric advanced life support, intraosseous access for drug/fluid administration is recommended for pediatric age of : AIIMS 2002

A. < 1 year age B. < 5 years age
C. < 6 years age D. Any age

182. A 3-years old boy is brought to the casualty by his mother with progressive shortness of reatl for 1 day. The child has history of bronchial asthma. On examination, the child is blue, gasping and unresponsive. What will you like to do first : AIIMS 2002

A. Intubate
B. Administer 100% oxygen by mask
C. Ventilate with bag and mask
D. Administer nebulised salbutamol

183. A 5-years old child presents with confusion, increased salivation, lacrimation, fasciculations, miosis, tachycardia and hypertension. Which of the following poisons can cause these manifestations : AIIMS 2002

A. Opium
B. Organophosphate insecticide
C. Dhatura
D. Organochlorine pesticide

184. Which one of the following disease is not developed by intrauterine growth retarded full term 'Low Birth Weight' infants in later life : UPSC 2002

A. Coronary heart disease
B. Hypertension
C. Diabetes
D. Malabsorption syndrome

185. A person working in hot environment who consumes more water without salt is likely to develop a condition called : UPSC 2002

A. Heat stroke B. Heat exhaustion
C. Heat cramps D. Heat hyperpyrexia

186. What is the correct sequence of the following while resuscitating an infant with Foreign Body airway obstruction : UPSC 2002

1. Chest thrust
2. Tongue-jaw lift
3. Back blows

Select the correct sequences from the codes given below :

Codes :

A. 1,3,2 B. 3,2,1
C. 3,1,2 D. 2,1,3

187. A 40 year old lady delivered a full term baby. On examination of the baby, the neonatologist noted certain urogenital abnormality. He took the picture. The most likely diagnosis in the question is : AI 2003

A. Urogenital sinus B. Hypertrophied clitoris
C. Micropenis D. Vulval hematoma

Ans.	174. A	175. A	176. A	177. D	178. D	179. A	180. B	181. C	182. C	183. B
	184. D	185. C	186. C	187. B						

188. Which one of the following is the most common cause of abdominal mass in neonates : UPSC 2003
A. Neuroblastoma
B. Wilm's tumor
C. Distended Bladder
D. Multicystic dysplastic kidneys

189. Transient myeloproliferative disorder of the newborn is seen in associated with : AI 2003
A. Turner's syndrome B. Down's syndrome
C. Neurofibromatosis D. Ataxia telangiectasia

190. An albino girl gets married to a normal boy. What are the chances of their having an affected child and what are the chances of their children being carriers: AI 2003
A. None affected, all carriers
B. All normal
C. 50% carriers
D. 50% affected, 50 carriers

191. An eight yrs old boy presents with back pain and mild fever. His plain X-ray of the dorsolumbar spine reveals a solitary collapsed dorsal vertebra with preserved disc spaces. There was no associated soft tissue shadow. The most likely diagnosis is : AI 2003
A. Ewing's sarcoma B. Tuberculosis
C. Histiocytosis D. Metastasis

192. In triple screening test for Down's syndrome during pregnancy all of the following are included except : AIIMS 2003
A. Serum beta hCG
B. Serum oestriol
C. Maternal serum Alfa fetoprotein
D. Acetyl cholinesterase

193. The following statements regarding Turner's syndrome are true except : AIIMS 2003
A. Occurrence of Turner's syndrome is influenced by maternal age.
B. Most patients have primary amenorrhoea.
C. Most patients have short stature.
D. Edema of hands and feet is an important feature during infancy.

194. The most common leukocytoclastic vasculitis affecting children are : AIIMS 2003
A. Takayasu disease
B. Mucocutaneous lymph node syndrome. (Kawasaki disease).
C. Henoch Schonlein purpura
D. Polyarteritis nodosa.

195. A 13-years old boy is referred for evaluation of nocturnal enuresis and short stature. His blood pressure is normal. The hemoglobin level is 8g/dl. Urea 112 mg/dl, creatinine 6 mg/dl, sodium 119 mEq/dl, potassium 4 mEq/l, calcium 7 mg/dl, phosphate 6 mg/dl and alkaline phosphatase 300 U/I. Urinalysis shows trace proteinuria with hyaline casts; no red and white cells are seen. Ultrasound shows bilateral small kidneys and the micturating cystourethrogram is normal. The most likely diagnosis is : AIIMS 2003
A. Alport's syndrome
B. Medullary sponge kidney
C. Chronic glomerulonephritis
D. Nephronophthisis

196. Regarding neonatal circumcision, which one of the following is true : AIIMS 2003
A. It should be done without anaesthesia, as it is hazardous to give anaesthesia.
B. It should be done without anesthesia, as neonates do not perceive pain as adult.
C. It should be done under local anaesthesia only.
D. General anaesthesia should be given to neonate for circumcision as they also feel pain as adult.

197. Webbing of neck, increased carrying angle, low posterior hair line and short fourth metacarpal are characteristics of : AI 2004
A. Klinefelter syndrome B. Turner's syndrome
C. Cri du chat syndrome D. Noonan syndrome

198. Retardation of skeletal maturity can be caused by all except : AI 2004
A. Chronic renal failure
B. Hypothyroidism
C. Protein energy malnutrition (PEM)
D. Congenital adrenal hyperplasia

199. Bone marrow transplantation can be used as a treatment for all except: AI 2004
A. Osteopetrosis B. Adrenoleukodystrophy
C. Hurler's syndrome D. Hemochromatosis

200. What is the term used for babies born as a result of retarded intrauterine foetal growth? UPSC 2004
A. Pre-term babies
B. Low birth weight babies
C. Small for date babies
D. Retarded babies

201. Which one of the following is not an indication for intravenous Gammaglobulin : UPSC 2004
A. Idiopathic thrombocytopenic purpura
B. Kawasaki disease
C. Acute infective polyneuritis
D. Systemic lupus erythematosus

Ans. 188. D 189. B 190. C 191. C 192. D 193. A 194. C 195. D 196. D 197. B 198. D 199. D 200. C 201. D

202. Consider the following conditions : UPSC 2004
1. Mental retardation
2. Stunting of growth
3. Hypotonia
4. Congenital heart disease

Which of the above are the features of Edwards syndrome:
A. 1 and 3 B. 2 and 4
C. 1, 2 and 4 D. 1, 2, 3 and 4

203. A baby girl presents with bilateral inguinal masses, thought to be hernias but are found to be testes in the inguinal canals. Which karyotype would you expect to find in the child? AIIMS 2004
A. 46, XX B. 46, XY
C. 47, XX D. 47, XYY

204. The most common malignant neoplasm of infancy is : AI 2005
A. Malignant teratoma B. Neuroblastoma
C. Wilms' tumor D. Hepatoblastoma

205. A new born presented with bloated abdomen shortly after birth with passing of less meconium. A full-thickness biopsy of the retum was carried out. Which one of the following rectal biopsy findings is most likely to be present : AI 2005
A. Fibrosis of submucosa
B. Hyalinisation of the muscular coat
C. Thickened muscularis propria
D. Lack of ganglion cells

206. The major use of sulfonamides is in the treatment of : Orissa 1991
A. Streptococcal pharyngitis
B. Urinary tract infection
C. Pneumonia
D. Otitis media

207. Restricted fluid intake and a diet low in salt and protein is given in : UPSC 1984
A. Hepatitis
B. Oliguric phase of acute nephritis
C. Nephrotic syndrome
D. Kwashiorkor
E. Congestive cardiac failure

208. A 4 kg infant with severe dehydration (10% dehydration) needs the following amount of intravenous fluid in the first 24 hours : PGI 1983, 92, 94
A. 500 ml B. 800 ml
C. 1000 ml D. 1200 ml
E. 1400 ml

209. Which of the following inborn errors of metabolism is associated with mental retardation: AMC 1982; AIIMS 1983, 92, 97, 98
A. Alkaptonuria B. Homocystinuria
C. Pentosuria D. Galactosemia

210. A 3 years old child is seen with coma, weakness, salivation and one sided constricted pupil. The most probable diagnosis is : AMC 1981; TN 1989, 92, 94
A. Tetanus
B. Organophosphorus poisoning
C. Phenobarbitone poisoning
D. Electrolyte imbalance

211. Regarding the management of acute rheumatic fever, which one of the following statements is correct: CSE 2006
A. Give antibiotics for the treatment of active Group A streptococcal infections.
B. Give antibiotics for prophylaxis against Group A streptococci.
C. Give both those mentioned above at (a) and (b).
D. Antibiotics have no role.

212. The following are characteristic of autism except : Maharashtra 2006
A. Onset after 6 years of age
B. Sever deficient in social interaction
C. Repetitive behaviour
D. Delayed language development

213. Macrocephaly is seen in which of the following syndromes ? AIIMS 2008
A. Metachromatic leucodystrophy
B. Adrenoleukodystrophy
C. Canavan's disese
D. Krabbe's disease

214. A down syndrome patient is posted for surgery, the necessary preoperative investigation to be done is : AI 2009
A. Echocardiography B. CT brain
C. X-ray cervical spine D. USG abdomen

215. A child presents raised sweat cloride levels and suspicion of cystic fibrosis, which other test would you do to exclude the diagnosis of cystic fibrosis? AI 2009
A. Repeat sweat chloride measurements
B. Nasal electrode potential difference
C. Fat in stool for next 72 hours
D. DNA analysis for delta F-508 mutation

216. Staging for Wilms syndrome : AI 2009
A. Chadwick
B. International staging international society of pediatrics (ISOP)
C. AJCC
D. TNM

Ans.									
202. C	203. B	204. B	205. D	206. B	207. B	208. B	209. D	210. D	211. C
212. A	213. C	214. A	215. B	216. B					

EXPLANATIONS OF MISCELLANEOUS

1. Ans.— B. Autism

Onset occurs before 3 years of age.

Diagnostic triad of features is :

* Impaired social interaction
* Impaired communication
* Impaired imagination

Language development is delayed

Rigid repetitive pattern of behavior is seen.

2. Ans. B 46 XY

Individual with 'androgen insensitivity syndrome' are XY individuals (male karyotype) with a female phenotype.

Mutation in the androgen receptor causes resistance to androgen action and the androgen insensitivity syndrome results.

3. Ans. A. Gaucher's disease

The t/t of choice for Gaucher's disease is enzyme replacemnt therapy. A recombinantly produced mannose terminated enzyme called cerezyme is used in the t/t of Gaucher's disease.

4. Ans. B 36 weeks

Fetal Hb —> $(\alpha_2\gamma_2)$

Adults Hb —> $(\alpha_2\beta_2)$

* During the initial fetal life, the major hemoglobin synthesized in the body is fetal hemoglobin, because in fetus, the chain synthesized predominantly is the γ chain.
* β chain is present in only trace amount in early embryos.
* The rate of synthesis of γ and β chains and the amount of HbA and HbF are inversely related during introauterine stage.
* As the age of the fetus increases, the synthesis of β chains and the amount of adult hemoglobin in the blood increases.
* At 36 weeks of gestational age the rate of synthesis of β chain exceeds that of γ chain. This is called switch over.

What exactly is switch over :

Switch over is the point at which the rate of synthesis of β chain exceeds the rate of synthesis of γ chain.

Don't confuse it with the concentration of hemoglobin remember that despite having higher rate of synthesis of β chains it is not, HbA, but HbF, which is present in greater concentration when switch over occurs.

When does it begin and end :

* Switch over occurs at 36th gestational week, so that may be taken as the beginning of switch over and after that β chains remains the predominant chain synthesized.

5. Ans. A. Check pulses

An orderly sequence of events in resuscitation is (A, B, C) airway, breathing and circulation.

If the patient has no spontaneous respirations, steps should be immediately taken to breathe for the child. Airway should be opened and rescue breathing should be provided.

Rescue breathing is done by

Mouth-to-mouth

Mouth-to-nose

Mouth-to-mask

Bag mask respirations

Successful rescue breathing will provide good chest rise and relief of deep cyanosis.

Usually after bag and mask ventilation it should be checked whether spontaneous ventilation is present or not.

This is assessed by watching the chest movements.

If these do not indicate adequate ventilation, immediate intubation is the next step.

But in the question they have not specified, whether the ventilation is adequate or not (after the oxygenation).

If they wanted to know this, it would have been specifically mentioned in the question that the patient remained in apnea after the bag & mask ventilation.

So, we can assume that the ventilation becomes normal after bag and mask ventilation.

Once the respiratory system is taken care of cardiovascular system needs attention.

Circulation should be first assessed by checking the pulse.

If there is no pulse or if the pulse is less than 60 beats/m with poor perfusion chest compression must be given.

6. Ans.— D. Decerebrate rigidity

7. Ans.— C. Steatorrhoea.

8. Ans.— B. Hyperammonemia

9. Ans.— C. Pellagra

There is Diarrhoea, Dermatitis, Delirium and Dementia.

10. Ans.— C. Staphylococcal infection

11. Ans.— B. Beyond 6 months of age

12. Ans.— C. Bullous lesions

13. Ans.— D. Gardner's syndrome

14. Ans.— B. Klippel-Feil syndrome

15. Ans.— A. Infantile convulsions

16. Ans.— D. Juvenile rheumatoid arthritis

17. Ans.— B. CALLA Ag +ve

18. Ans.— A. Enteritis

19. Ans.— A. 1% Atropine ointment

Homatropine is used in adults and middle aged whereas in elderly, phenylephrine is used.

20. Ans.— D. Amyloblastoma

21. Ans.— B. Rheumatic fever

22. Ans.— A. Down's syndrome

23. Ans.— D. Inadequate rest

24. Ans.— B. Hypothyroidism

25. Ans.— D. Hypothermia

26. Ans.— A. Genetic short stature

Bone age is delayed in constitutional delay, hypopitutarism, hypothyroidism and Turner's syndrome.

27. Ans.— B. Renal Colic

28. Ans.— A. Wilm's tumour

29. Ans.— A. Amyloidosis

30. Ans.— C. Sodium bicarbonate

31. Ans.— B. Nalorphine

32. Ans.— C. Atropine

33. Ans.— D. Cyanide poisoning

34. Ans.— B. Atropine poisoning

35. Ans.— C. Strabismus

There is also mydriasis, dryness of skin, and delirium.

36. Ans.— B. Substitute ampicillin with cotrimoxazole

37. Ans.— D. Marked jaundice

38. Ans.— A. Face

39. Ans.— B. Coproporphyrin-III

Lead poisoning is common in Pica (children eating point or pencil lead).

40. Ans.— A. Hemophilia

41. Ans.— D. Henoch-Schonlein syndrome

42. Ans.— B. Glomerulonephritis

In Henoch Schonlein purpura, there is mild renal involvement, indicated by microscopic hematuria and slight proteinuria. Serum IgA levels are transiently raised and macromolecular IgA complexes are usually present in circulation. Most patient completely recover without any specific treatment.

43. Ans.— D. 47, XYY—Klinefelter's syndrome

44. Ans.— D. Possible association with Reye's syndrome

45. Ans.— D. Codeine

Lithium, anticonvulsants and anticoagulants (Warfarin etc.) are also contraindicated.

46. Ans.— D. Nystagmus

47. Ans.— A. Diarrhoea

48. Ans.— C. Liver

49. Ans.— B. Growth of blood vessels into vitreous followed by fibrosis.

50. Ans.— A. PAM (Pyridine aldoxime methiodide)

51. Ans.— A. Kayser-Fleischer ring

52. Ans.— D. All of the above

Ceruloplasmin levels are low. In cornea, there is Kayser Fleischer ring. Proximal renal tubules are affected. There is hemolysis and neurological symptoms. Liver content of copper may reach levels of 500-2000 mg/g.

53. Ans.— D. Upward slanting of eyes

54. Ans.— D. Leukemias

55. Ans.— A. Down's syndrome

56. Ans.— A. Phocomelia

57. Ans.— C. Tetracycline

There is permanent yellow or brownish staining.

58. Ans.— D. Not treated with steroids

59. Ans.— C. Death by time of puberty

60. Ans.— D. Vertebra

61. Ans.— B. Luxation of lens

Marfan's syndrome is a disorder of connective tissue (elastin). The gene fibrillin is in chromosome 15. Inheritance is autosomal dominant. There is ectopic lentis, long thin fingers, hyperextensible joints and aortic dilatation. It differs from homocystinuria which presents as ectopia lentis but has associated mental retardation. In Marfan's syndrome IQ is normal.

62. Ans.— B. Hyperaldosteronism

63. Ans.— D. Splenomegaly

64. Ans.— C. 28

65. Ans.— B. Semiquantitative test for foetal haemoglobin

66. Ans.— B. Jaundice

67. Ans.— C. Back

68. Ans.— D. Cleft palate and hare lip

69. Ans.— C. 245 gms

70. Ans.— A. Isovaleric acidemia

71. Ans.— A. Cafe-au-lait spots

72. Ans.— C. Atleast one quart of milk of a day

73. Ans.— D. Pendred's syndrome

74. Ans.— B. Achondroplasia

75. Ans.— D. Essential hypertension

Diuretics (Thiazide, frusemide) and not hypertension can result in hypokalemia.

76. Ans.— D. Undescended testis

77. Ans.— B. 60 meq/L

78. Ans.— B. Muscle phosphorylase

79. Ans.— B. Trisomy 21

80. Ans.— A. 24

81. Ans.— A. Galactokinase

82. Ans.— A. Tall stature

Stature is not tall and chromosome pattern is commonly XO.

83. Ans.— B. Cleft palate

84. Ans.— A. Asthma

85. Ans.— B. 1-4 weeks

86. Ans.— B. Respiratory alkalosis

87. Ans.— D. Premature closure of epiphysis

88. Ans.— D. AML

89. Ans.— B. Beckwith Wiedemann syndrome

90. Ans.— D. Penicillin and estrogens

91. Ans.— B. Staphylococcus

Spread is usually haematogenous

92. Ans.— C. Turner's syndrome

93. Ans.— A. Guthrie test

94. Ans.— B. ASLO titre

95. Ans.— A. Growing pains

96. Ans.— D. Lactic acidosis

97. Ans.— A. Kwashiorkar

98. Ans.— C. Hypothyroidism

99. Ans.— A. Establish airways

100. Ans.— A. Engleman disease

101. Ans.— A. Surfactant

L : S ratio of more than 2 indicates fetal lung maturity.

102. Ans.— A. Ringer's lactage

103. Ans.— A. Congenital idiopathic nephrotic syndrome

It is common in non-seminomatous testicular tumor (i.e. teratoma).

104. Ans.— A. Pierre Robin syndrome

105. Ans.— C. Oxygen therapy

106. Ans.— B. Enterobious vermicularis infestation

107. Ans.— C. Skin lesions

108. Ans.— A. Rheumatoid arthritis

Most common initial joint involved is knee. Iridocyclitis type.

109. Ans.— D. Glucose without salt

110. Ans.— B. Ingestion of belladonna
111. Ans.— A. Phenytoin
112. Ans.— D. Down's syndrome
113. Ans.— D. Aortic root dilatation
114. Ans.— B. Self-mutilation
115. Ans.— A. Pigmentary degeneration
116. Ans.— C. Both A & B
117. Ans.— A. Evanescent rash
118. Ans.— A. Fever 39°C
119. Ans.— C. Filaria
120. Ans.— D. Protein loosing enteropathy
121. Ans.— C. 5 4 2 6
122. Ans.— D. Scurvy
123. Ans.— D. A B C D
3 1 2 4
124. Ans.— D. Copper poisoning
125. Ans.— B. Iron
Iron deficiency anaemia is commonly associated with pica.
126. Ans.— C. Ganciclovir
127. Ans.— C. II, III and IV are correct
128. Ans.— B. Posterior subcapsular cataract
129. Ans.— A. Microscopic haematuria
130. Ans.— A. Organic aciduria
131. Ans.— B. Blond hair with MR
132. Ans.— A. HMD
133. Ans.— B. Nothing should be done
134. Ans.— A. Risk of HIV upto 90%
135. Ans.— A. Lactase
136. Ans.— A. Decreased Nuchal fold thickness
137. Ans.— A. Rhabdomyosarcoma
138. Ans.— D. Constitutional
139. Ans.— A. Birth
140. Ans.— C. Both a & b
141. Ans.— D. 16 yrs
142. Ans.— A. DM
143. Ans.— D. L4, L5
144. Ans.— D. 16
145. Ans.— A. Rheumatoid factor positive
It may not be always positive. It usually starts with fever.
146. Ans.— A. Start diet therapy immediately with complete restriction of phenylalanine.
Phenylalanine is not completely eliminated as it is required for normal growth.
147. Ans.— C. A B C D
3 2 4 1
148. Ans.— A. Alkaptonuria
149. Ans.— C. HCO_3^-
150. Ans.— B. Clomiphene
151. Ans.— E. Death occurs usually in infancy
152. Ans.— A. Duodenal atresia
Brushfield spots on iris are also seen. Leukemia is 20 times more common. Thyroid dysfunction and retarded sexual development are also seen.
153. Ans.— B. Neck X-ray
154. Ans.— D. No dehydration
155. Ans.— D. Ultrasound
156. Ans.— A. Stomach lavage
157. Ans.— B. Serum ceruloplasmin
158. Ans.— A. ESWL
159. Ans.— C. Spinal muscular atrophy
160. Ans.— B. Send urine for culture and sensitivity and start I.V. antibiotics immediately.
161. Ans.— D. Excessive intake of sodium
162. Ans.— D. Chondrodysplasia punctata
163. Ans.— C. Histioxytosis-X
This syndrome has three classes, the most common childhood histiocytosis is histiocytosis-X or Langerhans cell histiocytosis.
164. Ans.— C. IV Ig
Intravenous gamma globulin and aspirin are recommended for treatment of Kawasaki disease (a systemic vasculitis of unknown etiology).
165. Ans.— B. Multiple carboxylase deficiency
It is often biotin responsive.
166. Ans.— A. Involvement of hip, ankles
167. Ans.— B. 8
168. Ans.— B. Hurler's disease
169. Ans.— A. Isotretinoin
170. Ans.— B. Foreign body
171. Ans.— A. Acetazolamide
172. Ans.— B. Refsum's disease
173. Ans.— C. Erb's palsy

174. Ans.— A. Congenital myopathy

175. Ans.— A. Recurrent urinary tract infection

176. Ans.— A. Organic aciduria

177. Ans.— D. Observe for progression of symptoms

The snake may be non-poisonous.

178. Ans.— D. Skin pinching is not reliable in making a diagnosis.

The severity of dehydration and disturbances of electrolytes and pH are assessed clinically.

179. Ans.— A. Diarrhoea

180. Ans.— B. Ear lobe to the umbilicus

181. Ans.— C. < 6 years age

182. Ans.— C. Ventilate with bag and mask

183. Ans.— B. Organophosphate insecticide

184. Ans.— D. Malabsorption syndrome

185. Ans.— C. Heat cramps

186. Ans.— C. 3, 1, 2

187. Ans.— B. Hypertrophied clitoris

188. Ans.— D. Multicystic dysplastic kidneys

- MC cause of abdominal mass in neonate is Multicystic dysplastic kidneys.
- MC abdominal tumor in child below 1 year of age is neuroblastoma.

189. Ans.— B. Down's syndrome

- "Children with Down syndrome are suspectible to MDS and a family history may indicate a hereditary form of sideroblastic anemia or Fancony's anemia".
- The Physical examination is remarkable for signs of anaemia about 20% of patients have splenomegaly some unusual skin lesions, including Sweet's syndrome have been associated with MDS.

190. Ans.— C. 50% carriers

- Albinism AD disease
- If mother affected father unaffected then chances of carrier is 50%

191. Ans.— C. Histiocytosis

- Nelson clearly states "They may asymptomatic or painful.
- Local swelling with involvement of the spine. Which may result in collapse of the vertebral body, which can be seen roentgeno graphically and may cause secondary compression of the spinal cord in flat & long bones evidence exists of reactive new born formation (until the lesions begin to heal)"

192. Ans.— D. Acetyl cholinesterase

193. Ans.— A. Occurrence of Turner's syndrome is influenced by maternal age.

194. Ans.— C. Henoch Schonlein purpura

195. Ans.— D. Nephronophthisis

196. Ans.— D. General anaesthesia should be given to neonate for circumcision as they also feel pain as adult.

197. Ans.— B. Turner's syndrome

198. Ans.— D. Congenital adrenal hyperplasia

Linear bone growth can occur as long as the epiphyses are separated from the shaft of the bone, but such growth ceases after epiphyses unite with the shaft (epiphysical closure).

- Children with cong. adrenal hyperplasia have early onset of puberty and advanced osseous maturation. Early closure of epiphyses leads ultimately to short stature.

(Note: Retardation of skeletal maturity and retardation of skeletal growth is opposite thing so do not confuse).

- Children with hypothyroidism show growth retardation and delayed skeletal maturation, dental development and puberty.

Retardation of bone maturation (Delayed bone age).

- Hypothyroidism
- Hypopituitarism
- Malnutrition
- Chronic diseases (including ch. renal failure)
- Cushing's syndrome

199. Ans.— D. Hemochromatosis

200. Ans.— C. Small for date babies

201. Ans.— D. Systemic lupus erythematosus

202. Ans.— C. 1, 2 and 4

203. Ans.— B. 46, XY

The initial step in evaluating an infant with ambiguous genitalia is a, locate the urethral meatus, palpate the scrotum or labia and the inguinal regions for testes (palpable gonads almost always indicate the presence of testicular tissue and thus that the infant is a genetic male), and look for any other anatomic abnormalities. Ultrasonography is helpful in demonstrating the presence or absence of a uterus and can often locate the gonads. A rapid karyotype (such as fluorescent in situ hybridizatin of interphase nuclei for X and Y-chromosomes) can quickly determine the genetic sex of the infant.

204. Ans.— B. Neuroblastoma

"Neuroblastoma is the most common intra-abdominal solid tumour in childhood accounting for 7-8% of all pediatric cancers."

- Wilm's tumour is the most common malignant tumour of the kidney.
- Leukaemia is the most common form of childhood malignancy, accounting for approx. 30% of all child-hood cancer.
- "Leukaemia is followed by brain tumour, lymphoma neuroblastoma, Wilm's tumour, soft tisue sarcoma and tumour of bone and eye."

205. Ans.— D. Lack of ganglion cells

- "Failure to pass meconium within first 36 hours of life, abdominal distension, vomiting and poor feeding are the usual symptoms of Hirschsprung's disease (Aganglionosis)."
- *Feature of Hirschsprung's disease :*
  - Congenital absence of ganglion cells in the submucosal and myenteric plexses of the distal intestine.
  - Distal rectum is always aganglionic and the aganglionosis extendes proximally usually ending intransition zone in the rectosigmoid colon.
  - Empty rectum on digital examination or rectal impaction.
  - Rapid expulsion of faces often follows examination.
  - Barium enema : Narrow aganglionic bowel with dilated proximal bowel.
  - Diagnosis is confirmed by rectal biopsy.
  - Hypertrophied nerves are observed in the aganglionic segment.
    - Treatment :
    - Surgical
    - Initially colostomy in the ganglionic bowel.
    - Subsequently : Excision of aganglionic segment with a pull through procedure enabling an anastomosis to be performed between the ganglionic colon and the anus.
    - Name of the surgery : Duhamel, Swenson

206. Ans.— B. Urinary tract infection

207. Ans.— B. Oliguric phase of acute nephritis

208. Ans.— B. 800 ml

209. Ans.— D. Galactosemia

210. Ans.— D. Electrolyte imbalance

211. Ans.— C. Give both those mentioned above at (a) and (b)

212. Ans.— A. Onset after 6 years of age

213. Ans.— C Canavan's disease

Canavan's disease

* Autosomal recessive disorder.
* Caused due to deficiency of the enzyme N-Aspertoacylase.
* This leads to accumulationof N-Acetyl Aspartic acid in brain and urine.

214. Ans.— A. Echocardiography

All patients with Down syndrome must have a echocardiograph in the first year of life to rule out CHD as there high incidence of CHD in them.

215. Ans.— B. Nasal electrode potential difference

Diagnostic Criteria for CF

Presence of typical clinical featurs OR CF in a sibling OR + ve newborn screening test

+ (And)

Two elevated sweat chlorides on separate days Or identification of Two CF mutations OR an abnormal nasal potential difference.

216. Ans.— B. ISOP

ISOP has provided Guidelines regarding staging and therapeutic management of ns/ms tumor

Staging is based on the results of physical exm, imaging tests (untrasound, CT scan etc.) and on the results of surgery, if it has been done.

ENTRANCE EXAMINATION IN HAEMATOLOGY

Book Contains :—

* Factual Data
* Important Points for Viva/MCQ's
* Important Text from Haematology i.e Factual data, Biochemical, Physiological, Pharmacological, Pathological and Clinical Aspects .
* Clinical Aspects & Recent Advances
* Helpful for MBBS, BDS & Entrance Exams

Useful for MBBS, BDS & Other Exams

- Edited by **Dr. M.S. Bhatia** (MD, Wip WPA), DNB and **Dr. Nirmaljit Kaur** (MD) experienced editors, examiners & paper setters.

CBS PUBLISHERS & DISTRIBUTORS PVT. LTD.

4596/1-A 11 DARYA GANJ, NEW DELHI-110002 (INDIA)

E-cbspubs@vsnl.com • Website : www.cbspd.com

Branch ; 2975, 17th Cross, K.R. Road, Bansankari 2nd Stage, Bangalore-70

REVIEW PAPER—I

(Based on Difficult & Important MCQ's)

GROWTH & DEVELOPMENT

1. **In a 7 year old child of weight 23 Kg, surface area is ——— m²:**
   A. 0.73 B. 0.80
   C. 0.87 D. 0.93
2. **Child death rate is maximum in —— year of life :**
   A. 1 B. 2
   C. 3 D. 4
3. **Child survival index is calculated from deaths under -- ---------years of age :**
   A. 3 B. 5
   C. 7 D. 12
4. **Natal teeth can occur in following except :**
   A. Hallerman Streiff syndrome
   B. Pierre-Robin syndrome
   C. Ellis-van Creveld syndrome
   D. None of the above
5. **Mottling of enamel but no enamel hypoplasia is seen in :**
   A. Hypothyrodism
   B. Irradiation
   C. Fluorosis
   D. Vitamin D resistant rickets
6. **Infants turn to sounds above the ear at —— months :**
   A. 3 B. 6
   C. 8 D. 10
7. **Following reflex is normal in infant :**
   A. Magnus and de kleijn reflex
   B. Grunfelder reflex
   C. Babinski
   D. All of the above
8. **Subcutaneous tissue increases to a peak at —— months :**
   A. 6 B. 9
   C. 12 D. 18
9. **The children of the same weight have the same food requirements regardless of their ages is ——— law :**
   A. Baer's B. Camerer's
   C. Coutard's D. Ewald's
10. **Each parent contributes on an average, one half, of an individual's heritage, each grandparent one fourth or each grandgrand parent one eight etc is ——— law :**
    A. Godelier's B. Galton's
    C. Dollo's D. Gudden
11. **In a child of 15 months, average increase in head circumference per month is :**
    A. 0.6 B. 0.4
    C. 0.25 D. 0.15
12. **Teeth development begins at —— week of intrauterine life :**
    A. 8 B. 10
    C. 12 D. 14

NUTRITION

13. **Excess of following vitamins is not known to produce any disorder except for :**
    A. B2 B. Biotin
    C. Folate D. C
14. **Corner sign is seen in :**
    A. Rickets B. Scurvy
    C. Hyperparathyrodism D. B2 deficiency
15. **Deficiency of which mineral may result in hypothyroidism :**
    A. Chronium B. Cobalt
    C. Cu D. Zinc
16. **Rickets may be often seen in :**
    A. Down's syndrome B. Edward's syndrome
    C. Lowe syndrome D. Reye's syndrome

Ans. 1. C 2. C 3. B 4. D 5. D 6. C 7. D 8. B 9. B 10. B 11. C 12. D 13. B 14. C 15. C 16. C

17. **Low osmolality dialysate differs from high osmolality dialysate by difference in :**
A. Lactate B. Dextrose
C. Magnesium D. Calcium

18. **In a 3 day old preterm baby, the fluid requirement is ——ml/kg/d :**
A. 60 B. 75
C. 90 D. 120

19. **In scurvy, following phenomenon may be seen :**
A. Porret's B. Pool
C. Lewis D. Lust's

20. **A bottle-fed baby should not take more than one tenth of its own weight of cow's milk per day is —— rule :**
A. Jackson's B. Rolleston
C. Budin D. Allen

HAEMATOLOGY

21. **For converting arterial blood gases in kPa to mm.Hg, it is multiplied by factor :**
A. 3.5 B. 5
C. 7.5 D. 9

22. **For obtaining, an approximate estimate of arterial pH from a mixed venous sample, the following procedure is done :**
A. Add 0.01 B. Substract 0.3
C. Add 0.25 D. Substract 0.03

23. **For Paroxysmal cold haemoglobinuria, test used is :**
A. Farber's test
B. Eisberg test
C. Donath-Landsteiner test
D. Davidsohn differential absorption test

24. **"Alice in Wonderland" may be seen in :**
A. AML
B. ALL
C. Infectious mononucleosis
D. Beta Thalassemia

25. **Mentzer index is :**
A. MCV + RBC count B. MCHC + RBC Count
C. RBC Count + MCH D. RBC count + MCV

26. **No clinical symptoms have been identified to deficiency of blood coagulation factor :**
A. VI B. XI
C. XII D. XII

27. **In sickle cell anemia, life of RBCs is about —— days :**
A. 7-10 B. 17-20
C. 60-65 D. 85-90

28. **In Thalassemia, Mentzer index is below :**
A. 7 B. 10
C. 13 D. 17

29. **In iron efficiency anemia, Mentzer index is :**
A. < 10 B. > 10
C. < 13 D. > 13

30. **Owren disease is due to deficiency of coagulation factor :**
A. III B. V
C. VII D. XIII

31. **MCV is maximum in :**
A. New born B. 3 months old
C. 6 years old D. 12 years old

32. **Cyerny's anemia is due to defective :**
A. Diet B. Chromosome
C. Metabolism D. Absorption

33. **Anaemia pseudoleukemia infantum is —— anemia:**
A. Cyerny's B. Fanconi's
C. Jaksch's D. Leaderer's

34. **Normal Lymphocyte count is maximum in—— :**
A. New born B. 1 year old
C. 6 years old D. 10 years old

35. **Initial acidosis in newborn is corrected within —— hours :**
A. Half B. 6
C. 24 D. 72

36. **Peroxidase positive leukemia is :**
A. Lymphocytic B. Myelocytic
C. Erythroleukemia D. Monocytic

37. **Antitubercular drugs which can be used in G-6-P deficiency :**
A. Steptomycin + INH + Rifampicin
B. Ethambultol + INH + Rifampicin
C. Ethambutol + Rifampicin + Ethionamide
D. PAS + Ethambutol + Streptomycin

38. **Gunther's disease is :**
A. Congenital erythropoietic prophyria
B. Erthyropoietic protoporphyria
C. Epidermolysis bullosa
D. Impetigo contagiosa

39. **If production of delta chain is suppressed, hemoglobin impaired is :**
A. HbA B. HbA2
C. HbF D. All of the above

40. **HbD disease is more commonly reported among :**
A. Tamils B. Assamese
C. Punjabis D. Bengalis

Ans.									
17. B, C	18. C	19. D	20. B	21. C	22. D	23. C	24. C	25. A	26. C
27. B	28. C	29. D	30. B	31. A	32. A	33. C	34. B	35. C	36. B
37. C	38. A	39. B	40. C						

41. **Arterial pO2 reaches the adult level by ——— years of age :**
A. 1 B. 2
C. 5 D. 10

42. **Non-specific immunosuppression to an antigen induced by administration of large doses of an unrelated antigen is ——— phenomenon :**
A. Hoffmann B. Lewis
C. Liacopoulos D. Liesegang

43. **The blood and serum of an immunized person, when transferred to another subject, will render the latter immune. This is ——— law :**
A. Barfurth's B. Behring's
C. Ewald's D. Fajan's

44 **A palmer crease correlated with an increased risk for leukemia and other malignancies in children is ——— line :**
A. Poupart's B. Poirier
C. Sydney D. Thompson

45. **Preleukemia or myelodysplastic syndrome is associated with abnormalities in chromosomes :**
A. 4 and 6 B. 5 and 7
C. 5 and 8 D. 6 and 7

46. **In hemoglobin E disease, there is abnormality of lysine at position —— of beta chain :**
A. 6 B. 12
C. 24 D. 26

DISEASES & IMMUNITY

47. **Mumps skin test detects ——— to mumps :**
A. Susceptibility B. Infection
C. Immunity D. Carrier

48. **Tuberculin test may be negative in the presence of following acute disorders except :**
A. Pertusis B. Measles
C. Leukaemia D. Nephrotic syndrome

49. **Schwartz stain is used in vaccine for :**
A. TB B. Measles
C. Mumps D. Rubella

50. **Paratyphoid fever is also known as —— disease :**
A. Cavare's B. Brion-Kayser's
C. Bostock's D. Barlow's

51. **TB of spine is also known as —— disease :**
A. Corvisart's B. David's
C. Eulenburg's D. Flegel's

52. **Foetal skin scarring is seen with following congenital infections except :**
A. Cytomegalovirus B. Syphilis
C. Herpes D. Varicella

53. **Cataract is seen in following congenital infections except :**
A. CMV B. Rubella
C. HSV D. Toxoplasmosis

54. **Increase in severity of an infectious disease when a small dose of chemotherapeutical remedy is given is called ——— phenomenon :**
A. Gartner B. Hata
C. Hecht D. Pool

55. **The appearance of minute subcutaneous petechiae below in area at which a tourniquet is applied not too tightly for ten minutes upon the upper arm; characteristic of scarlet fever and hemorrhagic diathesis. This is —— phenomenon :**
A. Liesegang B. Porret's
C. Rumpel-Leede D. Rust

56. **The severity of a malarial attack depends upon the number of parasites in the blood is —— law :**
A. Knapp's B. Kahler's
C. Golgi's D. Gudden's

57. **A redline observed on the gingivae in pulmonary tuberculosis is ——— line :**
A. Brucke's B. Czermak
C. Thompson D. Topinard

58. **A generalised lymphadenopathy that occurs during the incubation period of various exanthematons fever on children is :**
A. Weil sign B. Vipond Sign
C. Wartenberg sign D. Zaufal sign

59. **The existence of albumin in the sputum, indicating T.B. is ——— reaction :**
A. Nadi B. Posner
C. Roger's D. Russo

60. **'A-80' antigen may be used in the diagnosis of following except :**
A. T.B. B. H. influenza
C. Nocardiasis D. Leishmaniasis

Ans.									
41. C	42. C	43. B	44. C	45. B	46. D	47. C	48. D	49. B	50. B
51. B	52. A	53. A	54. B	55. C	56. C	57. C	58. B	59. C	60. B

GIT

61. Lactose intolerance is a recognised finding in all except:
A. The majority of Indians and orientals
B. Coeliac disease
C. Severe malnutrition
D. Post-infective diarrhoea

62. Hypersenstivity to cow's milk is important in :
A. Hamman Rich syndrome
B. Heiner syndrome
C. Young syndrome
D. Good Pasture syndrome

63. Dance's sign is present in :
A. Appendicitis B. Intussusception
C. Meconium ileus D. Necrotising colitis

64. Early vomiting (day 1) is characteristic in :
A. Adrenogenital syndrome
B. Inborn errors of metabolism
C. Necrotising enterocolitis
D. Duodenal atresia

65. Small left colon syndrome is commonly seen in the following except :
A. Twins
B. Premature infants
C. Delivered by caesarean section
D. Infants of Diabetic mother
E. Infants of Anaemic mothers

66. Sahli Nencki test detects ——— of pancreas :
A. Lipase B. Peptidase
C. Diabetes mellitus D. Malignancy

CVS

67. In infants, external cardiac massage is given at the rate of——— beats/min :
A. 120 B. 100
C. 80 D. 60

68. In a 2-year old child, the hypertension is diagnosed if there is consistent elevation of systolic B.P. from ——— mmHg (atleast) :
A. 90 B. 100
C. 110 D. 120

69. Bulging of epigastrium due to extensive pericardial effusion is ——— sign :
A. Boyce's B. Auenbrugger
C. Boston's D. Abraham's

70. In hypertelorism and moon facies, most likely congenital heart disease is :
A. PS B. MR
C. ASD D. VSD

71. A2 heart sound in delayed in following except :
A. PDA B. AR
C. LBBB D. VSD

72. Plesch test is positive in :
A. AS B. MS
C. PS D. PDA

73. CHF without cardiac enlargement occurs in all except:
A. Cor-triatriatum B. TGA
C. Congenital MS D. Rheumatic MS

74. PR interval in a neonate is —— sec :
A. 0.06-0.12 B. 0.10-0.14
C. 0.14-0.18 D. 0.12-0.20

75. Traube-Hering waves are similar to :
A. Wilson waves B. Korotkoff's waves
C. Mayer waves D. Marey waves

76. R/S ratio in V1 in 3-6 months old child is :
A. 6.5 B. 5.0
C. 4.0 D. 2.4

77. Most common tachyarrythmia of childhood is :
A. Premature atrial contractions
B. Sinus bradycardia
C. Paroxysmal supraventricular tachycardia
D. First degree heart block

78. When B.P. rises, pulse rate falls. This is ——— law :
A. Fajan's B. Flint's
C. Kahler's D. Marey's

79. In an infant, chest compression on external cardiac massage should be ——— inches :
A. 1/4-1/2 B. 1/2-1
C. 1-1.5 D. 1.5-2

80. In a 5 year old child, blood volume is —— ml :
A. 1200 B. 1500
C. 2000 D. 2400

81. Fall of systolic blood pressure on assuming an erect posture from the lying down position is ——— phenomenon :
A. Meirowsky B. Orbeli
C. Schellong-Strisower D. Simonsen

82. 'Egg on side' appearance of heart is typically seen in :
A. VSD B. TOF
C. TGA D. ASD

Ans. 61. A 62. B 63. B 64. D 65. E 66. A 67. B 68. C 69. B 70. A
71. D 72. D 3. D 74. A 75. C 76. C 77. C 78. D 79. B 80. B
81. C 82. C

83. **A faint murmur heard with the stethoscope over the lower-end of the sternum for a short time after death is ——— phenomenon :**
A. Negro B. Orbeli
C. Hering D. Hata

84. **Term 'Warm shock' is a variety of :**
A. Cardiogenic shock B. Hypovolemic shock
C. Distributive shock D. Hypotensive shock

85. **In oxygen saturation monitoring, a level of ——% indicates an oxygen tension of 6-7 kpa :**
A. 50 B. 60
C. 75 D. 85

RESPIRATORY SYSTEM

86. **Total lung capacity in newborn is ——— to that of an adult :**
A. 1/60 B. 1/35
C. 1/20 D. 1/10]

87. **Surfactant can be detected in lung exudate from human fetuses as early as ——— week :**
A. 20 B. 24
C. 28 D. 32

88. **Tidal volume in a 3 kg infant at respiratory rate of 28 per min is approximately —— ml:**
A. 6 B. 16
C. 28 D. 38

89. **Normal newborn requires about ——— ml of oxygen/min/kg :**
A. 5 B. 7
C. 12 D. 16

90. **A deterioration in both perfusion and ventilation is seen on V-Q scanning in :**
A. Congenital lobar emphysema
B. Sequestrated lung segment
C. Pulmonary embolism
D. Bronchietasis

91. **PEFR below ———% is considered abnormal :**
A. 50 B. 60
C. 75 D. 90

92. **Arrest of breathing before stoppage of the heart's action in certain fatal brain conditions is ——— phenomenon :**
A. Collie B. Duckworth
C. Becker D. Cushing

93. **The tympanic note of skodaic resonance in pleuritis with effusion varies in pitch during inspiration and expiration, being raised on inspiration is ——— phenomenon :**
A. Aschner B. Aubert
C. Felton's D. Friedreich's

94. **In penumonia, if pulse pressure in millimetres of mercury does not fall below the pulse rate, the prognosis is good, it is ——— rule :**
A. Budin B. Bastedo's
C. Cowling D. Gibson's

95. **In a 5-year old child, the vital capacity is ———% of that of an adult :**
A. 15 B. 25
C. 35 D. 40

96. **A child with pale colour, PCO2 38 mmHg, pulsus paradoxus of 12 mmHg, O2 saturation of 92% is suffering from ——— type of asthma :**
A. Acute, mild B. Acute, moderate
C. Acute status D. Chronic

97. **The tympanic note of skodaic resonance in pleuritis with effusion varies in pitch with the opening and closing of the patient's mouth is ——— phenomenon :**
A. Lust's B. Porret's
C. Wedensky D. Williams

98. **If respiratory distress does not appear within —— hours, then hyaline membrane disease is unlikely :**
A. 1-6 B. 6-12
C. 12-18 D. 36-48

99. **In esophageal atresia, pneumonia is most common in :**
A. Right upper lobe B. Left upper lobe
C. Left upper lobe D. Left lower lobe

100. **Electromechanical dissociation is seen with :**
A. Tension pneumothorax
B. Severe hypokalemia
C. Severe hypovolemia
D. Pulmonary embolism

101. **Neonatal apnoeic attacks are seen in following except :**
A. Hyperglycinaemia
B. Maple syrup urine disease
C. Hypercalcaemia
D. Isovaleric acidaemia

Ans.									
83. C	84. C	85. D	86. B	87. B	88. B	89. B	90. A	91. C	92. B
93. D	94. D	95. B	96. B	97. D	98. C	99. A	100. B	101. C	

RENAL SYSTEMS

102. Normal value of TRP (Tubular Reabsorption of Phosphorus) is ——— or more :
A. 60 B. 70
C. 80 D. 90

103. Orthostatic proteinuria usually does not exceed —— gm :
A. 0.5 B. 1.5
C. 2.0 D. 2.5

104. Hypernephroma may be associated with :
A. Sturge Weber disease
B. von Hippel-Landau disease
C. Little disease
D. Tay Sachs disease

105. Which of the following is nephrotoxic :
A. Propranolol B. Paracetamol
C. INH D. None of the above

106. In a young child, the most frequent cause of proteinuria is :
A. Physiological B. Lipoid nephrosis
C. Ac. GN D. DM

107. In Turner's syndrome, following congenital renal defect may be present :
A. Polycystic kidney
B. Horseshoe kidney
C. Cleft or double renal pelvi
D. Bladder diverticulum

108. Urinary porphyrins are normal in :
A. Congenital erythropoietic porphyria
B. Erthyropoeitic protoporphyria
C. Porphyria cutanea tarda
D. None of the above

109. Creatinine clearance is --------- ml/min/1.73m^2:
A. 110 B. 120
C. 130 D. 140

CNS

110. Stickler syndrome includes manifestations of Pierre Robin syndrome with following except :
A. Myopia B. Seizures
C. Hearing loss D. Arthropathies

111. Lissencephaly has :
A. Elongated brain B. Widened brain
C. Smooth brain D. Absence of meninges

112. Hickey-Hare test may be positive in :
A. Medulloblastoma
B. Tuberculoma
C. Craniopharyngioma
D. Neurocysticercosis

113. Cardinal feature of Landau-Klefner syndrome is :
A. Agnosia B. Apraxia
C. Aphasia D. Alexia

114. In Hallervorden-Spatz disease, prominent pathology lies in :
A. Temporal lobes B. Basal ganglia
C. Pons D. Thalamus

115. Joubert syndrome is autosomal recessive anomaly of :
A. Pons B. Basal ganglia
C. Cerebellum
D. Midbrain

116. An effusion of blood in the region of fourth ventricle of cerebrum as a result of slight injury is — lesion:
A. Ebstein's B. Blumenthal's
C. Baehr-Lohlein's D. Durets's

ENDOCRINE

117. In Kocher-Debre-Semelaigne syndrome unusual presentation of hypothyroidism is :
A. Premature closure of fontanelles
B. Muscular hypertrophy
C. Normal osseous development
D. Long extremtities

118. Hypoglycemia in the newborn period is a recognized feature of all except :
A. Prematurity B. Post maturity
C. Intracranial injury D. Adrenal haemorrhage

119. Commonest presentation of Phaeochromocytoma is :
A. Diabetes mellitus B. Hypertension
C. Loss of weight D. Fainting

MISCELLANEOUS

120. Chinese paralytic syndrome typically mimics :
A. Multiple sclerosis
B. Guillain Barre syndrome
C. Strychnine poisoning
D. Lathyrism

121. Primary defect in Wiskott-Aldrich syndrome is believed to be in surface sialoglycoprotein :
A. gpL 65 B. gpL 87
C. gpL 115 D. gpL 123

Ans.									
102. C	103. B	104. B	105. A	106. B	107. B,C	108. B	109. C	110. B	111. C
112. C	113. C	114. B	115. C	116. D	117. B	118. D	119. B	120. B	121. C

122. **Wokman's disease (deficiency of lysosomal lipase) is :**
A. Autosomal dominant B. Autosomal recessive
C. X-linked dominant D. X-linked recessive

123. **Weill-Marchesani syndrome is characterized by the following except :**
A. Short stature B. Arachnodactyly
C. Ectopia lentis D. Spherophakia

124. **Schinzel-Giedion syndrome is characterized by following except :**
A. Hypertrichosis B. Renal anomalies
C. Cardiac anomalies D. Brain anomalies

125. **Jarcho-Levin syndrome is characterized by the following except :**
A. Short neck B. Short trunk
C. Short extremities D. Rib defects

126. **A child who has swallowed writing ink is at great risk of developing :**
A. Encephalopathy B. Cardiac arrythmias
C. Methemoglobinemia D. ARF

127. **Dermatographism is seen in :**
A. Ichthyosis vulgaris B. Epidermolysis bullosa
C. Kwashiorkor D. Urticaria

128. **Telecanthus (hypertelorism) is a recognized feature of all except :**
A. Renal agenesis (Potter facies)
B. Cranio facial dysostosis
C. Acrocephalosyndacyly (Apert)
D. Waardenburg's syndrome

129. **Davidsohn test is used for :**
A. ITP
B. Infectious mononucleosis
C. Beta thalassemia
D. AML

130. **Gordon's biological test is used for :**
A. Congenital Adrenal hyperplasia
B. Hodgkin's disease
C. von Willebrand disease
D. Tetralogy of Fallot

131. **Levinson test will be positive in :**
A. Resistant typhoid B. Resistant malaria
C. TBM D. CML

132. **Mehu's test will be positive in :**
A. ITP B. Porphyria
C. Nephrotic syndrome D. Obstructive Jaundice

133. **Moretti's test is used in :**
A. Rabies B. Hydatid disease
C. Typhoid D. Congen, Pyloric stenosis

134. **Silver Russel syndrome is characterized by following except :**
A. Low birth weights
B. Frontal bossing
C. Growth hormone level usually normal
D. Long and incurved 5th fingers

135. **Cori's disease is same as :**
A. Pompe's disease B. Forbe's disease
C. Anderson disease D. Her's disease

136. **In Tarui's disease, there is inborn error of :**
A. Alpha galctosidase B. Phosphofructokinase
C. Muscle phosphorylase D. Acid maltase

137. **Duke's disease is which of exanthematous number illness:**
A. First B. Third
C. Fourth D. Fifth

138. **Tom cat urine odour is due to :**
A. Maple syrup disease
B. Methionine
C. Trimethylominuria
D. Methyl crobomyl glycinuria

139. **In asplenia, most infections are because of pneumococci and :**
A. Staphylococcus B. E. coli
C. H. influenzae D. Klebsiella

140. **In Usher syndrome, there is retinitis pigmentosa with :**
A. Cataract B. Deafness
C. CSOM D. Antrochoanal polyp

141. **Hurler's syndrome closely resembles :**
A. Hunter's syndrome B. Schieie's syndrome
C. Morquio A D. Sanfilippo A

142. **Cardinal symptom of Kinsbourne syndrome is :**
A. Ichthyosis B. Ataxia
C. Seizures D. Cataract

143. **Least common symptom in Young syndrome among the following is :**
A. Azoospermia B. Clubbing
C. Bronchiectasis D. Sinusitis

144. **Rockerbottom feet may be seen in :**
A. Patau's syndrome B. Edwards syndrome
C. Turner's syndrome D. Down's syndrome

145. **All of the following are features of Alport's syndrome except :**
A. Nephritis B. Deafness
C. Proteinuria D. Rickets

146. **Following drug may produce peripheral neuropathy :**
A. Cephaloridine B. Thiabendazole
C. Lincomycin D. Griseofulvin

Ans.									
122. B	123. B	124. D	125. C	126. C	127. D	128. A	129. B	130. B	131. C
132. C	133. C	134. D	135. B	136. B	137. C	138. D	139. C	140. B	141. B
142. B	143. B	144. B	145. D	146. B					

147. Following drug is contraindicated in G-6-P deficiency:
A. Tolbutamide B. Penicillamine
C. Doxycycline D. Griseofulvin

148. Sniffing position is used for :
A. Neurosurgery on putuita.y
B. Airway obstruction
C. TOF
D. Doing nephrectomy

149. In Pierre Robin syndrome, baby is test put in ——— position :
A. Sitting B. Prone
C. Supine D. Left lateral

150. In a 2 year old child, the size of tube required for intubation is :
A. 2.0 B. 3.5
C. 4.0 D. 6.0

151. Following substances are very efficiently adsorbed by activated charcol except :
A. Aspirin B. Primaquin
C. Ferrous sulfate D. Phenol

152. THAM is used in the treatment of :
A. Metabolic acidosis
B. Respiratory acidosis
C. Metabolic alkalosis
D. Respiratory alkalosis

153. Waugh's syndrome most commonly presents as :
A. Jaundice B. Intussuception
C. Appendicitis D. Pyloric stenosis

154. Gorham's syndrome involves :
A. Kidneys B. Liver
C. Skeletal system D. Pancreas

155. Peripheral neuropathy may be produced by :
A. Albendazole B. Flumebendazole
C. Mebendazole D. Thiabendazole

156. Among the following malignancies, least common in childhood is :
A. Leukemia B. Tumors of CNS
C. Neuroblastoma D. Lymphomas

157. In Tangier's disease, treatment of choice is :
A. Cholesterol free diet
B. Anticholesterol drugs
C. Low triglyceride
D. Splenectomy

158. In Fabry's disease, lipid accumulates in the following except :
A. Heart B. Pancreas
C. Kidney D. Ganglion cells

159. Penicillamine therapy should be stopped in Wilson's disease if there is presence of following except :
A. Immune complex GN
B. SLE like syndrome
C. Adenopathy
D. Nephrotic syndrome

160. Tuberous sclerosis is also called ——— disease :
A. Little B. Boureneville
C. Leigh D. Canavan

161. Drowning in childhood may result in :
A. Hyponatremia B. Hypokalemia
C. Hyperkalemia D. Hypermagnesemia

162. In children with atopic eczema —— is most commonly involved :
A. Face B. Neck
C. Chest D. Legs

163. Chromosomal abnormality in Prader Willi syndrome is :
A. del 8q 24 B. del 13q 14
C. del 15q 11 D. del 22q 11

164. The following are causes of low set ears except :
A. Hellermann Streiff syndrome
B. Seckel's syndrome
C. Turner's syndrome
D. Lawrence Moon Biedle syndrome

165. 'Circus phenomenon' is associated with :
A. Volvulus B. Focal seizures
C. ADHD D. PSVT

166. In Langer-Gideon syndrome, there is following chromosomal abnormality :
A. del 8q 24 B. del 11 p 13
C. del 11p 15 D. del 22q 11

167. Term 'Cytogenetic noise' is used for :
A. Chromosomal abnormality in malignancy only
B. Iatrogenic chromosomal abnormality
C. Random chromosomal abnormality
D. Tendency to develop congenital deafness

168. Increase in per C° temperature, there is altered fluid requiremnet of about ———% :
A. 7.5 B. 8.5
C. 1.0 D. 12.5

169. A masculinized female with elevated plasma 17 alpha hydroxyprogesterone androgens, and urinary 17-ketosteroids but there is fall of aldosterone levels. She has :
A. 21 hydroxylase deficiency, simple type
B. 21 hydroxylase deficiency salt-wasting type
C. 17-hydroxylase deficiency
D. 11-hydroxylase deficiency

Ans.									
147. A	148. B	149. B	150. C	151. C	152. A,B	153. B	154. C	155. C	156. D
157. D	158. B	159. C	160. B	161. B	162. A	163. C	164. D	165. D	166. A
167. C	168. D	169. B							

170. **Term "Nil" disease is used for :**
A. Hemolytic uremic syndrome
B. Measles in incubation
C. Lipoid nephrosis
D. Congenital AIDS

171. **Attention reflex of pupil is known as —— reflex :**
A. Philippson's B. Piltz
C. Puusepp's D. Remak's

172. **Term `Nyxis' means :**
A. Nystagmus B. Paracentesis
C. Floppy D. Hyperactive

173. **Relaxation of overlying abdominal muscles following ingestion of food is —— reflex :**
A. Schaffer's B. von Hering's
C. Weiss's D. Throckmorton's

174. **Dancing eyes seen together with "dancing hands and feet' are seen in :**
A. Wilm's tumor B. Neuroblastoma
C. Fallot's tetralogy D. Head injury

175. **A full slow and soft pulse said to be characteristic of jaundice is —— pulse :**
A. Monneret's B. Allorhythmic
C. Trip-hammer D. Vermicular

176. **Lisch spots are seen in :**
A. Seckel dwarfism
B. Engelman's syndrome
C. Neurofibromatosis
D. Ellis-van Crevel syndrome

177. **Pitted enamel is seen in :**
A. Hypothyroidism B. Fluorosis
C. Tuberous sclerosis D. Irradiation

178. **Parrot's atrophy of newborn is another name :**
A. Congenital adrenal hyperplasia
B. Duchenne's muscular dystrophy
C. Primary marasmus
D. Down's syndrome

179. **When an infant is held in the prone position, the entire body forms a convex upward arc; gentle pressure on the head or gravity flexes the neck and hip, reversing the arc. This is —— reflex :**
A. Haab's B. Hughes
C. Landau D. Loven

180. **Delayed respiratory distress syndrome in infants may be seen in :**
A. Dandy Walker syndrome
B. Wilson-Mikity syndrome
C. Down's syndrome
D. VSD

181. **Floppy infant syndrome is seen in following glycogenoses type :**
A. I B. II
C. V D. VI

182. **Secondary hyperlipidemia in children is seen in the following types of glycogen storage disease except :**
A. Type I B. Type III
C. Type V D. Type VI

183. **Organisms age fastest when young. This is —— law :**
A. Barfurth's B. Kahler's
C. Minot's D. Pojot's

184. **Absence of measles rash at the site of infection of convalescent measles serum which has not prevented the appearance of the eruption is —— phenomenon:**
A. Ashman's B. Aubert's
C. Debre's D. Duckworth's

185. **A reaction which appears in infants in cases of starvation after the starvation is relieved; it consists of a slight gain in weight elevation of temperature and appearance of watery stools containing a large number of cells is —— reaction :**
A. Bittorf B. Gubler
C. Morelli D. Zed

186. **The law that regeneration is more complete in younger individuals than is older ones is —— law:**
A. Ricco's B. Rosa's
C. Spallanzani D. Teevan's

187. **Thickening of calvarium may be due to which of the following condition :**
A. Dandy Walker syndrome
B. Brain atrophy
C. Universal cranio-synostosis
D. Untreated hydrocephalus

188. **Thymic atrophy may be produced by:**
A. Thyroxine B. Corticosteroids
C. Procarbazine D. Methotrexate

189. **Pressure on the inner side of the biceps muscle produces closure of the fist in tetany is —— phenomenon :**
A. Goldblatt B. Hektoen
C. Hochsinger D. Lust

190. **Sail sign helps in identification of normal :**
A. Spleen B. Kidney
C. Pancreas D. Thymus

Ans.	170. C	171. B	172. B	173. B	174. B	175. A	176. C	177. C	178. C	179. C
	180. B	181. B	182. C	183. C	184. C	185. D	186. C	187. B	188. B	189. C
	190. D									

191. Thymus is usually small or absent in all of the following conditions except :
A. Prematurity
B. Congenital rubella
C. Adenosine deaminase deficiency
D. ALL

192. Rectosigmoid index is useful in the diagnosis of :
A. Diverticulosis B. Crohn's disease
C. Aganglionosis D. Meconium ileus

193. The lines of the face in young children, described as being indicative of specific types of disease are ——— lines :
A. Kilian B. Jodelot
C. Moyer D. Morgan

194. Prayer test may be useful in predicting complication due to :
A. Diphtheria B. Measles
C. Juvenile DM D. Cretinism

195. Hochsinger's sign in present in :
A. Measles B. Childhood TB
C. Thalassemia D. Enteric fever

196. "Squashed faces" and low set ears are seen in ——— syndrome :
A. Down B. Potter
C. Crouzen D. Apert

197. Lobster hands are seen in :
A. Crouzen syndrome B. Acromegaly
C. de Lange syndrome D. Potter's syndrome

198. Heaped up ridges of bones are seen in :
A. Hydrocephalus B. Craniostenosis
C. Down's syndrome D. Potter's syndrome

199. Metabolic acidosis is a recognized complication of parenteral nutrition in the neonate following intravenous administration of all except :
A. Glucose B. Fructose
C. Sorbitol D. Amino acids solutions

200. Robinson Kepler test is positive in :
A. Cushing's syndrome B. Addison's disease
C. Cretinism D. Myxoedoma

201. Sucrose lysis test is positive in :
A. Giardiasis B. Diabetes mellitus
C. PNH D. Hereditary spherocytis

202. Thormablem test detects —— in urine :
A. Urobilinogen B. Globulins
C. Melanin D. Haemoglobin

203. Duret lesions are seen in :
A. AIDS
B. Diabetic kidney
C. Cerebellar herniation
D. Infectious mononucleosis

204. If ———% or less of ears are above horizontal line joining at level of medial canthi to ears are called low set years :
A. 5 B. 10
C. 20 D. 25

205. The aetiology of "Caker sores" is :
A. Staph. infection B. Congenital syphilis
C. Herpangina D. Autoimmune

206. MCV is minimum in following age group :
A. At birth B. 1—6 months
C. 6—24 months D. 2—6 years

207. Absent reflexes are a feature of following except :
A. Kugelberg-Wilander disease
B. Down syndrome
C. Ducheme Muscular dystrophy
D. Decerebration

208. Following are methods used to look for rearranged DNA except :
A. Northern blotting
B. Southern blotting
C. Polymerase chain reaction
D. Finger printing

209. The most common cause of neonatal hemoperitoneum is :
A. Necrotising enterocolitis
B. Hemorrhagic disease
C. Trauma
D. Exchange transfusions via umbilical catheter

210. High arched polate may be seen in the following except :
A. Treacher Collins syndrome
B. Ehlers-Danlos syndrome
C. Seckel's syndrome
D. Marfan's syndrome

211. Which of the following resembles frog's belly :
A. Mixed parotid tumor
B. Bifid Uvula
C. Ranula
D. Ileocolic intussusception

Ans.										
	191. D	192. C	193. B	194. A	195. B	196. B	197. C	198. A	199. A	200. B
	201. C	202. C	203. C	204. B	205. D	206. C	207. D	208. A	209. C	210. C
	211. C									

12. PEDIATRICS

References Quoted

S.N.	Books
1.	Ghai's **Essential Pediatrics.** Interprint, New Delhi.
2.	**Current Pediatric Diagnosis and Treatment**, Prentice-Hall International, Inc., NewYork.

Unforgetable Supplement

PSYCHIATRIC NURSING

(Dr. M.S. Bhatia, M.D., Dip. W.P.A)

About this book

- **This book : a must for :**
  - All Nursing Paramedical Students
  - Psychiatric Nursing
- This new book is specifically written for easy grasping of Psychiatry in a clearent, pointwise, simple and easy understandable language and is exclusively based on the examination and practice oriented pattern.
- Each chapter is followed by important Facts and Review Questions.
- A section on the general principles of psychiatry with a special emphasis on the **historical aspects,** aetiology, sympto-matology, psychiatric examination and **Glossary** has been included.
- An updated section on psychiatric treatment —including newer advances has been added.
- **Important topics** on Indian Psychiatry (Contributions of various Psychiatrists, Epidemiology of various disorders, manpower, National Mental Health Programme of India, Forensic Psychiatry etc.) have been explained.
- An important list of appendices include list of Psychotropic Drugs (Alphabetically, trade name wise, main indications, dosages and preparations) and a list of psychological tests commonly used in India.
- This concised textbook aimed at important **comprehensive theoretical** and **practical skills** in psychiatry and allied disciplines.

CBS Publishers & Distributors Pvt. Ltd.

NEW DELHI • BANGALORE • PUNE • CHENNAI • COCHIN (INDIA)